ENCYCLOPAEDIA OF WOMEN HEALTH

ENCYCLOPAEDIA
OF
WOMEN HEALTH

PARVESH HANDA

GYAN PUBLISHING HOUSE
New Delhi - 110002

Encyclopaedia of Women Health

ISBN: 81-212-0902-1

Reprinted in 2012 in India by
Gyan Publishing House
23, Main Ansari Road, Daryaganj,
New Delhi - 110002
Phones : 23282060, 23261060
Fax : (011) 23285914
E-mail : books@gyanbooks.com
Website: gyanbooks.com

Printed at: G. Print Process, Delhi

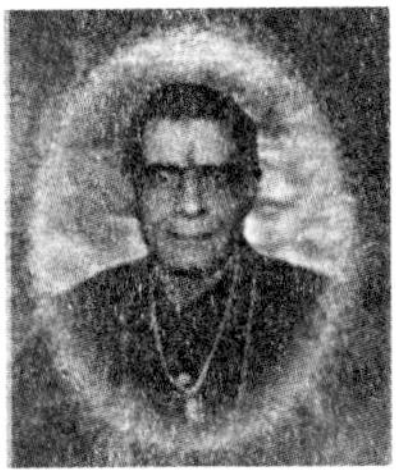

This book is lovingly dedicated to

Respected Guru Dev

(Dr.) Pt. Manmohan Shastri Ji

of Babyal (Ambala)

for his constant Gifts of Light, Life, Inspirations and Divine True Love

Contents

Preface

This encyclopaedia is the result of my effort to provide a complete guide of women health. Every family's first and foremost preference is a healthy woman. I have made special effort to provide a personal approach. A woman should follow the philosophy that 'a single gram of prevention is worth a kilogram of the cure'. The lesson, of course is that we would be wise to guard our health.

My primary aim in writing this book is to provide sufficient knowledge to women about sufferings from medical disorders. Having over 30 years of wide experience in cosmetology, I have described in detail on skin disorders/diseases commonly seen among women. My experience of dermatology was insufficient to allow me to write on medical field. I gladly acknowledge the help, which has been given to me most willingly by medical colleagues. I would like to acknowledge the courtesy of renowned medical experts Dr. D.S. Jaspal (President IMA-Haryana), Dr. Suresh Sharma MD (Obs and Gynec) and Dr. Rajeev Gupta MD (Radiology) an PGI specialist for their whole-heartedly assistance in writing this Encyclopaedia.

Ms. Parvesh Handa

Acknowledgements

Sincere gratitude for the exceptional co-operation and contributions for assisting in preparing this book to

Dr. D.S. Jaspal
President, Indian Medical Association–Haryana

Dr. Suresh Sharma
MD, (Obs & Gynec), Haryana Civil Medical Services

Dr. Rajeev Gupta
M.D. (Radiology), PGI MS Rothak

1
Women's Guide to Health, Tests and Screenings

Menstruation and Menopause

Menstruation cycle is the term applied to the recurrent series of changes in a woman's reproductive system of which menstruation is the outward manifestation. The term menstruation (also called monthly periods or the menses or the catamenia) refers to the discharge of blood and mucus from the uterus, which recurs in woman from puberty to the menopause at regular intervals of about a month, except during pregnancy and sometimes during lactation (breastfeeding). Most of the girls start to menstruate between the age 12 to 15 years (the average being a little over 13 years). The onset of puberty is accompanied by a number of other changes, both bodily and mentally. These are the growth of pelvis and its assumption of the adult female shape, the development of external genitals, the appearance of hair on the pubes and in the axillae, the development of the breasts, a general development of a graceful rounded contour in the body and the awakening of the sexual sense. These changes come on gradually, and the body does not become that of a fully developed woman until the age of about 20. Clinically, the start of menstruation may be quite sudden, or may be preceded for several months by periodic headaches and general upsets of health, without any actual discharge of blood.

Menstrual Habit: This term refers to the duration of menstruation, and indirectly to the amount of loss. The average duration is five days, but it varies greatly in different persons. The extremes are cases where it only lasts for an hour or so, and in cases where it goes on for more than eight days. However, anything below two hours or above eight days is abnormal. It tends to be greater in hot climates, less in cold, greater in urban dwellers and those living in luxuries and eating stimulating food. Sexual stimulation and habits of thought tend to increase it.

Amenorrhoea: This means the absence of menstruation during the active sexual period of life from puberty to the menopause. Amenorrhoea is one of the early symptoms of pregnancy and it persists in 60% of the women during the first few months of lactation.

Menorrhagia: It means excessive hemorrhage at the menstrual period.

Metrorrhagia: It means bleeding from the uterus in the intervals between menstrual periods.

Dysmenorrhoea: It means painful menstruation.

Leucorrhoea: It means a discharge of a white or yellowish nature, not blood. Recent investigations have shown that the secretion from the uterus and upper portion of the vagina flow down and are reabsorbed in the lower part of the vagina. This is normal, constant flow within the female organs. The presence of infection in any of these tissues usually causes whitish discharge (called leucorrhoea) that may continue for weeks or for months continuously. This discharge may arise from Trichomonas vaginalis, an infection due to a small parasite that normally inhabits the bowel. Other causes of leucorrhoea are pelvic congestion, endocrine disturbances, lacerations, injuries and atrophy of the vaginal tissues following the menopause. In young girls the discharge may be due to the following reasons:

1. An irritation of the labia or external genital organs due to soiled undergarments, dirt, intestinal worms and masturbation.
2. The irritated tissue may become infected with staphy-lococcus germs, which are generally present in the skin.
3. When the girl reaches puberty, due to over-activity in her sex glands and organs, it results excessive white discharge.
4. There is slight discharge at the time of ovulation. However, it does not indicate the presence of any disease.
5. In mature women a profuse, yellowish discharge is associated with burning, intense itching on urination die to a serious infection (usually due to an venereal disease).

6. A thin watery discharge may be due to the presence of cancer in the uterus or cervix.
7. A creamy discharge, slightly blood-stained may be due to Trichomonas or some other infection.

Menopause or Change of Life

Menopause is the time when menstruation ceases to recur. It is often called as the 'climacteric' or the 'change of life'. It usually occurs between the age 40 to 50, generally after the age 45. The menopause, sometimes, occur before the age of 40 and occasionally in females in their twenties. The female reproductive time of life begins at adolescence in the early teens and continues until the end of the menopause. The early symptoms of menopause are increased nervous tension, menstrual disturbances, hot flashes, chilly feelings, excitability, easy fatigue, depression, crying spells, sleeplessness, palpitation, dizziness, headaches, numbness and tingling, and other annoying symptoms. All these miseries arise from the fact that ovaries are no longer producing their normal amount of estrogen or female hormone. Lack of normal hormone balance may result in a constant backache, due perhaps to osteoporosis(or thinning of the bones) arising from low level of estrogen in the blood stream. Unless properly treated, this may eventually lead to a collapse of one or more of the vertebrae, causing the woman to lose weight because of bending and deformity of the spine.

A General Guide to Health Tests

Test	*Purpose*	*Age*	*How often to be tested*
Blood Pressure	To detect hypertension- a major risk factor for cardiovascular disease	21+	Annually, more frequently if over 140/90
Breast Self-Examination	To detect changes in breast tissue or its appearance	20+	Monthly, 7-10 days after onset of period
Cholesterol Test	To check cholesterol content of blood is too high-a mojor factor in heart disease	45+	Every 5 years or as advised by the doctor

(contd.)

Colorectal Exam.	To detect signs of colorect cancer, which can be cured if detected early.	50+	Fecal Occult Blood Test annually. Flexible Sigmoidoscopy with Digital Rectal Examination (DRE) every 5 years. May have Colonoscopy and DRE every 10 years.
Mammogram	To detect changes in breast, breast tissue that are too small to be felt.	40+	Annually.
Pap Smear	To detect cervical abnormalities, including cancer.	21+	Annually or if referred by the doctor.
Pelvic Exam.	To detect uterine abnormalities, including cancer.	30+	Annually
Professional Breast Exam.	To detect changes in breasts that remain unnoticed.	20-40	Every three years.

Treatment of Common Women Health Problems

Health Problem	*Usual Symptoms*	*Treatment*
Dysmenorrhea	Painful cramping during periods usually caused by high levels of prostaglandins. Symptoms of headache, nausea and diarrhea.	Exercise and high-fiber diets. Have medicines to reduce prostaglandins or to reduce pain.
Endometriosis	Caused by bits of the uterine tissue growing outside the uternus. This	Hormones therapy helps some patients, whereas it needs to have the excess tissue surgically

	condition can cause severe, steady pains few days prior to periods, which goes away after menses.	removed.
Osteoporosis	Loss of bone mass occurs in both sexes, but is more severe in post-menopausal women due to hormone changes. Loss of body height, back pain and hunch back are common symptoms.	Regular weight-bearing exercise and a calcium rich diet help. Hormone therapy can stop loss of bone mass.
Pelvic Inflamm-atory Disease (PID)	PID is an extremely serious infection of the uterus, fallopian tubes and ovaries. Symptoms include severe lower abdominal pain, unusual bleeding, vaginal discharge, fever and chills.	Oral/intravenous antibiotics and a bed rest is the only best treatment for PID. Better consult a doctor.
Pre-menstrual Syndore (PMS)	Women experience PMS one or two weks prior to their periods. The condition have depression, confusion, sleepessness, weightgain, breast tenderness and food craving.	Low-fat, low-sugar diets, vitamin supplementation, adequate rest and regular exercise relieve PMS.
Sexually Trans-mitted Diseases (STD)	STD include syphilis, gonorrhea, chlamydia, herpes	Treatment depends upon the STD, but often antibiotics are

	and AIDS. It usually occur due to sexual contact. Symptoms include discharge, pain, sores etc.	recommended. However, there is no cure for AIDS. Practise safe sex.
Vaginitis	Caused by bacterial or yeast infections of the vaginal tissue. Symptoms include yellowish, white or curdled looking discharge, burning, itching, soreness and/ or a painful intercourse.	Oral medication (antibiotics) or a vaginal suppositories or creams are usually suggested by the doctor. An early treatment is advised.
Stress	It is a physical and psychological reaction to change. Persons under stress may have changed sleeping or eating patterns, feel fatigued, irritable and generally anxious.	A stress management class can help you learn coping and relaxation techniques. Yoga and meditation helps to alleviate stress.

More serious symptoms of the menopause are quickly brought under control by the use of estrogen. The usual dosage is 2 mg. (20,000 units) injected every week with the consultation of your doctor. However, Estrogen tablets, (1.25 mg) may be given daily as a maintenance dose (with the consultation of doctor). Remember, larger amount of estrogen may produce bleeding and soreness in the breasts.

(The author thanks to the experts of renowned Fortis Heart Hospital at Mohali for advising above women health guidance tips for this Encyclopedia)

Today the world is on its wheel. Scientific and technological research has become the watch-ward of progress. New discoveries and inventions have brought radical changes in human life. In the field of medicine and surgery miracle drugs and treatments have been introduced to alleviate the suffering of human being. On the other hand incidence of diseases has shown an upward trend in decline of human health due to general negligence and fast changing culture in our society. According to a medical survey more than 50 percent females today are suffering from the genital disorders for one reason or the other.

Negligence is the root of general decline of human health. Women in particular, it is observed, have the origin of their diseases, in some disorders in their genital organs. But these women blame their fate, keep suffering under the veil of superstitions. Ignorance and superstitions cause too many casualties and mishaps. A timely treatment, however, may control such mishaps to large extent.

It is quite true that the instinct of motherhood is too strong in a woman yet she is shy and disturbed usually at the time of her first sexual relations with male partner. Lack of proper knowledge on the subject and general ignorance lead many newly married couples to commit such mistakes, which keep them repenting the rest of their life. Subjects like pregnancy, expectant mother's care, maternity, stages of labor, various sexual diseases, breast-feeding, postnatal care and taking care the baby are the subjects have been widely described in coming chapters of this book.

Periodic Health Examination

Generally people want to know how often should periodic health examinations be performed? In people under 45 years of age a periodic health examination be performed once a year – after that a check up twice a year is advisable. In case you feel perfectly fit, it is most important to have yourself examined, as many conditions of serious nature can exist for a long time without producing symptoms. Diseases can sometimes be spotted in its very early stages, when it is easier to cure. One should go to the family physician for periodic health examination, who may refer to specialists if he thinks additional tests or examinations are required. Total body scanner (also known as CAT scan) test is valuable, but the test is very expensive is possible for those who are suspected of having a serious disease such as cancer.

Adolescence and Puberty?

The teenage period between the ages of 12 and 25 is considered the adolescent period. It is the time when there is the most rapid growth and the most sudden changes in physical, psychological and physiological development.

The period when sex functions mature, roughly between 12 and 15 years of age in girls, and 13 to 16 years of age in boys is considered the puberty.

The major evidences of puberty in young girls :
are the following:-

1. Breast development.
2. The appearance of pubic and axillary hair.
3. The assumption of the female type of figure.
4. The onset of menstruation.

The major evidences of puberty in a boy :
are the following:-

1. Increase in the size of the external genitals.
2. The appearance of pubic and axillary hair.
3. The appearance of hair on the face and upper lip.
4. Change in voice, with deepening in tone.
5. The development of muscles and masculine figure.

Irregular menstruation in young girls :

Girls tend to mature one or two years earlier than boys. Usually, at the onset of menstruation, a girl will be the same age as her mother was when she began to menstruate. In warmer climates the girls tend to mature and to menstruate at an earlier age. When menstruation starts, usually it is irregular for initial few months. It may occur every two to three weeks or may occur only once in two to three months. Also the amount of the flow varies widely. Anywhere a period from one to three years is required for regular menstruation cycle and it requires no treatment. If a young girl is irregular in her periods for a year or two, it is wise to have herself examined. A rectal examination will give the necessary information as to the state of the uterus and ovaries. It is not necessary to do the vaginal examination on young girls.

Development of breasts in young girls:

Breasts usually begin to develop about one year before the onset of menstruation. It is common for one breast or one nipple to develop before the other in most of the young girls. It is perfectly normal. Both the breasts will eventually catch up in its development and will be approximately the same size. There is sometimes pain and tenderness in the developing breasts; this requires no treatment unless it is very severe. At about 10 to 12 years of age all girls should be told about menstruation so that they are prepared for its onset. The child's mother should instruct girls about the adolescence, puberty and sexual changes. It is best that she should get the information factually from an older person rather than from her friends, who may be misinformed.

Organs responsible for the onset of adolescence?

The pituitary gland, the ovaries and the testicles begin to secrete larger quantities of the sex hormones and thus bring on the changes seen in adolescents. Both boys and girls tend to develop pimples and blackheads during this period. This condition is called acne. Special diet, special methods of keeping the face clean and medications prove helpful.

Increased sexual urges of children during adolescence?

This is a natural phenomenon during adolescence and parents need not be discouraged. It is normal for boys and girls to want to get to know one another and to want to get along with each other. Sexual curiosity is part of that desire to learn more about the opposite sex and doesn't necessarily lead to complete sexual relations. During this period, sexual curiosity should be controlled gently, and children should be directed so that their curiosity doesn't result in harmful pursuits.

When to begin sex education?

A child should be educated about sex gradually from his or her earliest years when he or she first evinces interest in sex. By the time adolescence is reached, children should know a great deal about sex so that they are better able to manage their sexual urges. Ignorance about sexual matters, of ten result in unwanted pregnancies or venereal infections among young ones. Generally, there are so many myths about boys and girls to masturbate during adolescent period. It is important not to make them feel guilty about this practice. In majority of cases, in both boys and girls, late or delayed adolescence requires no treatment. Eventually, all children reach physical maturity without the need for medical treatment. A hormonal treatment if there is faulty menstruation, would be safe to wait until she is 16 or 17 years of age. Better consult a gynecologist.

2
Genital Problems of Teenagers and Adults

1. Post-natal depression

Depression is common among women after the childbirth as a result she usually loses sexual and other interests besides feeling irritability and fatigue. The depression is more likely to occur if a woman feels isolated and inadequate support from her husband and other members of her family.

2. Post-natal check up

The mother should pay a visit to the doctor for check up between six and eight weeks after delivering the child, which gives the mother the opportunity to discuss any problem faced by her.

3. Post-natal sex

After childbirth, a woman's sexual desire and activities are conditioned on several factors such as strain of parenthood, reduced sexual desire and arousal and because of a painful episiotomy scar. Sexual intercourse can be resumed whenever a woman feels comfortable about having sex. Woman who breast-feed are usually more sexually aroused and responsive than woman who choose to bottle-feed their baby. If intercourse continues to be painful, consult your doctor.

4. Post-natal menstruation

If the mother is breast feeding, menstruation usually doesn't return for about six months, but approximately 10-15% women start to menstruate by two to three months after childbirth and 25-30% by three to four months and remaining by six to seven months. Ovulation is useful before the 20th week after the childbirth, but very few lactating women ovulate before this period. However, pregnancy rarely occurs in the first four to five months of puerperium. Continue breastfeeding, even if periods have started. The periods leave no ill effect over the quality of breast milk.

5. Post-natal body care

If you have gained weight, your tummy must have put on extra flesh after the childbirth, as your skin and muscles must have grown to hold the constant weight of body in womb. Do not worry as the muscles will gradually tighten up again, but do not forget gentle exercises. Breast feeding helps the stomach get back to shape as it encourages the uterus to contract and after two months of delivery the uterus should be in its non-pregnant size.

6. Post-natal health problems

Sometimes, few days after the childbirth, the discharge changes to pale brown. Some women have a rush of blood when the baby breast-feeds. If you pass blood clots or fresh blood or the lochia smells unpleasant, consult your doctor immediately, these are the signs of the part of placenta has left inside the womb or there is an infection. After giving birth to a baby, women are often prone to infections. Make sure to keep vaginal area clean and wash the area with a mild soap and water after every trip to the toilet.

Once the lochia has stopped, a breast-feeding mother may not have periods for several months, After childbirth, the mother often have painful contractions. Suckling breast nipples causes the uterus to contract to its normal size. Post-birth pains are common and these stop after few days. If there is continuous pain or bleeding, consult your doctor. Constipation, too, can be a problem if you have stitches. Do not push or strain while in toilet. Take care if you suffer from backache after the childbirth. Do not lift heavy weights during this period.

7. How to plan for a healthy child?

Child's health does not start after the birth, even before the baby is conceived in the mother's womb. Planning of children can be considered in three parts such as before conception, during conception and after conception. Oral contraceptives have harmful side effects and are no longer advised. Start treatment under acupressure therapy at least three months prior to conceiving. The couple should drink a glass of charged water (Health Drink) daily and female partner must have three regular menses before conceiving in order to have a healthy fully developed uterus. A daily massage on both sides of two wrists for five minutes by female partner proves beneficial for healthy pregnancy.

To prepare charged water (Health Drink), mix 300 gm. of Amla powder to 100 gm. of ginger powder. Take one teaspoonful of this powder with water in the morning and evening. Another way is to add two teaspoonful of above powder of Amla and ginger in four glasses of water. Use fresh Amla and ginger (if available). Boil, till it is reduced to three glasses. Filter the water and add to it salt or honey. Amla is concentrated vitamin C. It has 16 times more vitamin C than lemon and helps to give protection to the body against cold and increases digestion power. The Health Drink is beneficial especially for the convalescing people, old, growing children and the expectant mothers.

8. Acupressure therapy for pregnant

Nature has provided the body with proper regulators and protectors. These are our endocrine (ductless) glands, which secrete hormones directly into our blood. And so the proper functioning of these controllers of our body is very important and most vital for sound health-not only in the development of our body and mind but also in the development of our looks and even character. Malfunctioning of endocrine glands effect the reproductive organs in the body. Pineal gland controls sex system and water in the body which leads to premature sex development. Malfunctioning of ovaries, testes and sex glands control heat of the productive side of the life, which damage reproductive organs (cause problems of menses, self-abuse and less/more sex desire). Applying pressure on the palms play an important role for healthy pregnancy. Here are few important tips to be kept in mind during, before / after conception, pregnancy and post-natal period :

The couple must start the treatment under acupressure therapy at least three months prior to conceiving to ensure proper creation of hormones. Drink a glass of Health Drink (Gold/Silver/Copper/Iron charged water) every day to ensure female partner must have three regular menses before conceiving.

9. Tips to have a healthy child?

- According to Ayurved, if the intercourse is made during the later dates 10th to15th the day on which the menses is seen, is to be counted as the first day, there is better possibility of conceiving and the child to be born (if conceived) will be healthy. During the period of menstruation flow, the couple should avoid intercourse, if there is conception during this period, there is possibility of the child being born with physical and mental defects.
- The problems of menstruation (early, irregular, scanty, painful, excessive), the treatment of pressing and rubbing on both wrists will leave amazing results to regulate menstruation and cure leucorrhoea (white or yellow vaginal discharge).
- During first pregnancy the expectant mother is usually much worried and has great tension. This adds to the labor pains, which also vitally effects not only the body but also mind. Even in case of the use of forceps at the time of delivery or caesarean operation, the child's body may get damaged and even the mother is hurt.
- To have a painless childbirth, roll grooved wooden roller vigorously on the back of both arms from nail to elbow for about 15 minutes. If roller is not available, rub palms and soles with two metal combs vigorously from nails to wrist for 5 to 10 minutes. For painless childbirth, apply continuous pressure on the back part of the tongue beyond the teeth for a minute and repeat few times with an interval of three minutes.
- To avoid difficult labor, press hard on the inner side above the ankles for two minutes. Pause and press again and again till the child is born. There is often severe pain after the birth of child due to accumulation of milk (not fed on breast milk). Press on the middle portion of the back of both the palms. It will relieve breast pain and inflammation.
- After the delivery of the baby or operation for sterilization there is great possibility of the lady putting on fat (obesity) because sex glands are disturbed. Press on the palms, which help in maintaining of good physique.
- Applying pressure on palms help enough production of milk for the baby. This helps in curing impotency in males. Men and women if disturbed by erotic dreams and discharged in sleep can successfully try this treatment.

- In case of suffering from syphilis or other venereal diseases, massage ice on the affected part for two to four minutes. Here is another treatment for those not suffering from diabetes. Take first urine and add to it one to two teaspoon of Soda bicarb. Boil the urine, allow it to cool, remove upper crust with cotton, soak in the urine and massage the affected part and area around it for five to six minutes. Now clean the area with an antiseptic liquid.

10. How to get child of desired sex?

The couple will be in a position to have a child of desired sex if the day on which the menses is seen is to be counted as the first day. The couple should avoid sexual intercourse during menses. Otherwise if there is conception in this period, there is possibility of child born with physical and mental defects. For getting a male child, on the even dates such as 4,6,8,10,12, 14 day, the husband should lie with his wife on the left side during sleep for 15 minutes to enable him to breathe with his right nostril before they indulge in sexual intercourse. For getting a female child, it is suggested that on odd dates such as 5,7,9,11,13,15 day the husband should lie with his wife on right side for 15 minutes to enable him to breathe with his nostril before preparing for sexual intercourse. If the intercourse is made during the later dates between 10th to 15th day there is possibility of conceiving immediately and the child to be born will be healthy.

After the baby is conceived, the mother should take proper care about her nourishment. Eat plenty of seasonal fruits and drink enough milk to get maximum natural calcium. The expectant mother should have acupressure therapy treatment and have some light exercises including walking throughout pregnancy period to ensure healthy growth of baby in womb. Remember, the child starts learning from the mother's womb. The husband should keep his wife happy during the vital period.

11. Marriage between blood relations

Marriage between blood relations should be avoided. Such marriages are genetically unhealthy as both may carry the same type of genes which could intensify the unhealthy manifestation in the issue. I know a couple, both suffering from diabetes. The first baby they had was mentally retarded. The couple had normal second baby and the third issue was a premature, died at birth. The fourth baby the mother delivered was diabetic since birth.

12. Foreplay- a secret of sex pleasure

The sexual arousal of the partners is known as foreplay. To increase a woman's cooperation in sex, the male stimulate the erotic zones such as breast nipples, lips, face, neck, genitalia (the clitoris), thighs and back stipulated by foreplay provide satisfying release to the women. Female orgasm is the acme of pleasure, associated with spontaneous spasms of the muscles in and around the genitalia (mainly the clitoris and vagina). Such contractions come in waves and this sexual release of female corresponds to the climax experience by male partner at the time of ejaculation. Women attain an orgasmic spontaneous release through manual practice than through an intercourse, some others get an orgasmic spontaneous release during sleep (similar to night emissions in males). For most women sexual gratification is an overall feeling of satisfaction at the end of the act.

13. How to strengthen sex glands?

Malfunctioning of ovaries, testes, sex glands is seen generally among those children who start getting mature at the age of 12 to 14. Usually, each girl have disturbances of menstruation-late or painful or too little or sometimes too much, which leads to resulting in retardation of the body's growth. As for the boys, they usually turn to self-abuse and start getting dreams pertaining to sex-love and their overall growth is disturbed. Moreover, this creates psychological problems, which if not solved immediately, usually become the root cause of unhappiness in couples in early married life. Proper functioning of glands help in maintaining heat of the body and play an important role in developing attractiveness of a teen-aged girl or boy.

To strengthen sex glands/organs, females are advised to apply pressure on pressure points on palms of both hands regularly, during and after the pregnancy as these glands secrete sex hormones. It also causes problem of sex rigidity or over-sex desire. A couple had no issue even after ten years of their marriage. Both started acupressure treatment applying pressure on palms of both hands to strengthen their glands. Surprisingly, the wife became pregnant within ten months.

14. Night emission

Involuntary discharge of semen during sleep or emission during night dreams is common among male and female youths. There is misconception based on the traditional teaching that semen is manufactured out of the blood. Semen is, in fact the fluid produced by testicles and its emission during the intercourse or in an involuntary discharge during sleep.

15. Fetal Death

The first trimester fetal death is technically an embryo until eight weeks after fertilization. Nearly 40% of pregnancies end in failure due to abortion during this trimester. The incidence of fetal loss in the second trimester is observed about 7%. Death of fetus in the third trimester are generally identified about one percent.

16. How to bath genital organs?

Take off your clothes. Sit on a stool in a water tub filled with cold water in summer and lukewarm water in winter. The level of water should be 1-2 inches above the stool. Take a piece of cloth, in water and gently rub your abdomen for two minutes. In case of men, take hold of the foreskin of male organ in two fingers and rub in lightly with soft piece of cloth dipping in cold water followed by rubbing the entire spine with a wet towel.

In case of women, they should rub their abdomen as in case of men. Pull the lips of the vagina and rub slowly with a wet piece of cloth. In the end rub the spine. Genital bath as well as a hip bath should not be taken at the time of menstruation. If the tub is not available, genital bath can be taken in the sun as stated above.

17. Cancer in Women

In women two most likely places where cancer may develop are the breasts and the uterus. Both areas are easily examined. Every young woman should be taught to examine her own breasts after each menstrual period. In case of detection of a tumor or anything unusual, she should take advice of a doctor. Any kind of abnormality (feel of the breast tissue outlining the curves within the breasts and up in the armpit) should be examined thoroughly. Cancer of the cervix, breast or uterus are the most common in women. Over 40% females suffer from cervical cancer, nearly 12% from breast cancer and the remaining patients suffer from vaginal or cancers of the other parts of body.

18. Breast Tumor and Cancer

If there is only one single nodule or lump in the breast, painful or without pain, it should always be removed. In case the cancer appears

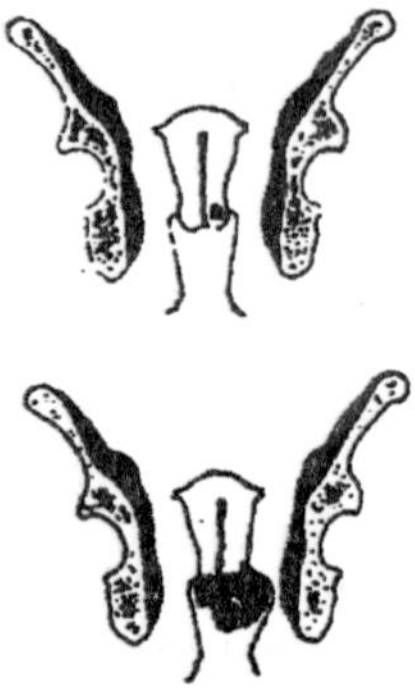

Cancer in Cervix

to have extended into the neighboring lymph nodes, the patient should be given extensive radiation therapy. Great majority of breast cancer occurs in either the upper portion of the breast, towards the shoulder or close to the nipple. Breast cancer is common between the age 35 and 65 years.

19. Cancer in cervix

It is a vicious killer of woman today. Every woman after the age 20 should have a pelvic examination and a Pap smear at least once a year or after six months. Any water discharge should be investigated, as it could be a cancer. Be careful, if the bleeding or spotting follows intercourse or douching. Modern treatment for the uterine cancer consists of implanting a small amount of radium within the cervical canal followed later by heavy dose of radiation therapy to the whole area. Performing a hysterectomy, removing the uterus, cervix, ovaries and tubes are the treatments.

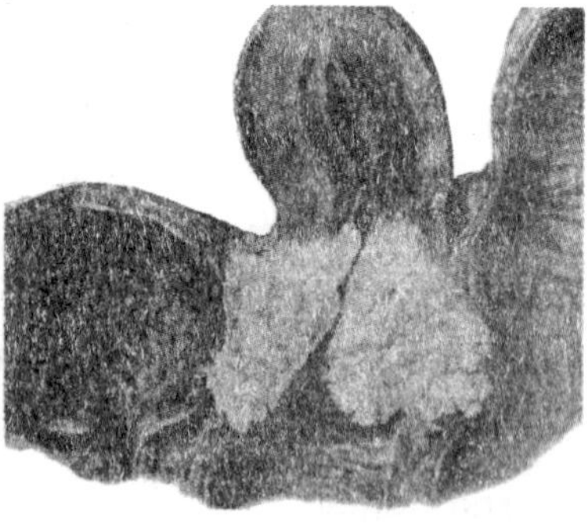

Cervical Cancer

20. Cancer in uterus

It is less common type of cancer, known as fundal carcinoma, may sometimes develop within the cavity of uterus itself. This is less malignant than cancer of the cervix. Can be detected by Pap smear. If cancer is found, a hysterectomy should be done without delay. The cancer cells find their way into the abdominal cavities and may spread to the pelvis and eventually in the whole body.

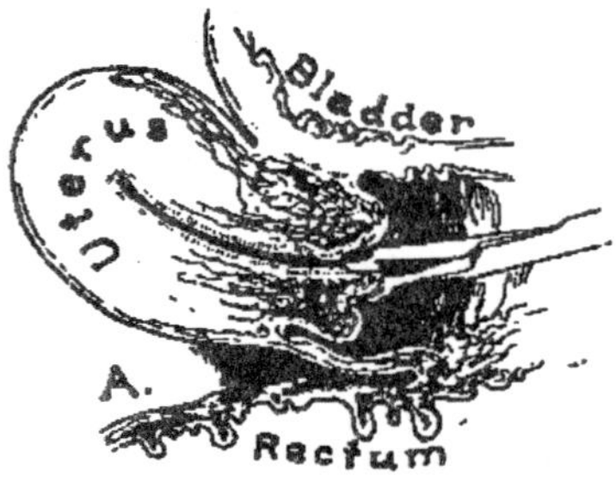

Uterus Cancer

21. Ovarian cysts and cancer

They are most frequent tumors in the body. Every woman has a small cyst on the ovary, which may disappear spontaneously. The ovarian cyst causes distension of the abdomen and pressure on the organs such as the bladder or rectum. It should be removed by surgery without delay. Cancer may develop in the wall of ovarian cyst, may spread to other nearby organs causing obstruction of the bowel.

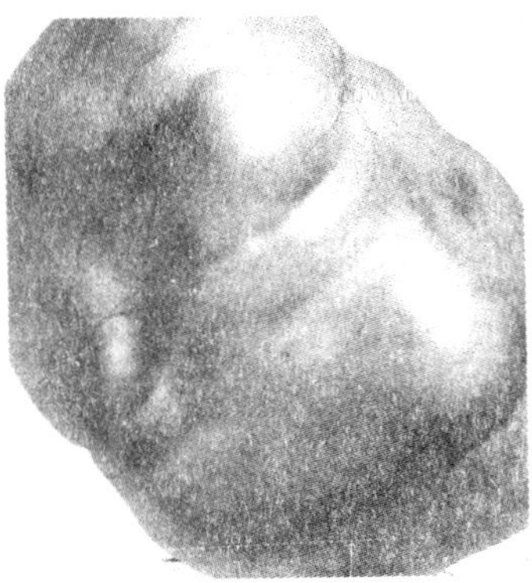

Ovarian Cyst

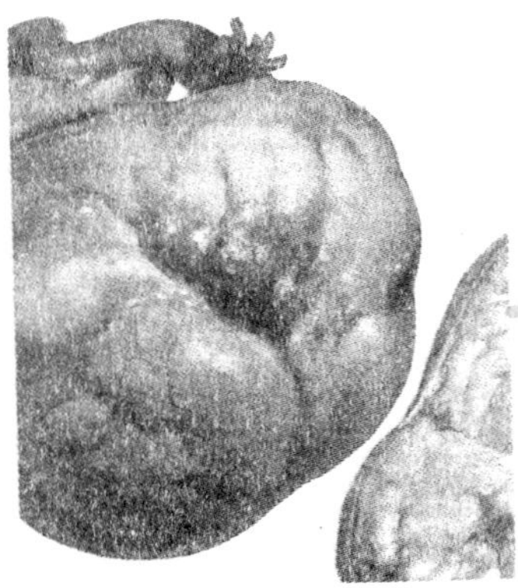

Ovarian Cancer

22. Masturbation

Teenage boys and girls have certain sex problems that never seemed to exist in early childhood. The rapidly growing sex organs are easily stimulated, often to be embarrassment of the young person. Unless the young person is careful, harmful habits may be formed. The act of self-stimulation, known as masturbation, is often a real problem to the young person. These secret acts of sexual excitement can be harmful, especially when carried to excess. Often the individual tends to become secretive. Frequent masturbation with its tendency to day time dreaming can be harmful. Youth wants to enjoy life should avoid all such practices. However, an occasional emission of seminal fluid during sleep is not unusual in any young man or a woman. There is no reason for him or her to feel anxious and guilty about this

23. Closed hymen

Sometimes, sexually well-developed female do not have menses in spite of good health and without psychological disorders. Sometimes, she may experience periodic pain in the lower belly. Such women are found to have completely closed hymen. After ultrasound examination, in many cases when surgically operated and the dark blood was let out, her periods started.

24. Varicose veins

Varicose veins are enlarged superficial veins into the leg due to increased pressure on the veins cause to lose elasticity and they

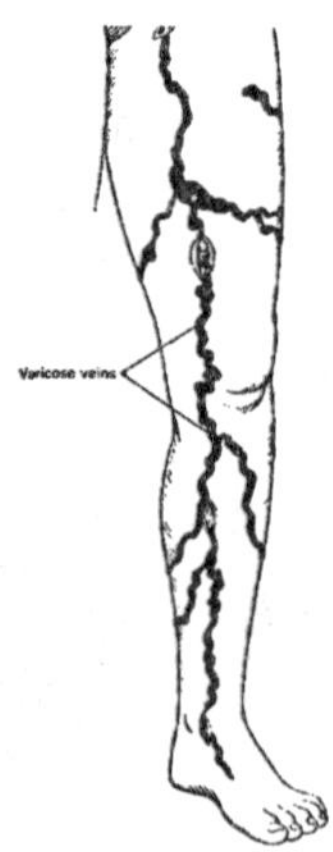

Varicose Veins

become elongated. Varicose veins look like an snake-like appearance. The valves in the varicose veins are incompetent to prevent backflow of blood resulting in stagnation, followed by swelling and pain in the legs, around the ankles and the calves, when the person suffering from varicose veins has been standing for a long time usually lead to reduced blood supply to the muscles. The following measures are suggested to treat varicose veins :

1. Check your weight as extra weight increases pressure on your venous circulation.
2. Blood sugar should be kept within prescribed limits.
3. Avoid prolonged standing.
4. Wear comfortable padded low-heel shoes.
5. Wear varicose vein stockings available at a chemist or surgical store.

25. How to choose a contraceptive?

It is a personal decision depending on the couple. For a newly married couple on way to plan their family, the best options are condoms and spermicides (seek medical consultation). In case of a woman who has never conceived before using an IUCD could result in infection of the tubes or uterus, which may lead to infertility. The couple blessed with one child would like to space out the other, birth control pills are the best option but these have to be taken daily. The permanent method of conception is recommended in case the couple doesn't want any more children. But it is prudent to wait till your child/children are five years of age. So depending upon the economic background, weight and education choose the right contraceptive for yourself. IUD prevents pregnancy by its copper action, which prevent embryo implantation in the uterus. On expiry, its efficiency is decreased. The IUD needs to be changed on its expiry. You should get the old one removed and new one inserted within a week of your periods.

26. Yellow discharge

Yellow discharge from vagina can be due to infection- fungal or bacterial conditions. Candid V6/V3 is used for treating fungal infection. For bacterial infection get a high vaginal swab for culture sensitivity done.

27. Loose vaginal muscles

Loose vaginal muscles cannot prove that you are not a virgin, nor these muscles will fail in satisfying the male partner. Regular practive of VAJROLI MUDRA- a Yogic posture, however, helps to tighten and strengthen loose vaginal muscles. This yogic exercise strengthens the anterior and posterior parts of the pubic muscles. Do about 20 rounds of the Vajroli Mudra for good results.

In **Vajroli Mudra**, sit in Padma Asana (Lotus Pose) or any comfortable meditative asana. Place hands on knees, close eyes,

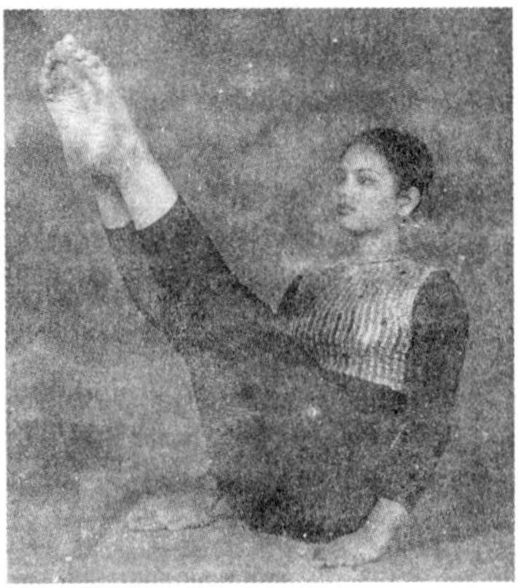

Vajroli Mudra

feel relax and breathe through nose. After a deep inhalation, hold breath and try to draw the sexual organs upward by pulling and tensing the lower abdomen contracting the pelvic muscles as if one has an urge to pass urine but want to hold one for some time as shown in the illustration. Now exhale, relax and repeat the posture. This posture helps those suffering from premature ejaculation and delay climaxing (orgasm) when involved in intercourse.

28. 'Aerola' and its purpose?

Aerola of female breasts is the pigmented area surrounding the nipple. Its size varies considerably from woman to woman and from breast to breast. The aerola consists of several oil producing Montromery's glands, which may form raised bumps and are sensitive to a woman's menstrual cycle. These glands act to protect and lubricate the nipple during lactation.

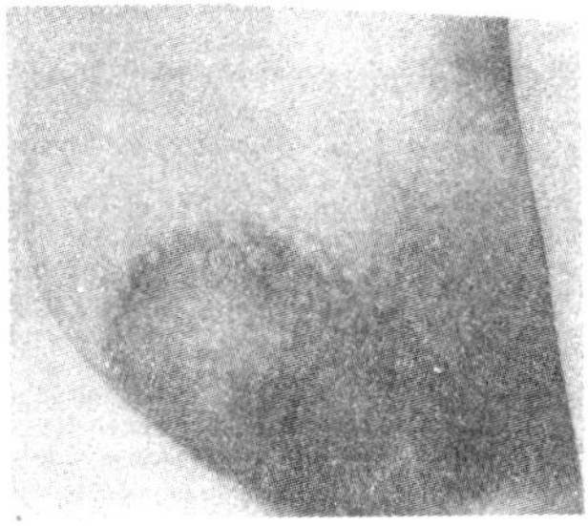

Aerola

29. Acidity during Pregnancy

Acidity, belching, gas: these occur because of the growing baby in womb. The enlarging uterus occupies more and more space in the abdomen as a result of which the stomach is pushed up. This leads to a reflux of the acid present in the stomach into the food pipe, causing heart burn. Take small frequent meals so that the stomach should not remain full. Avoid foods that cause acidity like tea, coffee, cola, spicy and sour foods. Take dinner at least two hours before bedtime. To cure heartburn, take a glass of milk with honey.

30. Marriage between blood relations

Marriage between close relations is genetically unhealthy. The father and mother may carry the same type of unhealthy genes, which could intensify the unhealthy manifestation in the offspring. Here is an example of a couple-both closely related. Their first baby was mentally retarded. They had an abnormal second baby. The third, a premature died at birth. The fourth was also premature and an abnormal baby.

31. Female Orgasm

Female orgasm is the acme of pleasure associated with spontaneous spasm of muscles in and around the genitalia (mainly the clitoris and vagina). Such contractions come in waves and the sexual release of the female corresponds to the climax experienced by the male partner at the time of ejaculation. Many women attain an orgasmic release easily through manual practices then through an intercourse. Some others, get an orgasmic spontaneous release during sleep as in case of night emission in males. For most women sexual gratification is an overall feeling of satisfaction at the end of the act.

32. How often to have sex?

Frequency of sex depends upon the couples to suit their mood and needs. The frequency of the relationship varies from couple to couple. Some need sex everyday, others on once or twice a month even in early stage of marriage. With increasing age there is decline in sex in many couples.

33. Lesbian

A lesbian is a female homosexual. Rather than being sexually attracted to the opposite sex, a woman is sexually attracted to her own sex. There are several women who have more than friendly relations with someone of their own sex, causing marital problems. Due to early marriage trend in India, most women do not stay single for years after adulthood. Early lesbian tendency in girls in adolescence or hostel life generally leads them to normal healthy homosexual act.

34. Puerparium

It is a medical term for the post delivery period when the genital passage and the uterus gradually get back to the original size and it takes about six weeks. Vaginal discharge, which is initially frank blood with mucous gradually become lighter in color till it finally stops. During puerparium, there are chances of uterus getting infected, A thorough hygiene condition after the delivery in women are to be maintained with a light nutritious diet supported with adequate vitamins and minerals.

35. Contraceptive Methods

These are mainly of three types:

1. ***Coitus interrupts*** : This is common but unreliable and unhealthy method of contraception usually practiced by traditional couples, in which the sex act is interrupted at the time of male ejaculation when the male organ is quickly withdrawn out of the vagina as soon as the semen is discharged out. However, long-term practice of coitus interrupts can cause pelvic congestion with the formation of ovarian cysts in the female.
2. ***Rhythm method*** : This method follows the natural ovulation pattern in women which takes place once a month on the 14th day of the cycle. The days immediately before and after this

day are the most fertile days, while the days following the menses and preceding the next period are the least fertile. The ovum is capable of getting fertilized for two or three days after its liberation. Discharged sperms remain vital for three or four days in the upper regions of the female genital tract. If the intercourse is avoided during ovulation and four days before and four days after, the chances of conception are minimal. The husband's cooperation is very necessary for the success of the method as he must completely avoid sex for about ten days in the mid cycle or use a condom.

3. ***Lactating the baby***: In many women, during total lactation the ovulation stops and menses doesn't take place. During this period she cannot conceive or has very low fertility. Lactation as a help to family spacing cannot be totally depended upon. There are instances, despite lactation, when the woman conceives even before menstruation restart. In some cases, menstruation and ovulation commence within three months. The early restart of sex brings on quicker menstruation and ovulation due to hormonal effect on the system with decreasing breast milk.

36. Female Sterilization and Male Vasectomy

Sterilizing the male or the female is the best way for permanent stop to pregnancy and childbirth, in males the operation is called Vasectomy. In this case the vas (the ducts carrying the sperms from the testes to the urethra in the penis) is cut on both sides and tied as it lies beneath the skin of the scrotum. Correctly done operation is 100% successful. Vasectomy has no fears about loss of sexual-pleasure and to perform the sex act and general debilitating effects. Vasectomy if performed un-hygienically can lead to an infection in the internal genital organs. In rare cases the operation causes nerve pain during erection.

In female the operation is known as tubectomy. The fallopian tubes on either side are cut and ligatured. The operation is most easily performed a week after delivery when the uterus is still high up in position and tubes easy to ligature. The operation is performed by laproscopic method (a pencil like instrument fitted with microscope and performs micro-surgery) performed with about an inch long cut into the abdomen.

37. Infertility

Nearly 60% female and 40% male are seen responsible for infertility. In women the causes of sterility are numerous : due to defect in the sex organs, ovarian problems, hormonal imbalance due to pituitary, thyroid or adrenal malfunction or due to chemical anti-sperm action of her genital secretions. On the other hand, in the male sterility is generally due to psychological or functional impotency, lack of sperm production by the testes, extremely frail sperms that lose their mobility and lack of vitality soon or due to an auto-immune reaction in the male's system that destroys his own sperms.

38. Artificial insemination

It is done with the husband's or donor's sperm, around the time of the wife's ovulation. The sperms are injected into the cervical canal to make sure the sperms have found their way up to the uterus. Even if the woman ovulates, if her tubes are blocked the sperm and ovum cannot unite. A donor's sample is required to find out the vitality of semen and the sperms.

39. Displacement of Uterus

The uterus or the womb is slung in the pelvic cavity and has great of movement in all directions. However, its natural position is upwards and forwards between the bladder and rectum. Displacement of uterus occurs because of several reasons and is usually accompanied by inflammation. The downward displacement of uterus is known as pro-lapse and in this condition the uterus slips downwards in the space between bladder and rectum. This condition is more common in older women.

The uterus distend during pregnancy when the fetus grows, its muscles get distended along with the advancing stage of pregnancy. The muscles, which support the uterus, must be strong enough to bear the burden of the growing child. After the delivery of child the uterus resumes its former shape and the muscles resume their former size. The symptoms, which indicate displacement of the uterus include backache or headache and heaviness in the bowels. Nerve centers are badly affected due to the displacement of uterus. The patient may be irritable and feel depressed. Doctors generally advise surgical interference for the treatment.

All body muscles (external or internal) if become lose, their tone and strength and their malfunctioning can result in such ailments. Lack of proper exercise and an inadequate diet lacking in essential vitamins and mineral substances can lead to weakness of the

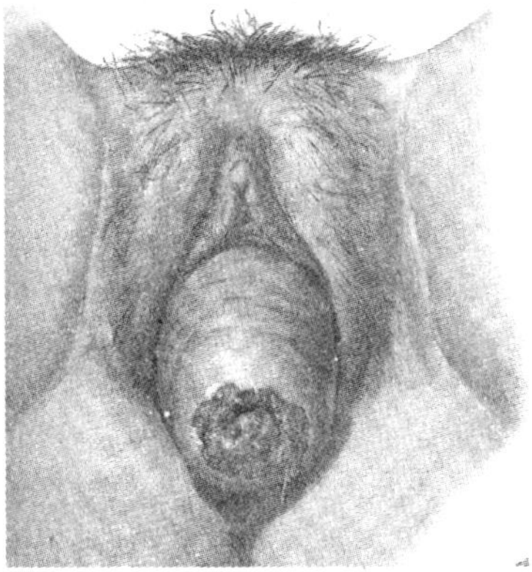

Prdapse Uterine

muscles of the body. A healthy woman doesn't experience any difficulty in childbirth and there are no complications afterwards. Remember, antenatal care and proper diet can ward off the danger of displacement of uterus. If the patient is weak and old, it could take long to put her back in shape. The following natural steps are recommended :

1. Take to fasting. Fasting should be continued for at least three days.
2. Have good diet containing fruits, milk and green vegetables.
3. Take bed rest, which provide relaxation. Relaxation drains out tension from the body.
4. Have a regular exercise plan designed to tone up the muscles supporting the uterus. Seek advise of a naturopathic doctor.
5. Rub the parts immersed in water while having Hip Bath.
6. Keep a hard pillow under the buttocks instead of under the head. This will help the uterus to return to its initial position.
7. Lie with your knees touching your breasts, that will help the uterus to resume its normal position.
8. Lie down after a meal with a pillow under your back.

40. Premature ejaculation

It is a malfunctioning due to psychological reasons generally in males who are sexually more aroused than the females who need a bit of foreplay to be ready for the intercourse. Too much anticipation of the sex act, too much of excitement can lead to premature ejaculation giving a feeling of failure or lack of fulfilment, which should follow the act of sexual intercourse. Apply Mud Pack on pubes before sleep at night.

41. Impotence

Impotence is the inability to perform sex - it may be partial or complete, temporary or permanent. Impotence can be in two categories – as a result of organic reasons or psychological reasons as described below :

Organic impotence : is caused by lesions of the external genitalia such as a tight foreskin, disturbances of endocrine glands like diminished activity of the gonads, thyroid glands or pituitary glands, diseases of the central nervous system and severe disturbance of health. Diabetes plays an adverse effect in this case. In case of treatment of impotency due to organic factors, deal with the disease, which has caused it.

Psychological impotence : is caused by the factors such as ignorance, fear, weakness or abnormality of sexual desire. The psychological treatment of impotence is to find the true reason and realize what has caused it.

Treatment : includes the following :

1. The best remedy for impotence is a healthy diet and exercise.
2. A wet pack (dipped in cold water) on the spine can help body to energize and strengthen the nervous system. Lie naked on the bed so that the wet bandage remains in constant touch with the spine.
3. Drink water in adequate quantity, it will draw away all the morbid matters poisoning the body system.

42. Frigidity

Frigidity is a condition in women, where she is unable to give her-self sexually to male partner and enjoy sex. This is usually due to the following reasons :

1. Psychological fear.
2. Wrong notions about sex.
3. Physical incapability.
4. Hormonal and genital defects.
5. Cultural taboos and social position.
6. Intellectual upbringing and emotional status playing a significant role in female sexual behavior.
7. Sexual indifferences (which is the major reason) or positive dislike for sex.
8. Physical causes such as inflamed vagina, a very rigid hymen, urinary problem or uterine infection.
9. Displaced ovaries.

43. Male sterility and sexual weakness

Failure to fertilize the ovum or female egg cells may be due to several causes as below :

1. An emotional factor (mental block) or obstructions in male genital organs.
2. Infection involving the male genital organs.
3. Production of weak or dead sperm cells.
4. Lack of normal sex desire or deficiency of hormones.
5. Emotional factors such as anxiety and worry, which may bring on feelings of guilt and weakness interfering normal male sex life.

Treatment : Male sterility may gets benefited by the following ways:

1. Take 50 mg. Vitamin E tablets three times a day (Seek medical advice).
2. Deficiency may be corrected by taking healthy diet full of vitamins.
3. In case the disorder is due to psychological reasons, consult a psychiatrist.

44. Nocturnal emission

Involuntary discharge of semen (the fluid produced by testicles in male) during sleep or nocturnal emission is one of the common disorder among youths or even in mid-age persons. Night emission among youngsters is generally due to excitement because of reading vulgar literature or seeing a motion picture or TV serials having exciting scenes. The following treatment are recommended to get rid of this psychological disorder :

1. Avoid thoughts of sex.
2. Eat rich food.
3. Have dinner three hours before sleep.
4. Have an evening walk followed by a bath.
5. Go to the bed early (not later than 9 p.m.).
6. Application of a Mud Pack on pubes during sleep at night.

45. Excessive sex

There are women who are extremely passionate and feel uncontrolled desire of sex. They are constantly attracted towards opposite sex. This is often due to the following reasons :

1. Deep sense of insecurity produced by neglect in childhood and adolescence.
2. Genetically, some females are hyper-fertile and highly sexual.

Excessively sexual women need psychotherapy. Hormone therapy, too, neutralizes the effect of estrogen by administering progesterone hormones help to large extent.

46. Painful intercourse

Also known as dyspareunia, which may arise from muscular spasm of the vagina. Sometimes, there is a superficial ulceration following some injury and the tissues are very painful to the touch. Bladder infections are common in such cases, and these may lead to further complications. Following are causes for a painful intercourse:

1. Tightness in the female genital area following surgery. In such case usually tissues may have been drawn too tightly together.
2. Any type of pelvic inflammation may cause pain during sexual intercourse.
3. Nervous tension due to unconsciously afraid of pregnancy.
4. Problems, such as body odours, halitosis etc.

5. Lack of understanding on the part of male partner may cause a female pain during marital relations.

47. Urine escapes when laughing

The disorder is due to weakness of urethral opening or weak vaginal muscles, sometimes due to repeated childbirths and prolonged labor. The overstretched urethral opening loses its elasticity. The urine usually escapes out with increased abdominal pressure due to short length of urethra in females. Special exercises to tone up muscles around the urethra and pelvic floor will be needed. Repeated pulling in by muscle contraction of the urethral clitoral part helps.

48. Premarital sex in women

Premarital sex is not common in Indian males as well as females due to early marriages. Sex life starts with marriage in most of the cases. Women feel the risk of pregnancy due to premarital sex. If the woman goes through an abortion, it has its physical risk to health and can produce hemorrhage, rupture of uterus, infection and other serious complications. It may also catch a pelvic infection, vaginitis or urinary infection and risk of sexually transmitted diseases.

49. Sex after menopause

Menopause is not the end of sex life and a woman can continue normal sex for years after she has stopped her menses and has passed child-bearing period. Many women enjoy satisfying sexual partnership even in old age. There are numerous couples in 60s who are involved in active sex life. Sometimes, menopausal women face problems having sex due to severe dryness of genital organs with pain during intercourse. Lubricating creams or estrogen ointments help to prevent the rapid atrophy of the vaginal mucosa.

50. Female hormones

Female hormones : estrogen and progesterone are produced in ovaries under the direction of the pituitary gland - the master endocrine gland of the body, which gives the woman strength, stamina, graceful curves and feminine shape of her body. Estrogen-the prominent female hormone gives her enormous drive, energy and great power. When a girl reaches eleven or twelve years of age, her ovaries start producing estrogen, causing her to grow and develop rapidly. The next 35 years are the reproductive period of her life when she can conceive and produce children. A young woman passes through ever changing monthly cycle. Progesterone has a special function of its own. As human life begins with production of some form of ovum or egg. Many thousands of developed egg cells are present in the ovary at birth, but only a few of these ever mature and become ready for fertilization (one each month of a woman's menstrual life).

51. Early start of periods

Sometimes, periods start even between the age of 10 and 11 due to hormonal imbalance. It has been observed that in few cases periods among teenagers do not stop until hormones are administered when her hemoglobin level starts decreasing drastically. Due to continuous intake of hormones, there are chances to put on lot of weight. Pelvic examination by Sonography is essential in such conditions. The patient should be given iron supplements to combat anemia and efforts should be taken to lose weight as obesity may further contribute to the hormonal imbalance.

52. Mid-cycle spotting

It can be due to hormonal imbalance. Get S, FSH, IH, T3, T4, TSH and prolactin tests done to rule out polyp or fibroid between periods.

53. Leakage of milk

Breasts are felt hard, sore and soaked because of milk secretion from breasts in early or mid pregnancy, often in the morning. Consult a gynecologist who will teach you how to take care of the breasts during pregnancy. Give a firm support to the breast using a good quality and correct-sized brassier which should be loose and supportive, but not too tight.

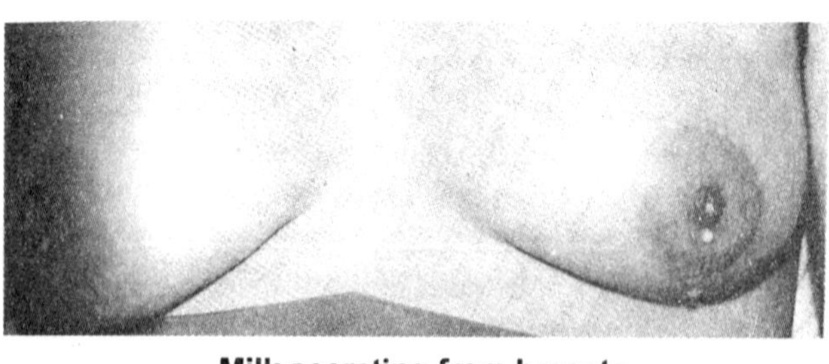

Milk secreting from breasts

54. Sex during pregnancy

Having sexual intercourse during pregnancy will not harm the fetus. You may continue right up to the onset of labor. As your abdomen enlarges, you may find intercourse more comfortable in positions that put less pressure on abdomen, like side-by-side position or the female on the top. If you have complications like bleeding or pain in abdomen, refrain from sexual activity and even nipple stimulation is to be avoided in such cases, as it can induce pre-term labor.

Doctors advise that intercourse should be avoided from the sixth to 12th week of pregnancy as it can cause miscarriage. Sexual intercourse is not recommended during the last two months of pregnancy too. At this time, there is risk of the essential amniotic fluid leakage during intercourse. However, the couple can and should engage in gentle love making, fondling and kissing. Intercourse during the first three months and the last two months of pregnancy is not advisable. During fourth to seventh month of pregnancy, intercourse is allowed unless there are medical reasons. Sexual act such as oral and anal sex should be strictly avoided throughout the pregnancy.

55. How to have male baby?

There is nothing much you can do to conceive a male baby except, perhaps use of Chinese calendar. Certain foods are said to change the pH of the vagina that, in turn promotes the longevity of the Y (male) chromosome containing sperms. Douching the vagina with various substances to change its pH is applicable in few cases but this is definitely not recommended. There are myths connected with the moon, such as if conceive during the waxlng moon you will have a male baby. And if during the waning moon a daughter. However, methods like ultrasound to detect sex of unborn baby in womb, are banned by the Government.

56. 4-D ultrasound

A 4-D Ultrasound is the latest addition in the armamentarium of an obstetrician. A 3-D Ultrasound gives a 3-D dimensional view of the baby. An ultrasound gives a 2D dimensional view, which makes the diagnosis of the malformations and the surface of the body of baby and internal malformations can be visualized clearly. A 3-D Ultrasound is like a still photograph whereas a 4-D Ultrasound is like taking video film of fetus malformation and the pregnancy, especially in case the mother is over thc age of 35 years and has delivered a malformed baby in past.

57. Rashes and pain in breasts

Rashes can be due to various reasons, the most common can be due to the reasons: allergy due to wearing synthetic brassiere, bacterial viral or fungal infections. A mammogram and ultrasound is done for lumpy, painful breast. If there are cysts found in the breasts, you can take any analgesic and wear tight bras to support them and relieve pain. 400mg of vitamin E or B taken over a period of time may lessen the pain. If the pain is severe, danazol or hormone therapy is recommended. Periodic examination of breast is also necessary.

58. Effect of copper-T

The effect after insertion of the Cu-T can lead to a change in menstrual flow for a couple of months. Some women experience backache, white discharge from vagina or heavy periods, spotting due to erosion and congestion and irritation around the cervix.

59. Stretch marks on abdomen during and after the pregnancy

Striae gravidarum or stretch marks appear on the lower abdomen in 50 to 90 percent of all pregnant women usually in the later half of pregnancy. These may also appear on thighs, hips, buttocks, breasts and upper arms of women, which appear as pinkish lines on the fair women and lighter than the normal skin in dark complexioned women. After delivery they acquire a silvery hue. The market is flush with creams and ointments to cure stretch marks. The stretch marks depend upon the family history, weight gain and nutritional status.

60. Severe cramps before periods

Between 30 to 50% women suffer cramps pain during or before menses, which differs from woman to woman .The cramps felt in abdomen before menses are difficult to cope but doesn't show that there is any abnormality in the genitals of the woman. About 10% women pass through severe pain and cramps during menses and are even unable to walk due to stress and strain as in case of delivery of child. During menstruation the pain in the lower back and pelvis is common and is called as 'initial pain'. The main reason for such pain is due to hormonal changes generally as a result of the contraction of uterus when it discharges blood.

A hot water bath of the lower part of the abdomen relieves pain. Consult a doctor if the pain is severe and doesn't stop for few days, the pain is different from menstruation pain and if you experience pain during and after intercourse. Smoking, sleeplessness and taking carbohydrates and fat foods worsen conditions. Bad sitting posture, headache, diarrhea, constipation, nausea or pain before menstruation further worsen the condition.

61. Sex in the morning

Morning is the better time for sex due to the following reasons:

1. The testoterone level in the male is higher in the morning.
2. Men and women have higher levels of growth of the hormone due to increased energy after a night of rest.
3. Often a man awakes with a full bladder, which compresses the venous blood return and prevents blood escaping from the penis as a result the male partner experience spontaneous erections in the morning.
4. Good sex act requires good blood flow towards sex organs and is achieved better in the morning with empty stomach.

62. Leakage of semen

The semen leaks out of vagina after the sex act, often women unable to conceive feel so. It is normal as a very small quantity of semen after the intercourse enters the uterus and rest of it has to come out of the vagina sooner or later. An adequate sperm count in semen may cause inability to conceive.

63. Ovarian cancer in Women?

It is generally caused due to rapid succession of childbirth, wear and tear of the cervical tissue and natural genital secretions. The

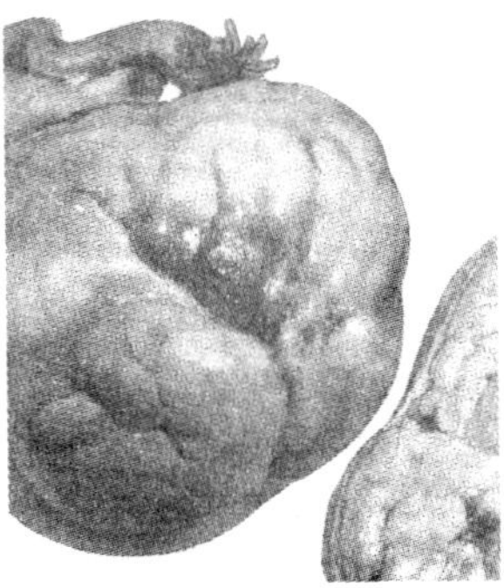

Ovarian Cancer

following symptoms are observed when patient suffers from cervical cancer :

1. Abnormal blood stained vaginal discharge.
2. Intermittent prolonged menstrual bleeding.
3. Intercourse bringing on bleeding.
4. Foul smelling vaginal secretion.
5. Pain in the lower abdomen running down the leg.
6. Constant backache.
7. Wear and tear of cervical tissues.

To treat cancer of cervix, measures such as surgical removal of affected part and destroying cancerous cells by radium or cobalt are adopted. If not treated at initial stage the cancerous cells may spread to liver and the brain.

64. Blood Tests during pregnancy

A blood test could reveal every disorder in your body. Everyone, from a pre-teen to a menopausal woman, will, at some time or the other, have to undergo for a blood test on the recommendation of doctor. The blood tests are usually of six types :

1. CBC-ESR Test : is required to test the erythrocyte sedimentation rate, which indicates the presence of an infection or an inflammatory process. The CBC test, which may count red cells in the blood. A high white blood count can also reveal the dreaded cancer of blood (Leukemia).
2. Follicular stimulating Hormones (FSH) Test : The doctor suggests FSH test to teens with irregular periods to rule out a condition known as the polyestic ovarian syndrome.
3. Haemogram : For women with excessive bleeding are required to go for Haemogram, which highlights anemic condition to check diabetes.
4. The Serum Beta HCG Blood Test : It is a test to confirm pregnancy and is usually recommended, if the woman has missed her period.
5. HIV Test : It is a compulsory for a pregnant woman to check sexually transmitted infections like Syphilis, Gonorrhea and Hepatitis-B, and to make decision about whether to continue the pregnancy.

6. RH factor : This concerns with pregnant women. If the mother is RH negative (RH-) the baby is usually delivered through a caesarean procedure.

65. Pre-elcamptic toxemia (PET)

PET is a combination of oedema e.g. swelling on the ankles and fingers followed by puffiness of the face and with increased blood pressure and presence of protein in the urine. The risk of PET is more in obese women and teenage girls. Women with family history of high blood pressure are prone to the risk. In case it is not treated timely there may be serious conditions of fits and the birth of a retard child. Infra-uterine growth retardation is a condition where the growth of a baby lags behind and it is more common in anemic and malnourished women.. For a healthy baby, it is essential to part with smoking and alcohol. Certain conditions like high blood pressure, chronic kidney diseases, heart ailments and some infections also affect baby's growth.

66. How to do a Pregnancy Tests?

Most pregnancy tests are based on hormonal concentration of bHCG in urine. This test is sensitive and become positive as early as 2 to 3 days before missed period in case of pregnancy. The accuracy is 98.5%. Collect the early morning urine sample in a clean bottle. Only a few drops are sufficient for a pregnancy test. 14 days after a missed period is the usual time to have a pregnancy test. A few doctors give hormone pills. Remember, you may bleed even if you are pregnant and this delay your finding out for sure pregnancy.

67. Abortion

Women with unwanted pregnancies have always resorted to abortion. With restricted law, an abortion is illegal. The pregnancy may be due to the following reasons :

1. Contraceptive failure.
2. Intercourse, when got drunk in parties or otherwise in higher society and fairly liberal families which sometimes end with sex.
3. Strong mutual attraction towards opposite sex.
4. Too shy to discuss contraception with the male partner, when a female becomes pregnant.

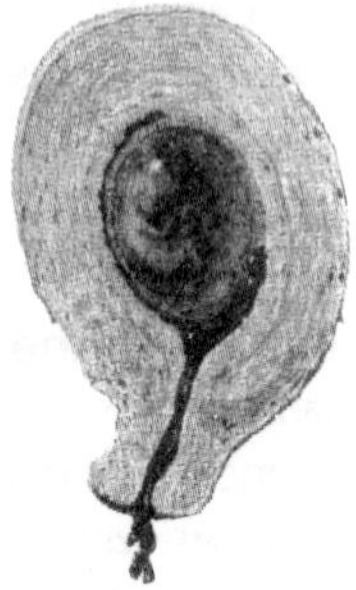

Threatened Abortion

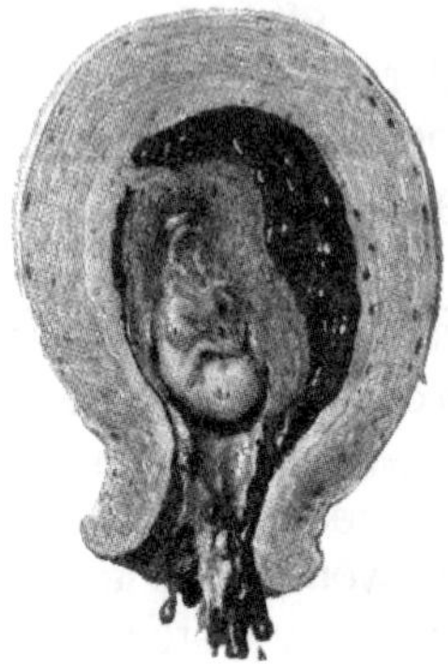

Inevitable Abortion

5. Urge to have sex with opposite sex in youth without thinking after-effect.
6. Fulfill the desire of boss at the place of work.

Most abortions are carried out before 12 weeks of pregnancy and by the commonest method called vacuum aspiration or suction. The cervix is dilated or widened carefully and the contents of the womb are sucked out using a suction apparatus.

Another method of abortion, instead of vacuum aspiration between 12 to 14 weeks of pregnancy is Dilation and Curettage by inserting prostaglandin pessaries or a substance called laminaria into the vagina. The contents of the womb are then removed by instrument called a curette made of soft wire rather than by suction. It cleans the womb and most of the tissues removed during abortion look like a very heavy period. If the bleeding persist and is very heavy, see a doctor immediately. Retained products in uterus lead to an infection. This sometimes happen about a week or ten days after the abortion.

68. Abortion after 12 weeks

Abortion after 12 weeks becomes more difficult although it is still a safe technique. In this process instead, after dilating the cervix, the doctor may insert instruments into the womb. The technique is called Dilation and Evacuation and is carried out under general anesthesia. Late abortions are conducted by Hysterectomy, a technique used very rarely, which involves removing contents of the womb by an operation very like a caesarean section. It is done under general anesthetic.

Any abortion done after 12 weeks is likely to cause pain and cramps, which may last several days and the womb shrinks back to its pre-pregnancy size. The bleeding will also go on for about a week. Avoid activities like swimming, soaking in a hot bath, wearing tampon or having sexual intercourse for six weeks.

69. Do and dont's about breast care

1. Keep your breast nipples clean and dry to prevent them from becoming sore and infected. Do not use soap to clean nipples and areola to avoid cracks.
2. Just wash breasts and nipples with water to remove traces of milk.
3. Make sure to change bra frequently. The secretion of nipples causes infection.
4. In case nipples are not soft and supple, apply some cream or oil. Avoid use of mustard oil, it irritates. Keep breasts exposed to air for sometime in a day.
5. Prevent engorgement of breasts to ensure frequent emptying and after a feed.
6. Breasts sag if the infant suckles while sitting or reclining in a faulty posture. Always let the baby suckles in a sitting position with the child in the lap and your hands under the head.
7. Remove the remaining milk with a couple of jerks after feeding the child.

70. Advantages of breast-feeding

Breast-feeding is the most perfectly balanced food that a baby needs for growth during first 3-4 months. It prevents many illness, infections and allergies. Lactation helps in controlling the bleeding after delivery, the womb returns to its normal position, sheds extra weight gained during the pregnancy, prevents cancer, helps in spacing children, convenient for mother during travel and the milk is more digestible as compared to cow's milk.

3
Skin Disorders

The human body has been given a most beautiful covering-the skin. Nothing is more lovely and attractive than a glowing healthy skin. Skin troubles often run in families. Everyone should be aware of the importance of keeping the skin healthy. Apart from enhancing beauty, your skin has several very important functions. It is your first line of defense against the germs that might enter the body. Enzymes on the surface of the skin quickly destroy germs, provided the skin is healthy and intact. But small breaks and tears in the surface of skin may open the way to infection within the skin and in deeper tissues as well.

Your skin has another important function; it helps to regulate the body temperature. When you exercise vigorously, you produce a lot of heat in the muscles. To keep the temperature of the body at a normal level, this heat must be removed quickly, otherwise you will soon have fever. To cool the body, large amount of blood is rapidly sent to the skin. Many tiny vessels within the skin open up, allowing much more blood to pass through and to be cooled by the outer atmosphere. The process of perspiration is very important. Tiny sweat glands within the skin pour out surprisingly large amount of water. At this perspiration evaporates, it carries off large quantities of heat and this perhaps helps to cool the body.

What is itching?

Itching is a unpleasant sensation, which we attempt to relieve by scratching. A certain amount of mild itching is normal for everyone.

Only when it is persistent and troublesome does it become serious. Many conditions contribute to itching. These include insect bites, hives, contact dermatitis, food allergies and heat rash. Other causes may be diabetes, uraemia, jaundice, pregnancy, menopause (the change of life). Persistent scratching may produce swelling in the skin with deep scratch marks and small ulcers into which germs have found their way, causing much more trouble. Itching due to drug reactions are common following the use of certain medicines such as aspirin, phenobarbital, pencillin and many others. Some medicines applied to the skin may also cause a certain amount of itching. Some people are allergic to nylon, others to wool, and still others to dyes and cosmetics. If the itching has spread over large areas of the body, try an oatmeal bath as described below:

Mix one cup of oatmeal with two cups of cold water and pour this into a tub of water. Lie in this tub for at least 20 minutes twice daily. When drying yourself, be careful not to increase the irritation. Gently pat the skin and then apply some soothing medicine in consultation with a doctor. If the itching around the rectal and genital areas, and around the face and eyes is severe, apply hydrocortisone ointment with the consultation of your doctor. Apply the following (self-made) ointment by mixing :

Camphor	1.0 gm.
Menthol	1.0 gm
Calamine lotion	100 cc.

Prickly Heat

Prickly heat or heat rash is an irritating eruption of the skin due to obstruction of the sweat gland over certain areas of the body. In this condition many tiny pin-head-size swellings occur in the skin, accompanied by severe itching. The most involved areas on the body are the chest, back, waistline, armpits and groins. Infants and overweight persons often suffer from heat rash.

Try to avoid scratching, for this may introduce germs into the deeper layers of the skin. Wear cool, light clothing and abstain from alcoholic drinks. Oatmeal baths twice in a day as described above under the heading 'Itching' may relieve the condition (itch). Be sure to drink plenty of water during hot weather. Keep the skin clean and avoid the use of harsh soaps.

Chafing of the Skin

When two skin surfaces rub together, such as under the breasts or between the thighs, one or both surfaces may become red and irritated. This opens the way for germs and fungi to infect the skin. Burning and itching often follow, especially in the armpits, around the anus, between the fingers and toes, and in the groins. Skin chaffing is always worse in those who are overweight, especially during hot weather. If the patient has diabetes, this increases susceptibilities to chafing.

Apply some good talcum powder several times a day. Wear cool clothing and avoid strenuous exercise in hot weather. Obese patients should definitely lose weight. Severely irritated skin may get relieved by applying cool, moist compresses containing a weak solution of potassium permanganate. Dissolve one tablet of potassium permanganate in one liter water. Wring out a small compress, such as a face cloth, and apply this to the irritated skin for at least 15-20 minutes three to four times in a day.

Excessive Sweating

A certain amount of sweating is normal for everyone. But excessive sweating is definitely abnormal. Many people are troubled with cold when, wet hands and feet, especially when under nervous strain. Remember, excessive moisture on the skin always raises the possibility of further infection with fungus and bacteria, especially on the feet, around the genital areas and under the armpits. If the armpits and groins are also involved, strong odors may arise. These odors usually arise from the breakdown of sweat and cellular debris, due to the action of germs on the skin.

Look for the cause. A complete physical examination is advisable to rule out presence of some other disorder that should be corrected. For localized areas, apply potassium permanganate compresses three times a day on affected area, followed by applying a good talcum powder. Frequent bathing is advisable for getting rid of odor. Superfluous hair should be removed from the underarm, armpits and groins to relieve the condition.

Acne, pimples and scars

Acne is caused by an increase in androgen hormone activity, which stimulates the functioning of the sebaceous glands. The shedding of dead skin cells cause blockage within the hair follicle, which become infected. An overgrowth of the skin over the pores is another prominent factor. Acne usually starts to develop around the adolescence in both male and female, which clears up after 5 to 10 years. In some older people acne can sometimes develop spontaneously. The face is the usual site of acne, although it can also appear on the chest, neck, shoulders, back, scalp, legs and upper arms.

Acne usually consists of the following:

- Blackheads : Blocked matter in the pores oxygenates and turns black.
- Comedones : Pores becoming blocked with mixture of sebum and dead skin cells.
- Nodules : Inflamed area cause scarring.
- Papules : Inflamed area without infection.
- Pustules : An inflammation, which contain pus.
- Macules (scarring) : Cause when the skin is treated incorrectly.
- Whiteheads : When pores have closed, trapping matter inside.

The hormonal imbalance, allergic reaction and poor diet are the major cause for the adrenal glands to be stimulated, leading to hormonal imbalances, which mostly occur during adolescence and occasionally during the menopause in women and also prior to periods. They may create the conditions under which acne erupt.

How to treat acnes and pimples by herbal ways?

1. Cleanse the skin thoroughly. Cleansing should consist of the products containing an anti-inflammatory substance being smoothed over the face with a disposable fabric or cotton wool.
2. Wipe the cleanser off with appropriate hydrolat such as thyme (ban ajwain), myrtle (mehndi plant) lemongrass, lavender (plant flower) or camomile german (babuna ka paudha) with disposable fabric or cotton wool. Repeat cleansing process twice.
3. Apply a compress of green tea (Camilla sinensis) on the face and leave for five minutes. Dry the face. Apply blend of essential oil in the appropriate base oil.
4. Gently press oil on the face, starting at the chin towards the forehead. Apply a warm, damp, green tea muslin compress over the top of the oil.

5. If there is no acne on the neck, gently place your hands on the trapezius muscle and in continuous flowing movement using long strokes, moving towards the occipital. Start with right hand, followed by the left hand. Repeat six times. Do not massage the face rapidly; this may cause further inflammation.
6. Now treat reflex points. Start at the forehead. Harmonize energy by holding the face in both hands for few seconds. If using a compress, leave for one to three minutes. If using a poultice, leave for five minutes. Now apply mask, leave it on the face for not more than ten minutes. Finish by wiping with a hydrolate. Relax for few minutes, and have a glass of water to drink. To complete treatment, rub hands briskly. Leave skin free for at least 24 hours.

How to get rid of pimples and acne by Ayurvedic treatments?

Pimple can mar many a lovely skins, besides permanently scarring. Pimples generally crop up on the cheeks, forehead and nose. The following home remedies can work wonder:

- Make a paste of the barks of neem and turmeric (haldi) and rub on the affected skin.
- Rub a piece of sandalwood on a clean stone using rose water or cucumber juice to make a paste. The pack gives a tingling fresh feeling and will discourage pimples.
- Multani mitti (Fuller's earth) pack is an effective means to control pimples. Dissolve multani mitti in water to make a thin paste. Smear over the affected skin and wash with cold water when it dries.
- Mix one part of slake lime with 20 parts water. Mix it to two parts pure sulphur powder. Boil the mixture till half the quantity is left. Apply a light coat of fluid to the pimples and acne.
- Take a spoonful of honey mixed with water and lemon juice daily in the morning.
- Crush mint to make a paste and apply the pack thrice a week. Wash the face after ten minutes with cold water.
- Mix gram-flour in a spoonful of coconut oil and rub it on the affected skin. When it dries, wash the face with mild hot water.
- Onion mask is used on blemished oily skin prone to pimples and acne. Mix together one tablespoon each onion juice and kaolin powder with a teaspoon of honey. Apply thick paste on the affected skin.

- A sulphur mask helps a lot. Mix together one teaspoon sulphur powder, two teaspoons Fuller's earth, one beaten egg white and a little rose water to make a paste. Apply pack on the affected skin, let it dry for 30 minutes, then wash off with luke-warm water. Make an allergy test before applying mask, because some skins suffer an adverse reaction to sulphur. To test, spread a little paste over the skin on elbows, leave for ten minutes to check reaction.

Precautions:

- Use sulphur soap to keep oil glands open.
- Steam your face once a week to clean skin pores.
- Cleanse stale make-up at night before going to bed.
- Do not peel-off pimples that cause septic and may leave behind permanent scars.
- Cut down on sweets, fats and spicy dishes.

Face Packs and Products for Skin Disorders

Face packs are used for toning of tired skin. Face pack has property similar to toner. A pack should be applied after applying a scrubber, which opens the pore due to scrubbing effect. Therefore, it is very essential to close down the pores with the help of a face pack. The following face packs are useful for a faulty skin:

- **Anti Sun Tan Pack** : Suitable for all types of skins for uniform complexion when used mixed with rose water and lemon juice.
- **Sandal Pack** : Suitable to tone up all types of skins and lighten the blemishes when used with rose water and glycerin.
- **Tulsi Pack** : Suitable for skins prone to acne and pimples.
- **Neem Pack**: Suitable for acne, pimple and scarred skin due to its antiseptic properties.
- **Cucumber Pack** : Suitable for dull, tired, tan skin (dry to normal skin) due to cleansing and toning properties when used with rose water.
- **Egg Pack** : Suitable for dull, wrinkled skin when used with rose water or a toner.
- **Orange Pack** : Suitable for excessive oily skin when used with astringent lotion.
- **Mint Pack** : Suitable for normal skin when used with rose water.

- **Skin Toner** : Tones the skin, reduces the pore size, prevents excessive sweating and sebum secretion.
- **Cleansing Milk** : Opens pores and draw out the dirt, dried sweat and sebum.
- **Astringent Lotion** : Used for oily skin and re-closes open pores.
- **Sun Screen Lotion** : Has the property to reflect back light and prevents rays from stimulating the production of melanin.
- **Moisturizer** : Essential for all types of skins.
- **Olive Oil** : Rich in vitamin E. Healthy skins need high proportion of vitamin E.
- **Rose Water** : Has natural toning properties.
- **Cold Cream** : Has good moisturizing property and prevents dryness.
- **Massage Cream** : A light weight, non-greasy and easily absorbable cream, which leaves relaxing effect on the facial/ body muscles and lot of glow is observed after massage.
- **All Purpose Cream** : Light in weight massage cream, which can be used to prevent dryness, provides softness and glow to the skin.
- **Almond Nourishing Cream** : Used as best remedy for any type of skin problem. Almond creams revives back the skin texture and brings glow.
- **Calamine Lotion** : Helps remove pimples, acne, scar and has sun-screening agents.
- **Tulsi Pomade** : Protects the skin from becoming dry. It heals dry, chapped and cracked skin. Has been known for its antiseptic and anti-bacterial properties.
- **Petroleum Jelly** : Protects the skin from drying and nourishes it.

Lesions of the Skin : A lesion is a structural change in the tissues caused by injury or disease. These are of two types: Primary lesions and Secondary Lesions.

Primary Lesions : These are the following :

1. MACULE : Small discolored spot or patch neither raised nor sunken on the skin.

2. PAPULE : Small elevated pimple without fluid or sometimes develop pus.
3. WHEAL : Itchy, swollen spot due to mosquito or insect bites.
4. TUBERCLE : Soiled lump projective above or under the surface of the skin.
5. TUMOR : External swelling varying in size, shape and color.
6. VESICLE : Small blister with clear fluid in it, beneath the epidermis.
7. BULLA : Large blister containing watery fluid.
8. PUSTULE : Pimply looking elevation with inflamed base containing pus.

Secondary Lesions : These develop in the later stage of the disease, which include :

1. SCALE : Dry or greasy epidermal flakes.
2. CRUST or SCAB : Accumulation of sebum and pus with epidermal material.
3. EXCORIATION : Skin abrasion produced by scratching or scraping due to loss of the skin.
4. FISSURE : Crack in the skin penetrating into the dermis.
5. ULCER : Mucous membrane of the body accompanied by pus.
6. SCAR : Usually forms after healing an injury or skin condition.
7. STAIN : Abnormal discoloration of skin.
8. ACUTE : A less violent skin disease.
9. CHRONIC : A long duration and recurring disease.
10. INFECTIOUS : A disease caused by pathogenic germs.
11. CONTAGIOUS : A disease communicable by contact.
12. CONGENITAL : Present since birth.
13. SEASONAL : Influenced by the weather.
14. OCCUPATIONAL : Afflicted by one's occupation.
15. PARASITIC : Caused by a vegetable or animal parasitic.
16. PATHOGENIC : A disease produced by bacteria.
17. SYSTEMIC : Over functioning of internal glands.
18. VENERAL : A disease acquired by contact with an infected person usually during sexual intercourse.

19. EPIDEMIC : A disease that attacks simultaneously large number of persons.
20. ALLERGY : Caused by contact with foods, cosmetics, medicines and tints resulting in itching, redness, swelling, blisters, oozing, pain, heat and scaling.

Treatment of Facial Scars and Blemished Skin with Essential Oils

It is not a surgery that can relieve from permanent scars, the cosmetic surgery is carried out to enhance the look of a person. Surgeons carrying out life saving procedures are not as concerned about the look of skin but most of the people, especially women are more concerned to rid of a treatment may eliminate the scars completely. Using essential oils before or after surgery treatment may lessen scarring and bruising. For the body, choose essential oils that have a relaxing effect. For the face, choose those that have energizing, toning effect.

New scars response very well to essential oil blends, which must be applied (not massaged) in the morning and evening for full effect. Choose essential oils that are anti-inflammatory and calming, as these are more effective. Camomile, yarrow, rose and geranium would be a good choice. Appropriate carrier or base oils would include camellia oil, macadamia oil, red carrot oil and rosehip seed oil. You may consult an herbal specialist, who may recommend use of a suitable essential oil according to the condition of your skin.

Treatment of old scars takes much longer to respond to treatment. Essential oils that help are frankincense, rose, geranium, fennel, lemon, orange and carrot seed. Very useful carrier or base oils are rosehip seed oil, borage oil, red carrot root oil and macadamia oil which are readily available at any herbal products store. Prepare massage oil for the scar area using the suggested essential oils and vegetable oils. On rest of the body, herbal ingredients such as camphor, sulphur, onion, garlic, curd, yeast, Fuller's earth (multani mitti) and vegetable juices are all useful in treating a blemished skin with scars. Here are few recipes (masks) very useful to eliminate scars. These have healing, soothing, astringent and tightening effect on the skin.

1. Mix together the ingredients such as ½ tablespoon oatmeal, ½ tablespoon camphor BP crystal and 2 tablespoons orange flower water. Apply the mask on the face and leave for 15 to 20 minutes, then wash off with lukewarm water.

2. Two drops of camphor spirit when added to one teaspoon each tomato juice and honey make a strong astringent skin tonic. This tonic should be left on the skin for about 15 minutes to relieve scars.
3. To improve your skin and cure scars apply home-made skin tonic, which can be prepared by mixing the following ingredients:

1 tablespoon	Glycerine
½ tablespoon	Borax Powder
5 tablespoons	Distilled Water

Blemished, Spotty, Wrinkled Skin during periods, pregnancy and postnatal

This is a serious skin problem for women during periods, pregnancy and after childbirth, which may become a permanent disorder if not treated timely. Rosemary flowers boiled in white wine lighten a sallow skin. A face wash with neat gin softens the wrinkles. Apricot oil rubbed into the most sensitive, soft skin every night before sleep fights ageing. An oily skin may benefit from a pack of mashed strawberries. Hard, leathery patches of skin can be softened with pineapple juice or a mash of papaya as both fruits contain enzymes. A tea made from fenugreek seeds purifies the blood. To clear minor blemishes, apply raspberry mask. Mix 25 gm. of mashed raspberries to a paste with 1 teaspoon each of plain yogurt and finely ground oatmeal. Leave on the face for 10 minutes, then rinse off.

Rubbing raw garlic on a spotty, blemished skin have a fine effect to kill spots. Comfrey, honey and garlic pack help to remedy for persistent pustules. Ground a handful of fresh comfrey leaves with enough honey to make a paste. For each teaspoon have one well-mashed garlic clove, apply on a piece of warmed cabbage leaf and tie on affected place on the skin and go to bed. To clear blemishes and spots, here are another ointments:

1. Melt 25 gm. of beeswax in a bowl on low heat. Add to it 100 gm. pure honey. Stir until cool, then pot. Keep in a cool place and apply to infected spots. Keep covered the area.
2. Collect the following ingredients :

1 tablespoon	Wheat-germ
2 teaspoons	Clear honey
1 teaspoon	Sunflower oil

1 teaspoon	Fresh lemon juice

Mix all ingredients together to make a thick paste. Apply in small circular rubbing movements to the face and neck. Leave for five minutes, then wash off with warm water. Splash with cold water and pat dry. Use this pack once or twice a week, but avoid use of soap in between. Wash your face in clear water only.

Red Cheeks

Sometimes, your skin react to products and shows signs of irritation or redness, you probably have hyper-reactive skin. There are two types of skin that fall into the 'sensitive skin' category: One that is susceptible to breakouts, and the other that is easily irritated. The irritation comes from an overdose of a product or using products that are too harsh. You have sensitive skin when:

1. You are prone to blotchy skin patches.
2. Products often cause redness and irritation.
3. Skin breaks out with exposure to household cleaners.
3. Alpha hydroxy acids and retinols irritate your skin.

The following measures should be taken to get rid of this problem:

- Choose make-up, moisturizers and sunscreens that are hypoallergenic and fragrance free.
- Minimize the amount of products you put on your face.
- Don't over-wash your face.
- Do not use exfoliants. Scrub instead with a mild, natural and gentle formula like sugar grains in olive oil. Don't use salt, as it may be too harsh.
- Use an astringent on oily areas only, but if redness occurs, discontinue using it.
- Use mild soap free cleansers.
- Opt for oil free make-up, especially foundation and blusher.
- Use a non-oily sunscreen daily.
- If you have breakouts, use a cleanser with salicylic acid to help exfoliate pores. There are also moisturizers that contain salicylic acid.

Red veins

The skin becomes red and thin, blood vessels seem very near the surface usually caused due to sensitive, neglected or ill-treated skin. Apply waxy cream, use moisturizer, avoid going from extreme of temperature to another and avoid rich, spicy foods, very hot drinks and alcohol.

Muddy Skin

The skin loses its radiance due to over-tiredness and lack of sleep. As a remedy the following measures are beneficial :

- Drink a glass of hot skimmed milk at night before going to bed
- Drink minimum four to six glasses of cold water everyday between the meals (not with the meals).
- Take fresh fruits, green vegetables as much as you can.
- Have cold drinks and fruit juices without sugar.

Red nose and prickly heat

Severe itching and burning are symptoms of red nose – a common trouble with hearty eaters and drinkers, and due to sudden change of temperature on delicate skin. Avoid sudden change of temperature and massage nose up and down with rose water mixed with glycerin. Red pustules of size of mustard grains appear on the body, especially on the chest, back and the abdomen due to profuse sweating during hot or rainy days and prickly heat. Apply green henna and leaves of 'neem' ground in water on affected skin. Pack of Fuller's earth (multani mitti) leaves a cooling effect on the skin. Avoid wearing heavy garments. Expose affected area to fresh air and have cool water bath twice a day during hot season.

Birthmarks

Dark brown patches to fleshy bumps and fairly small moles caused by scratching the pimples or due to small- pox disfigure the skin and sometimes leave a scar. Remedial measures include dealing minor scars with carbon snow, ray treatment and cortisone injections. Minor scars can be disguised temporarily by cosmetics or permanently by skin grafting or cosmetic surgery by a qualified skin specialist. Peeling treatment is the process, which cause deep cleansing by removing a thin layer of skin.

Boils and Pustules

Red, small, painful nodules start oozing pus and leave tiny scars. These generally occur in areas covered with coarse hair subjected to repeated mild friction on the neck, buttocks, knees and elbows.

Remedial measures include use of systemic antibiotics (only with the consultation of a doctor). Keep bowels clear and avoid fatty or

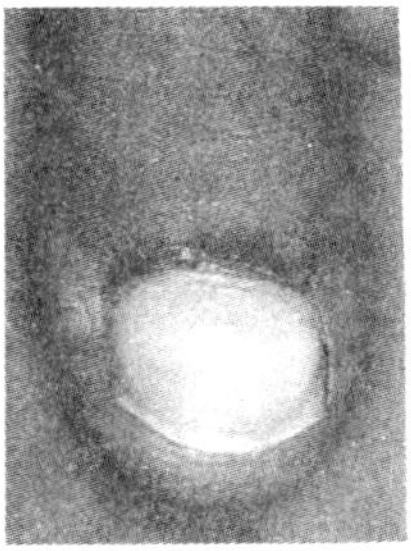

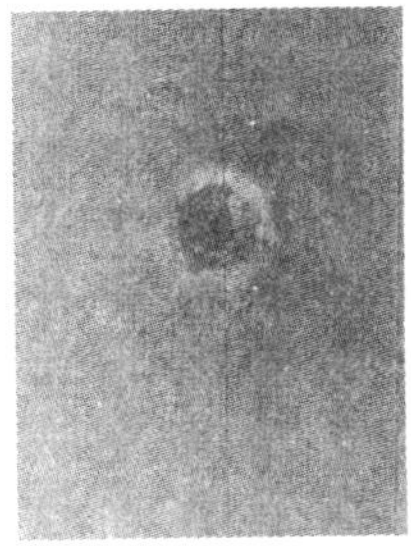

Boils and Pustules

sour products. Apply paste of 'neem' tree bark. Take melon, which keeps blood clean. Smear a leaf of 'peepal' tree with ghee and apply as a lukewarm bandage on the boil to enable it to burst.

Rhinoplasty (Deformed nose)

In this condition of a hump nose deformity, the skin of the upper part of the nose is free from the underlying bone and cartilage, which gives a saddle nose look. It may be treated surgically. The steps of operation include removal of hump, nasal curve, elevation of the tip of the nose and trimming of the lower part to suit the rest of the nose.

Leucoderma (White patches on skin)

Painless white spots or patches on the body, which expand if not treated. They are caused due to loss of pigmentation in the skin. To prevent the spread of leucoderma, protect from exposure to heat, have salt-free diet and apply 'chandan' pack on the patches. Soak seeds of 'babchi' in ginger juice for 72 hours, remove the husk, dry and powder, and apply on the patches. Apply the juice of the leaves of Goose Foot (bathua) to cure patches. The patient should be kept on salt-free diet.

The white patches on the skin are painless but a leucoderma patient is more embarrassed than a victim of any pain or discomfort. In addition to being a medical and beauty problem, it also becomes a social stigma. Remember, leucoderma is not a contagious disease. Darker skins have more patches, because such skins contain more melanin. It must be clarified here that white patches are not congenital, nor hereditary. Children are not affected if the mother has these patches. It is also erroneous to think that a woman who has leucoderma does not enjoy marital pleasures.

Crow's Feet

Lines and wrinkles appear on the face, skin hangs in folds and wrinkles appear around eyes causing ageing. Apply sesame or coconut oil over the face and neck before sleep. Remember, the anger and irritation add to the lines of age on the face. Douche with warm water and then cold water alternatively. Avoid rubbing the skin with towel but massage.

Cracked skin and open pores

The lips get chapped, the skin of the hands get cracks - generally occurs due to cold with the onset of winter or defective functioning of the sebaceous glands. Rub a little castor oil or olive oil on the skin. Apply hot milk cream on cracked skin. Use antibiotic cream and massage the affected skin at night. In case of open pores (when the face looks unattractive and the skin gives the appearance of enlarged pores) caused by the over-active glands, a poor diet and emotional disturbance the following treatments help :

Apply face pack twice a week. To make face pack, mix two tablespoons honey with ½ tablespoon lime juice and 1 tablespoon rose water. Another remedy is to apply a face mask. Mix cucumber juice with Fuller's earth (multani mitti) or gram flour and apply on the face. Let it dry for 10-15 minutes, then wash.

Sun Burn

Most sunburns are first-degree burns; you have roasted your epidermis-the outer layer of the skin, and its red, painful and hot. You can treat this sunburn easily as described below. If you have a second-degree burn, which involves the dermis or underlying skin

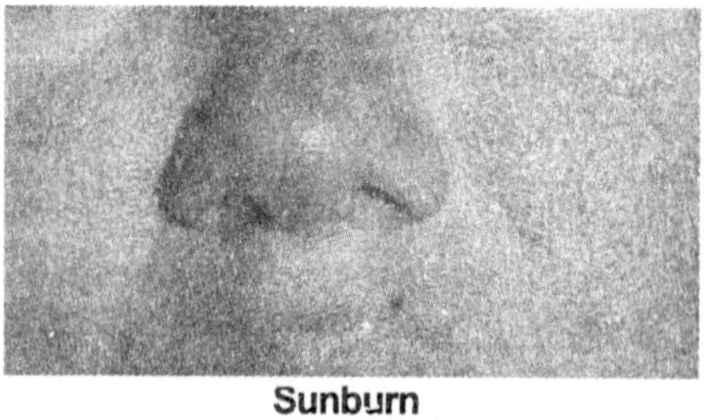

Sunburn

layer, which causes swelling, blisters, intense pain, and perhaps nausea, chills and fever as the body tries to cope with the shock, you need to seek immediate medical care.

Dryness of the skin due to dehydration causes scarring of the skin. It loses complexion and becomes dark, thick, leathery, wrinkled and patchy by the adverse effect of sun on the skin. Drink maximum quantity of water : at least 8 to 10 glasses a day in summer and 3 to 4 glasses a day during winter season. Apply sun tan lotion or cream. If the skin is dark, apply a mask of a mixture of bleaching powder and hydrogen peroxide. Aloe extract and lavender oil are excellent herbs to moisturize, cool and heal first-degree burns.

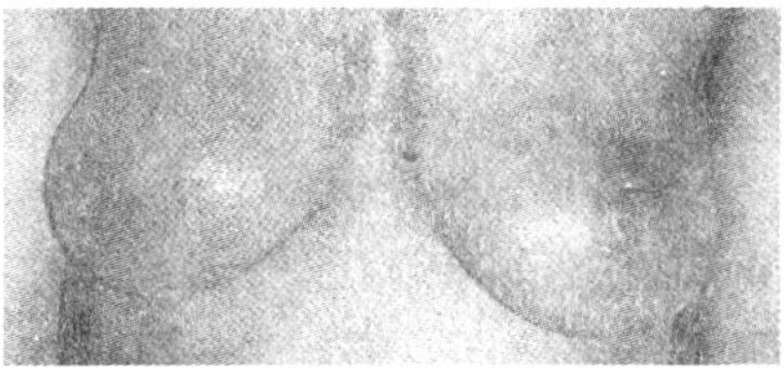

Scabies on the body

Contagious Diseases of skin

1. Scabies

Description : Scabies, also called sarcopties scabiei is a contagious disease caused by a mite, which lays eggs in burrows in the skin. The disease spreads through contact with infected individual, clothing and bedding. The commonly affected parts of the body are fingers, webs, palms, wrist, arm, skin around the breast nipples, buttocks, lower abdomen, area around female genitals and penis among males.

Signs and symptoms : Severe itching with excess irritation during night. Sometimes, a thin, slimy fluid oozes out of the scratched surface and then forms scabs.

Treatment : There are several ointments for the treatment of scabies. You may choose one as prescribed by your doctor. There are few herbal preparations for the treatment of affected skin as described below:

1. Boil the leaves of oleander (karbir) in 250 ml. water and massage the skin of affected parts with the thick oily liquid.
2. Mix lemon juice and jasmine oil in equal quantity and rub on the itching skin.
3. Ground in water poppy seeds, adding to it lemon juice. Massage the paste thus obtained on the affected skin to relieve itching and irritation.

4. Apply gamma benzene hexa-chloride (1% lotion or cream) on scabies.

2. Eczema

Description and symptoms : Eczema also called dermatitis or 'pama' in Ayurveda is an inflammatory disorder of the skin (causing dry, red, cracked or thickened skin), in which the scaly cuticles fissured with a sticky watery discharge are accompanied with itching and pain on the affected skin. The eczema may be dry or weeping (when it oozes). A dermatologist can only control the condition, not cure it.

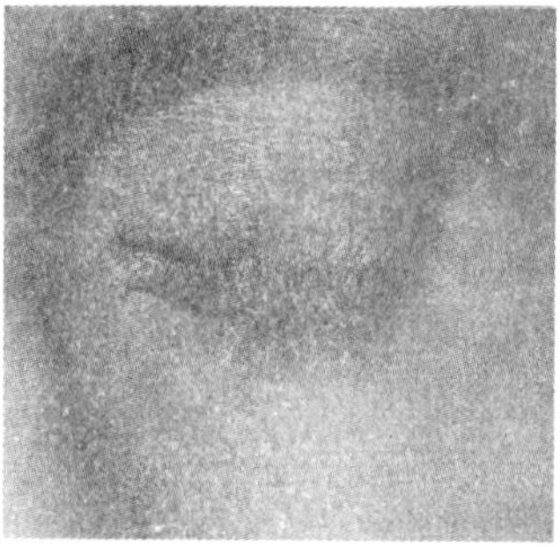

Eczema

Treatment : There are several ointments available in the market. You may select one after consulting your doctor. Most conventional treatments fall into either of the two categories: One is topical – a cream salve, or the other application that provides some degree of symptomatic relief. The other is oral – a prescription drug that suppresses bacteria or a virus that may be associated with the problem. The following home/ medicinal remedies cure the disorder:

1. Mix babchi powder with mustard oil and apply on the affected skin like an ointment.
2. Smear leaves of Indian butter tree (mahua) with sesame oil, warmed over heat and bandaged on the affected skin. Change the bandage after three to four hours.
3. Your doctor will recommend blood purifying drugs and foods. Certain components in oils, called fatty acids can help reduce inflammation and ease dermatitis (Perfect oils are available in the market). Follow the dosage according to the recommendations on the label or as prescribed by the doctor.

4. Antioxidants can help repair damaged skin by disarming free radicals, the unstable molecules that oxidize or destroy healthy cells. Free radicals can be produced as by-products of the body's fight against the inflammation of the dermatitis as well as by exposure to sunlight, smoking, eating fatty foods and many other lifestyle factors. Here are few most important antioxidants for the health of your skin and heal dermatitis (to be used strictly as per advice of a doctor). If the problem doesn't clear up within six weeks, consult your doctor:
   - Beta-carotene (recommended quantity 12 to 18 mg. daily).
   - Vitamin C (3,000 mg. to be taken in three doses a day at least 30 minutes before or 30 minutes after the meal, since stomach acid and the contents can destroy the effect of vitamin C).
   - Vitamin E (600 to 800 units daily).
   - Zinc (20 mg. a day for women and 30 mg. for men).
5. Fatty acids (certain components in oils usually omega-3, omega-6 and omega-9 oils from fish) and foods in your diet (dairy products, wheat, sugar, citrus fruits, corn, soy, peanut, butter, chocolate, coffee and alcohol) can help reduce inflammation and ease dermatitis. Watch their reaction and delete those that are triggering the problem, but at the same time supplement taking multivitamins.
6. Stress can cause or contribute to flare-ups of eczema. Meditation can help release the stress. Meditate daily for 15 minutes with closed eyes in a quiet room.
7. Aromatherapy : a first-rate relief including essential oils and herbs is a natural remedy to fight dermatitis. Apply three to four drops of each essential oil (borage or evening primrose) to the inflamed skin, which decrease the inflammation and irritation disappears. If the irritation worsens, discontinue use after three days and consult your doctor.
8. Horsetail is an ancient emollient herb that can be very useful in soothing the discomfort of eczema. To make a horsetail compress, put 1 teaspoon of dried or crushed fresh horsetail stems in 1 cup of water and boil for 10 to 15 minutes. Remove from the heat and let it cool until the liquid is just comfortably warm to the skin. Immerse a clean, soft, small cotton towel in

the boiled water and then squeeze out the excess liquid and wrap the towel around the inflamed area, and cover with another dry, heavy towel for at least ten minutes.

3. Freckles

Description and causes : Brownish spots on the skin due to precipitation of pigments or exposure to the sun caused by a melanin pigmentation in the skin. Freckles cannot be removed immediately but lightened temporarily.

Treatment : There are several home recipes used as skin lighteners as following :

1. Herbal lotions made with elder flower, lime flowers, lemon juice or castor oil when pressed into are used as skin lighteners.
2. Ground to a paste pumpkin seeds and mix to it olive oil keeps the skin soft and remove freckles when the paste is applied to brownish spots.
3. Ground yellow mustard in the milk and apply to the face at night. Wash thoroughly in the morning.
4. Ground turmeric and sesame seeds in equal quantity and mix to it little quantity of water to make a paste. Apply pack on brownish spots and wash when dries.
5. Grind leaves of 'tulsi' in water and apply paste to the face. It is a wonderful remedy to get rid of freckles.
6. Apply benzylbenzoate on all over the body (except face, neck and head) with a brush after consulting your doctor. The drug should be applied on dry skin after taking bath. Left on the body for 24 hours, followed by another application. Wash off the emulsion after 48 hours to enable all mites to kill.

4. Nettle Rash

Description and symptoms : In medical terms it is called urticaria and in Ayurveda termed as 'Sheeta-pitta'. It is a disorder of the skin in which wheals, red and pale rashes, edematous lesions and pink or white itchy and painful patches appear on the skin. Urticaria is caused by the following reasons :

1. Allergic conditions of the skin.
2. Physical factors like cold, heat, exertion, ultraviolet radiation.

3. Psychological stress generally resulting from sex problems.
4. Family problems (financial and employment etc.).
5. Hormonal imbalance, allergic reaction and poor diet.
6. Exposure to cold, taking bath in cold water.
7. Psychic situation and intestinal worms

The following are the measures to treat urticaria:

1. Mix three parts rose water with two parts vinegar and the mixture is applied locally to get immediate relief.
2. Ground together equal quantities of alum and red ochre (geru). The powder should be rubbed on wheals.
3. Grind 1 teaspoon 'jalneem' (lycopus europaeus) to 3 teaspoons beeswax and the mixture should be made into pills and taken with lukewarm water.
4. Avoid sour substances and non-vegetarian food (especially fish), but increase the quantity of turmeric in the food.

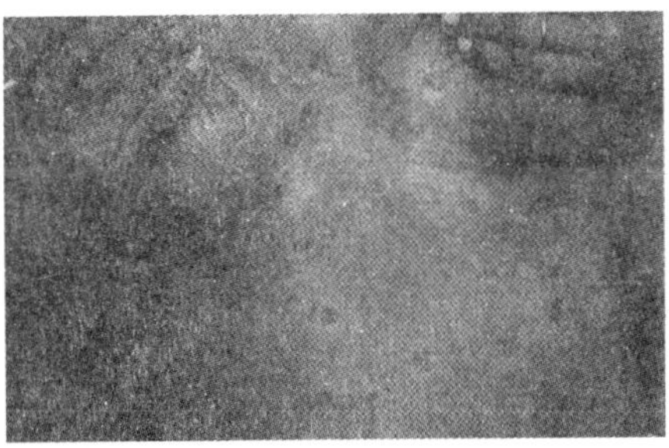

Psoriasis on breasts

5. Psoriasis

Description, signs and symptoms : It is called 'ekakushta' in Ayurveda. A skin disorder identified by silver-gray, dry, scaly papules on the skin generally on the soft inner side of elbows, knees and occasionally on scalp and forehead. They become rough and red with a silvery, soft, scabby appearance. Fair-skinned people suffer from it more often as compared to dark complexioned. The symptoms include scaling, itching, bleeding and disfigurement.

Causes : Psoriasis may be caused by use of detergents or as a result of allergic reaction.

Treatment : Psoriasis is a serious, often severe, condition that requires professional care. Usually. a dermatologist, who may not understand the cause of the disease or the cure, likely recommend treatments that provide only symptomatic relief. Usually, doctors recommend that patients should start with cotisone-based topical medication or light therapy before relying on nutrient-based topical medicines such as vitamin D or vitamin A based ointment, both of which can have long term side effect. The following treatments are recommended to relieve psoriasis :

1. A diet of raw foods including whey milk.
2. A diet including Vitamin A supplement and cold liver oil.
3. Application of extract of herbs such as witch hazel, nettle or calendula (marigold) with a clean cotton wool soaked in the solution relieves irritation.
4. In case of irritation on scalp, massage with the lotion prepared as below:

Boil four marigold heads in four cups of water for two minutes. Allow it to cool. Massage the lotion well into the scalp. Wash with a very mild shampoo or a solution of soapwort. Add lemon juice or cider vinegar to the rinsing water to ensure a thorough rinse.

5. Internal cleansing program : Cleanse your body of toxins by drinking six to eight glasses of pure water in a day.
6. Stewed fruits : Eat stewed figs, apples, raisins, apricots, pears, peaches or prunes; as their laxative effect will help clean your bowels.
7. Exercise is a vital part of the regimen for clearing psoriasis. It stimulates the internal structure of the body, increases circulation, activates the glands, oxygenate the blood, opens the pores and filters the blood through the liver and kidneys. A daily period of 30-40 minutes of any aerobic activity such as walking, swimming, cycling and playing tennis is very helpful.
8. Moisturize your skin with oil. Rubbing castor oil on thick skin lesions or applying a mixture of olive oil and peanut oil in equal quantity on thinner lesions can help moisturize the skin without any further irritating it.
9. Choose a regular deodorant over an antiperspirant, as antiperspirant block normal elimination through the sweat glands; whereas deodorants don't.

10. Hydrotherapy-generally known as a bath for healing skin crisis cleanses the body and begins to throw off your body toxins accumulating on the skin and your psoriasis starts getting better. To cope with the increased burning and itching, take a bath in lukewarm water, to which add 1 cup of apple cider vinegar (if your skin is not cracked from scratching) and 1 cup of rolled oats and ½ cup cornstarch powder. You may add to the water little baking powder for better results. Take bath in this alkaline mixture for 15 to 20 minutes in a day.

11. The food you eat should consist of 70 to 80% fruits and vegetable (containing leafy green salads) whose higher fiber contents help cleanse the colon or large intestine of toxins. The remaining 20 to 30% of your daily diet should be grains, poultry, fish and low fat, !ow sodium dairy products. Avoid taking processed foods, which contain hydrogenated fats and cause inflammation. Do not eat junk foods such as potato chips, pickles, ketchup, tomato juice, fried foods, alcohol, sweets, smoked foods, candies, pastries and pies. A little care in taking diet will help cure psoriasis

12. Yellow saffron tea helps heal the lining of the intestinal walls as it flushes the liver and kidneys of toxins. To prepare the tea, put ¼ teaspoon of saffron in a cup. Add to it boiling water and let stand for 15 minutes. Drink it till your psoriasis clears. The nutritional supplement lecithin helps alkalinize the body and is a natural laxative. Take 1 tablespoon of the granular lecithin three times a day to clear of psoriasis.

6. Fungal infection

Ringworm, moniliasis and candidasis are contagious fungal infections of the skin. In Ayurveda ringworm is called 'dadru' in which the patient notice circular scaly patches with severe itching on affected skin or scalp.

Treatments : The following treatments are recommended to cure ringworm infection :

1. Rub oil of lemon grass mixed with coconut oil or sesame oil, which is highly effective for quick relief.
2. Apply either the juice of marigold leaves or the paste of grounded leaves of 'genda' flower or 'tulsi' leaves.

3. Another remedy for ringworm is to scratch the patch and apply to it the paste of borax mixed to lime.
4. If the ringworm becomes chronic, it should be rubbed with a coarse cloth and applying to it a sap of swallow wort (Akh).
5. Avoid taking hot and pungent food and diet of milk and rice.

Candidiasis : is another form of fungal infection caused by candida albicans. Patients suffering from diabetes mellitus and hypothyroidism are usually prone to this infection. It may be associated with the use of oral contraceptives involving skin, intestines and vagina. Anti-fungal drugs along with antibiotics are usually prescribed by the doctors. Always take fatty diet with the treatment to allow maximum absorption.

Candidiasis includes thrush another common infection usually develops in the gastro-intestinal track and the skin of the individual persons. It is a disorder of candida in which whitish curd-like deposit appear on the tongue in infants as well as adult women with immune deficiency. Thrush infection of vagina is also called vulva vaginitis, is common in women with itching and discharge accompanied by redness in genital area or on the glans in male organ. The vaginal infection can be transmitted to the male partner and vice versa. A vaginal thrush usually clears with pessaries such as nystatin and clotrimazole. Contraceptive pills and use of antibiotics can create conditions, which encourage thrush. Avoid wearing nylon penties and tight jeans. Moist environments encourage this disease

7. Vaginitis

Description and causes : Vaginitis is a serious fungal infectious disease caused by bacteria, which invade the area causing one or

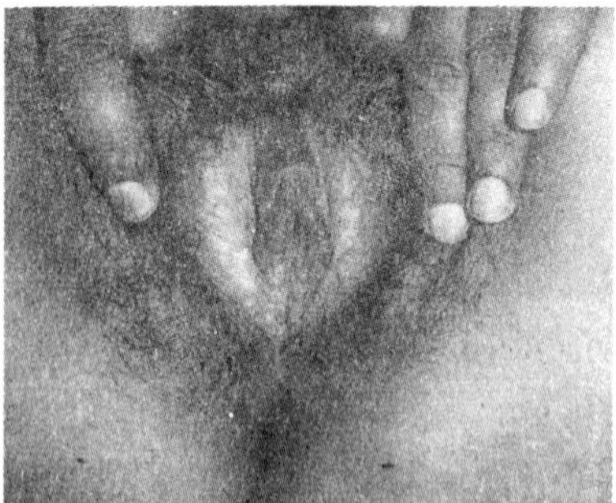

Vulva Vaginitis

more of the symptoms of infections such as soreness, irritation, inflammation, discharge, burning, swelling, redness, urinary discomfort and pain during sex. Untreated vaginitis can lead to pelvic inflammatory disease, which can result in infertility.

Signs and symptoms : See your doctor when you notice the following symptoms :

1. Pain or itching on your vagina or vulva (the area outside the vagina).
2. Reddening of your vulva.
3. Pain, when you urinate.
4. Pain when you indulge in sexual intercourse.
5. Greenish yellow, frothy, foul-smelling vaginal discharge.
6. Trichomoniasis – a sexually transmitted organism.
7. Foul-smelling, thin, white or blood-streaked discharge (which may signal atrophic vaginitis).
8. White or gray, fishy-smelling vaginal discharge (which suggests bacterial vaginosis).

The first and most important step in treating acute or chronic infectious vaginitis is, your doctor should know the type of infection you have and choosing a right treatment by your doctor or yourself. If you have a chronic infection that never completely goes away and you can have infections three times a year. You should immediately seek doctor's help if you are pregnant. Untreated vaginitis can lead to pelvic inflammatory disease, which can result in infertility.

Treatment : Conventional doctors try to solve the problem by killing bad organism with drugs, which is must if the infection is severe or chronic. These remedies help the good flora return to the vagina, restore the normal pH or chemical balance of the tissues and decrease inflammation and irritation as well as kill off the infecting organisms. Correct treatment depends on knowing which organism is causing you problem, usually due to the following reasons:

- Bacteria.
- The fungal yeast candida albicans.
- Trichomonas vaginalis.

The following remedies must be used to avoid vaginitis :

- Avoid sugar as well as refined carbohydrates and alcohol, both of which turn into glucose in the body.
- The most important food for healing vaginitis is yogurt. A woman suffering from vaginitis, candidiasis or trichomoniasis should eat daily about 100 gm. unsweetened yogurt with lactobacillus acidophilus bacteria and take three capsules of a supplement of the bacterium between the meals (having suggestions from your doctor). Generally, doctor advises that a woman suffering from vaginitis should use the capsule of L. acidophilus as vaginal suppositories by inserting one capsule into the vagina everyday in the morning in consultation with the doctor.
- Garlic is a strong anti-bacterial and anti-fungal infection fighter suitable for both vaginitis and candidiasis. The patient should take one garlic capsule once or twice daily till the condition cures.
- The chemical berberine in goldenseal fights off bacteria and candida in the mucous membranes of the vagina, which also strengthens the immune system.
- Use of boric acid suppositories for the treatment of candida (yeast) infection has surprising success rate. Regular use of the suppositories also helps prevent recurrences. If you have been diagnosed with an acute yeast infection, insert an 600 mg. capsule of boric acid powder into your vagina twice a day, in the morning and evening for a week. To prevent a recurrence, insert one capsule daily at bedtime for four times a week during your menstrual period to continue for at least three months. The suppository can cause burning in tissue that is already irritated by an infection. You can prevent burning sensation by coating the irritated tissues with vitamin E oil before inserting the suppository. Avoid using it if you are pregnant. Also do not forget to consult a doctor before this treatment.
- Using a gelatin capsule of vitamin E as a suppository is very soothing to vaginal tissue, decreasing irritation, redness, swelling and congestion. Insert a capsule once or twice daily for a week.
- Triphala - an Ayurvedic herb helps remove toxins from the body and restores a normal flow of body fluids. Both are important in treating a yeast infection. Soak ½ teaspoon of dried herb in 1 cup of hot water for five minutes, then drink the tea before sleep. If you don't like the taste, you can take two 500 mg. tablets or

capsules before going to bed. A once –a-month douche with triphala will help prevent recurrent yeast infections. Put a tablespoon of triphala in about ½ liter water and bring it to boil. Remove from the heat, let cool to lukewarm and strain. Use as a regular douche. The longer you keep the triphala in contact with the vaginal mucosa, the better it is. You must consult your doctor as douching can dry the vagina and upset its natural balance.

8. Skin allergy

Description : An everyday substance – may be the pollen from a tree, the dander from a cat or the dust or smoke is your enemy, an allergen. When you inhale the substance in your body, an antibody is created.

Signs and symptoms : The runny nose, the red and itchy eyes, the sneezing, the sinus headache, the scratchy throat, rashes and itching on the skin – all that you call allergy.

Treatment : Sensitivity to allergens may be concealed by taking antihistamine medication because antihistamine treat the symptoms, not the cause. Home remedies are very helpful to treat an allergic reaction. The following home remedies are suggested :

1. Use olive oil to soothe inflamed eyelids.
2. Melt 50 gm. white wax or paraffin wax or beeswax and 250 ml. olive oil together in a bowl held over boiling water. In another bowl gently heat 100 ml. Vinegar. Remove both bowls from the heat and beat the vinegar slowly into the oily mixture until it cools. Use the cream on skin affected by allergy.
3. A poultice made of raw grated carrots is a very old remedy for skin allergy.
4. Place 50 gm. dried bilberries in a stainless steel pan containing 900 ml lukewarm water. Leave for an hour. Then boil the liquid for 15-20 minutes. Remove from the heat and leave until it cools. Strain and use. Drink a small glass or a cup three times a day.
5. A detoxification bath helps to cleanse your immune system including allergens, infections, environmental toxins and stress. The detoxification baths relieve heat from the body and release stored toxins from fat cells into the blood. This bath can be very effective for decreasing and even preventing allergic symptoms, especially for those who are overloaded from chemicals.

For detoxification bath, first take a bath or shower to remove excess oil and dirt from your skin. Scrub with a rough washcloth or loofah, then rinse thoroughly. Next, fill the tub with water as hot as you can tolerate without discomfort and deep enough to immerse your body up to your neck. Sit in the tub, letting the water cover your entire body, including your hands and arms. Stay in the bath for five minutes, then take a brief but thorough warm shower to wash the toxins off your skin so they won't be reabsorbed.

9. Boils and Pustules

Description : A boil is a bacterial infection of a sweat gland or hair follicle, usually on the face, neck, in the armpit, buttocks, groin, knees and elbows that is caused by a skin pore or hair follicle being blocked by dead skin cells and other debris. These red, small, painful nodules start oozing pus and later leave a tiny scar. The immune system's white blood cells collapse, as a result creating large amounts of pus along with redness, swelling and pain.

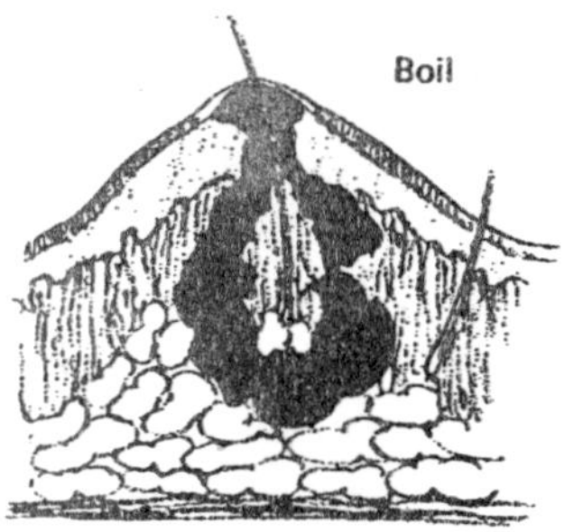

Boil

Carbuncle

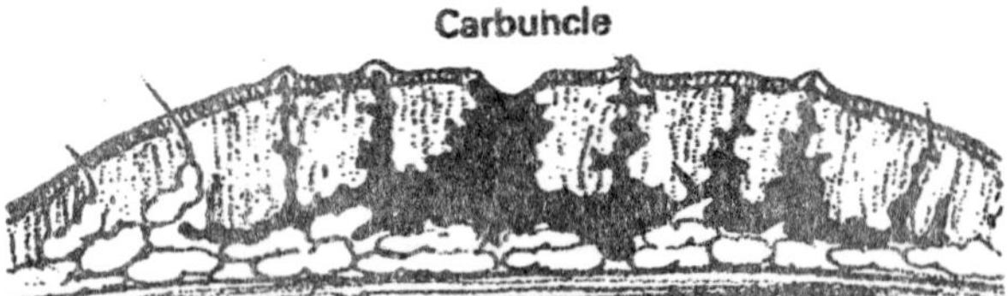

Pustule

Causes : However, recurrent boils are caused by gastrointestinal bacteria entering the blood stream and promoting skin infections. They are also caused by eating too much sugar (either refined sugar or sugar from fruit). Alternative medicines offer effective ways to heal small boils less than ½ inch across. Never lance or press a boil to open it, as this can spread the infection and may cause permanent scarring.

Treatment : If you have a boil that doesn't improve within a few days, see a doctor or a dermatologist for treatment, which may include antibiotics, draining or administering steroid injection. If you notice red lines radiating from the boil or if you have fever and swelling or if it is extremely tender or under a thick layer of skin, consult a skin specialist immediately. There are number of home preparations to cure boils:

1. Take a leaf of 'peepal' tree. Smear it with ghee and apply as lukewarm bandage on the boil. It will burst after some time.
2. De-pigmentation on forehead is caused by the adhesive of plastic 'bindi', on the breast by the plastic purse usually kept by women under the bra, on the fold of ear by spectacle frame, on the feet by rubber straps of the slippers and on the waist due to tight pressure caused by the petticoat string
3. Using hot compresses on a boil will bring blood to the area and may diminish bacteria. For an acute boil - one that pops up suddenly and is non recurrent – immerse a washcloth in hot water (as hot as you can tolerate, but not hot enough to burn), wring it out and place on the boil for 20 minutes twice a day.
4. Hot and cold compress drains out pus from the pustule. Treat the boil with just hot compresses Use alternating heat and cold to draw out the pus. Again soak a washcloth in hot water, wring it out and place it on the boil for 10 minutes. Then apply another washcloth, this time soak in icy cold water for 10 minutes. Repeat this cycle three times twice a day.
5. A herbal formulae with Echinacea and goldenseal will help kill the bacteria in the boil. Take 1 tablespoon of tincture of both herbs three times a day until the boil vanishes. Beware of the taste, it is very bitter.
6. In Ayurveda – the ancient natural healing system, boils are seen as 'pitta' disorder: an excess of fiber and heat. Turmeric is a cooling herb that can reduce the inflammation of a boil and help prevent recurrences. Look for a standardized extract of turmeric and take 450 mg. three times a day, or use it to make a skin paste that will quickly bring a boil to a head. To make paste, combine 1 teaspoon of turmeric powder, 1 teaspoon

Epsom salt and a baked onion in a blender to make a thick paste. Spread the paste on a piece of cloth to make a bandage and put the cloth over the boil. Wrap a plastic cloth over the bandage so that the yellow coloring of turmeric doesn't get over your bedding and the clothes. Leave poultice on overnight and clean in the morning. Repeat the process for two to three nights.

10. Herpes simplex

Description, symptoms and Treatment: The attack of herpes simplex is usually severe in which the lesions generally consist of multiple small vesicles or superficial ulcers on the upper lip on the face in women, and on the shaft of male organ (penis) in men. If the attack is mild, the lesions tend to heal in 10 to 14 days. If the infection is severe, an antibiotic treatment recommended by a doctor is essential.

11. Herpes zoster and genital warts

Description, causes and signs and symptoms: Herpes Zoster is a virus infection, commonly called 'blisters', which usually appear on genital area, thigh and buttocks (it is the variety of the virus that causes oral and genital herpes). It is a rashy infection caused by the varicella zoster. The group of little painful, tender and highly infectious blisters usually burst in the meantime. It is caused by the same virus as the chicken pox, usually caught while having sex with someone suffering from herpes (in case of genital herpes). In such case group of blisters appear on the genital area. There are three reasons that the virus can reactivate years – even decades – later and cause shingles.

Genital warts, also called candylomata acuminata, produce fungative growths on the glans in men, on the vulva in women and around the anus in both men and women. Genital warts are transmitted by contact in the sexually active persons. They may be related to the development of cervical cancer. So if you have genital warts, get them treated and have cervical smears.

Treatment of herpes and warts : Remedies to cure herpes zoster are as following :

1. Soothing with the essential oils of lemon, geranium, camomile

or lavender. The essential oils may be diluted in base oil and rubbed on the rash.

2. Take 25 gm. each of the herbs : dried mullein, mellow roots and marshmallow roots. Put them to simmer for three minutes in 3 liter of water. Strain and use on a compress throughout the day and night to reduce heat and irritation.
3. Common warts are treated by electro-cautery in which warts are removed with a cautery, which excises the wart with an electric current.

12. Warts

Warts are small epidermic growths caused by virus. These growths vary in size and shape and are commonly of three types: Plane warts, Common warts and Plantar warts. Plane warts are simplest of all warts. These are usually small, smooth and skin colored or brownish lesions, which are slightly raised from the skin. They usually occur on the face and outer surface of hands. The most affected are children and young adults. Common warts are larger and firmer elevations with a rough surface, and usually occur on the hands, forearm, knees and feet. Plantar warts are slightly different. They normally contain blood vessels and bleed because of this. The treatment of wart consists in eliminating them either by chemical lotion or physical means as described below:

1. Application of a peeling agent, like 4% sulphur calamine lotion or applying Retino A cream daily on the wart.
2. Freezing the wart with liquid nitrogen or carbon snow help a lot.

Warts caused by virus can take place anywhere on the surface of the body with unpleasant characteristics itching, burning and oozing. These should be diagnosed accurately and treated appropriately. Warts in genital area sexually transmitted, may be a risk factor for cervical cancer in women. Once the warts are diagnosed, they should be removed. It is important to treat them early rather than waiting until they spread and enlarge and become more difficult to eliminate. Warts are easily removed by cryosurgery or freezing with liquid nitrogen and electro-cautery (a procedure that burns the wart off with an electrified surgical tool). The easiest, best way to get rid of a wart is to have it frozen off by a doctor. Warts should be treated with natural methods as below :

1. Homeopathy treatment : Two homeopathic remedies to get rid of warts are to take medicines Thuja occidentalis and Antimonium crudum (both in 30 X potency). You may consult a homeopathic doctor for the treatment. If the wart is soft, fleshy and oozes or bleeds easily, use Thuja oocidentalis
2. Garlic oil is a traditional remedy for warts. Swab the oil on the wart or on a bandage applied to the wart.
3. Patient with warts should take a daily multivitamin/ mineral supplement that includes at least 200 micrograms of selenium.
4. Mind-body techniques such as self-hypnosis can be very effective for healing warts. You might sit comfortably in a chair. Relax the body with a few deep breaths, and form a mental picture of a patch of snow over your wart, which creates a pleasant, refreshing tingling in the area. Then melt the wart as it melts away. Do this visualization technique every day for five minutes or more.

13. Plantar warts

A plantar wart is a wart on the bottom of your foot. The result is a wart that's covered with calluses and can be as small as a pinhead or as large as a quarter. It has tiny brown, black or red spots, which are the blood vessels and it usually exists on the ball or heel of your foot, which can make walking painful. The following measures treat plantar warts

1. If natural methods have failed to remove your plantar wart or it is painful or bleeds, you should have it removed by a podiatrist. The most effective removal methods are application of liquid nitrogen, which freezes and kills the wart so that it falls off or a surgical laser.
2. Applying garlic : Putting garlic directly on a plantar wart can help to get rid of it. Mash a clove of garlic into pulp. Before you go to bed, put the pulp directly on the wart and cover it with a small adhesive bandage. In the morning, remove the bandage and clean the area. Within a couple of days, the wart starts shrinking and after ten days it usually dissolves. If the wart doesn't go away within 3-4 weeks, discontinue the treatment.
3. Tea tree essential oil : This essential oil is antiviral and can help get rid of plantar warts. Apply few drops of oil daily. Stop using the treatment after 3-4 months if the wart doesn't disappear.

4. Vitamin C : It strengthens your immune system. Take 1,000 mg. of vitamin C (an antiviral nutrient) daily.
5. An herbal cure to banish plantar wart : Astragalus is one of the best herbs to strengthen the immune system and defeating plantar warts. Follow the dosage recommendations on the label of the bottle you buy.

13. Shingles

There are many reasons that the virus can reactivate years – even decades – later and cause shingles. Shingles is a painful but relatively harmless infection that can usually be treated with either medications or home remedies. If you have shingles blisters anywhere on or near your head or you are immuno-compromised (meaning that you have AIDS, cancer or any immune-weakening disease) and have difficulty in eating or drinking, trouble with hearing and balance, you must consult a doctor immediately. These symptoms may mean that you have internal blisters, which can be very serious. Shingles show up as an itchy and sometimes painful, immediately followed by blisters that can break out anywhere above the waist. The blisters appear over a period of 3 to 5 days, during which you are likely to be feverish, headachy and weak. They take anywhere from two weeks to a month to heal. The following treatments are usually suggested:

1. Administering Vitamin B_{12}: Injections of vitamin B_{12} is a non-drug method for treating serious cases of shingles.
2. Acupuncture treatment: It relieves pain during an outbreak.
3. French clay and Tea tree oil: It is a topical treatment that helps dry up moist, weeping shingles blisters. To prepare a poultice, mix 1 teaspoon of water with enough French green clay to make a paste. Add to it one or two drops of Tea tree oil. Apply thin covering of the paste directly to the blisters. Leave the poultice on for two to three hours, then clean the area with a warm cloth. If you are applying poultice to someone, avoid touching the blisters directly with your hands or any other part of your skin.
4. Activated charcoal : A tremendously useful home remedy that draws the herpes virus out of the skin, quickly dry and heal blisters. Add enough water to a small amount of activated charcoal and equal quantity of corn starch or ground flaxseed to make a paste. Let stand for 15 to 20 minutes, then apply the

paste to blisters with a piece of muslin. Leave the paste on for minimum 12 hours, then wash it off. Keep reapplying it until the blisters are completely dry and healing.

5. Hydrogen peroxide: A gel of hydrogen peroxide contains high levels of oxygen, which is believed to kill viruses. Apply the gel to the blisters every two to three hours until they have dried and healed.
6. Homeopathic relief: The homeopathic remedy Rhus tox quickly reduces pain and speed up healing blisters.
7. Capsaicin ointment: Capsaicin cream is an outstanding treatment for postherapetic neuralgia, a condition that occurs mainly in people over the age 70.
8. Multivitamin/Mineral supplement: Vitamin and mineral contributes to the strength of immune system. They supplement if you have ever had a bout of shingles and want to prevent another.
9. Vitamin C: It is perhaps the most important immune booster for healthy immune functioning. Take 2,000 mg. twice a day.
10. Alpha-lipoic acid: It has powerful antioxidant properties and helps prevent shingles outbreak. Take 50 mg twice a day.
11. The amino acid lysine can help decrease the recurrence of shingles. Take 1,000 mg. a day.

(Note : Have treatment, after consulting a doctor/qualified practitioner)

14. Vitiligo

A pigmentary disorder of skin when the melanocytes in the localized areas of the body stop producing melanin. The lesions vary in shape and size on the skin of the body and spread quickly.

15. Cheilitis

In this condition, usually redness, scaling and swelling appear on both lips.

16. Chilblains

These appear due to exposure to cold, which cause lesions that consist pain, brownish-black discoloration on toes and fingers. Protect from cold and use vasodilators. Antibiotic treatment is recommended.

The area should be scrubbed, dried and smeared with ghee or mustard oil.

17. Leprosy

It affects not only the skin, but also the mucous membranes and the nerves. Leprosy is of two types: tuberculoid and lepromatous. The lepromatous leprosy is an infectious disease and in many cases it is hereditary. It cannot be cured with home remedies. The following treatments are recommended :

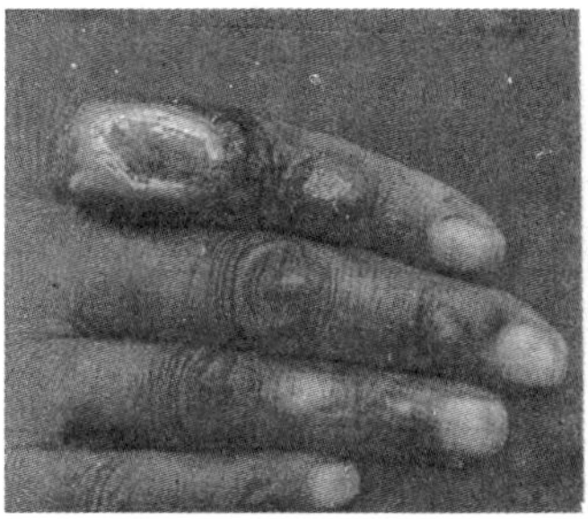

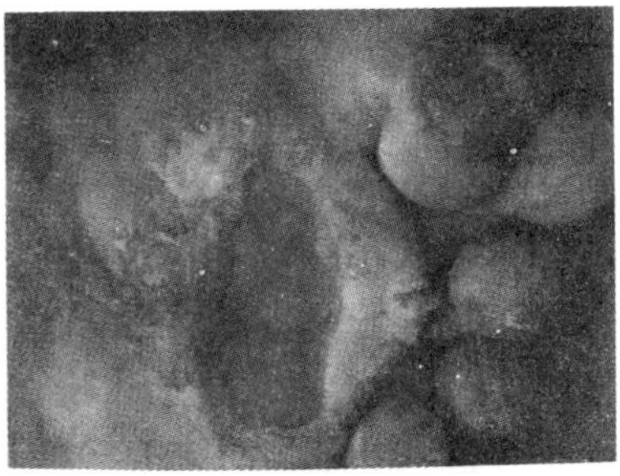

1. The body of the patient should be massaged with the sap of 'neem' tree. If the sap is not readily available, grind together five grains of pepper and 'neem' leaves in water and drink.
2. Massage with sesame or 'neem' oil helps to some extent.
3. The patient should be bathed with water in which leaves of 'neem' tree and 'amaltas' have been boiled.
4. Have salt-free diet or the salt in your diet should be as little as possible.
5. Avoid constipation and indigestion, as they aggravate the condition.

18. Dandruff

Dandruff is not a hair problern but a skin problem. The flaking and itchiness are the result of an over-production of a substance called sebum from glands in the scalp, and those glands are hyperactive because the scalp is excessively dry. Most dandruff shampoos have strong medications to control the symptoms of the dandruff.

Generally, dandruff shampoos contain aggressive cleansers that destroy the scalp's delicate balance of water and oil, which further irritates the glands and perpetuates the problem. There are many possible causes of the dandruff, including a yeast infection of the scalp or hormones imbalances. If you have tried self-care treatments for two to three months but your dandruff persists, see a dermatologist for the accurate diagnose and possible medical treatment for topical steroid medications. Here are several natural remedies effective to solve the problem of dandruff:

- **Aromatherapy treatment** : Aromatherapy formula for a shampoo that can help normalize the water-and-oil secreting glands of the scalp, helps to eliminate dandruff. Mix 10 drops of tea tree oil, 8 drops of cedar-wood oil, 6 drops each of pine oil and rosemary oil, 4 drops each of clary sage and lemon oil in two to three tablespoons of mild shampoo. These essential oils encourage your body systems to go into action to heal the problems that cause the formation of dandruff. Tea tree oil is an antiseptic helping to normalize the bacteria on the scalp. Rosemary and cedar-wood oils help to increase the circulation to the scalp. Pine oil and lemon oil eliminate the toxins from the skin of the scalp and promote internal cleansing. Clary sage helps regulate and balance oil production. Use the shampoo several times a week.
- **Rosemary essential oil treatment** : This essential oil helps to increase circulation, stimulate the scalp and reduce flaking. Put two to three drops of oil in a tablespoon of rich fatty carrier oil such as avocado oil, followed by massage into your scalp for 1 to 2 minutes daily.
- **Eucalyptus leaves treatment** : Eucalyptus tree leaves help fight infection and tone skin. To prepare a rinse with eucalyptus, put 4 teaspoons of dried leaves in ¼ liter of boiling water. Continue stirring and cover the utensil. Remove from the heat and steep for an hour. Strain the liquid into a large plastic bottle. Then add to it 1 tablespoon of apple-cider vinegar. After taking a shower, pour the rinse slowly over your hair. Don't rinse it out, just let it dry. Use this herbal rinse each time you shower.
- **Massaging the scalp** : Massage is the ancient system of natural healing to get rid of dandruff. Dandruff is a symptom of a body-wide condition of 'vata' or dryness. Massaging the scalp twice a week with warm sesame oil combats the excessive dryness. It is very calming and soothing to the system, since

dandruff is some time caused or complicated by anxiety, worry and hypertension. Massage the oil into your scalp for five to ten minutes before going to bed at night. Wrap your head in a hot towel and leave the towel for 10 minutes or for optimum moisturizing all night. Wash it out in the morning.

- **Minerals' cure for flaking and itching** : The mineral selenium can help relieve the flaking and itching caused by dandruff. Take 200-microgram supplement daily. Zinc rebuilds skin and can help your scalp heal from dandruff. Take 15-20 mg. daily.
- **Vitamin E** : Taking capsule of 400 international units of vitamin E a day balance the oils on the scalp and relieve dryness of hair.

4
The Three Trimesters of Pregnancy

The delivery date is usually 280 days after the first day of last period. This is, however, not accurate for a woman with a 28-day cycle. The 40th week period of pregnancy is usually classified into three trimesters. The first trimester is the period starting from 1 st to 12th week. The second trimester starts from 13th to 28th week and the period from 29th to 40th week is regarded the third trimester.

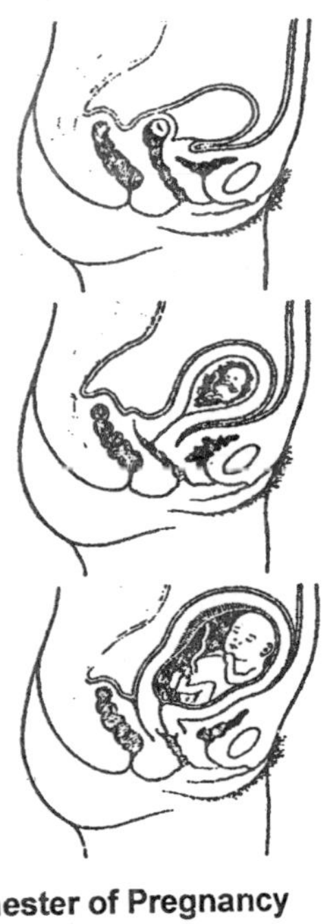

Ist Trimester

IInd Trimester

IIIrd Trimester

Three Trimester of Pregnancy

The symptoms of Pregnancy

- Missed period is regarded as the most obvious sign of pregnancy.
- Engorged and tender breasts.
- Nausea and vomiting.
- Exhaustion and tiredness.
- Excessive giddiness.
- Vaginal discharge.
- Change of taste.
- Strong liking and disliking for certain foods.
- Frequent urge to urinate.

Do not rely on a missed period. Go for the Urine Pregnancy Test. Sometime, women keep having their periods even for about three months after they conceive. It is the time to see your doctor who will want to carry out laboratory procedures such as complete blood count and urinalysis. You should see your doctor once a month for routine check up for the next five months and after that every two weeks until the baby comes. Each time your urine should be examined to make sure that your kidneys are functioning properly. It is natural that a woman feels a bit shy about medical examinations. But she should try to forget such feeling as she has no different from other women.

Formation of the embryo

- During week 1 to 2 : The pituitary secretes rising levels of follicle-stimulating hormone and, which cause the enlargement and differentiation of multiple primary ovarian follicles. The developing follicles produce estrogen. The estrogen level remains relatively low until four days before ovulation.
- During week 3 to 4 : The ovulation usually occurs on approximately day 14 of the menstrual cycle. If pregnancy occurs, continued production of progesterone results in more marked hypertrophic changes in the endometrial cells and glands to provide nourishment to the blastocyst. Fertilization occurs on or about day14 as the mature ovum and sperm unite to form the zygote. Implantation is complete by day 23.
- During the week 5 : The embryo is converted by the process of gastrulation. The formation of neural plate and its closure to form the neural tube. This process begins in the 5th week in the

thoracic region and extends caudally and cranially, resulting in complete closure by the end of 6th week.

- In six weeks, the embryo is 1.25 cm. long but doesn't look like a baby. If seen very minutely, the beginning of the limbs can be seen resembling like a large head having pits for eyes and a tail. In twelve weeks, the baby is around 9 cm. long.

What to do during the First Trimester of Pregnancy?

- Consult your doctor in case of severe nausea and vomiting. Avoid losing fluid.
- Have frequent small meals six to seven times in a day.
- Eat a dry biscuit or a rusk and sip lime water before leaving the bed.
- Take rest, as due to hormonal changes you will feel lethargic and exhausted.

Have 8 to 10 hours sleep during night and at least 3 to 4 hours sleep during the daytime.

- Restrict your fluid intake in the evening, otherwise frequent urination during the night will disturb your sleep.
- If there is pain or burning sensation while passing urine, consult your doctor. It may possibly due to infection.
- Eat hygienically cooked food. Relax for some time after taking meal.
- Sex can be continued except when there is pain in the abdomen or a miscarriage risk
- Light exercise is very important.
- Take your usual daily bath. A shower or a sponge bath is equally important.

What to avoid during the First Trimester of Pregnancy?

- Do not wear tight clothes.
- Avoid strong smells.
- Do not undertake over exertion.
- Avoid excess of tea, coffee and smoking. Tobacco smoke contains poisons.
- Do not stand for long period of time.

- Do not get up suddenly from a sitting position.
- Do not undertake long journeys.
- In case of fear of abortion, have bed rest.
- Avoid X-rays during this trimester, which are very harmful.
- Avoid contact with animals, especially cats and birds. There may be risk of an abortion or a pre-term delivery or birth of a sick baby.
- Medicines should be taken strictly on the prescription of your doctor during this trimester as the baby takes shape in this period.
- Consult your doctor immediately in case of bleeding or discharge through vagina, abdominal pain, painful burning urination, persistent vomiting, fever, rashes on the body and feeling of dizziness.
- Avoid drinking liquor. Alcohol causes added strain on your kidneys and liver. Even beer contains enough alcohol to leave harmful effects on both mother and the baby in womb.
- Do not use any vaginal douche without the recommendation of your doctor.
- Avoid tight band around waist. Wear low-heel shoes.
- Dental decay is common during pregnancy; see your diet doesn't lack Calcium.
- In case any time you feel sexual intercourse is uncomfortable, it is wise to refrain. In case you have pelvic infection, it should be cleared up without delay.

The Second Trimester of Pregnancy

The second trimester of pregnancy starts from the 13th week and continues up to the 28th week. It is the most enjoyable period as the discomforts of each pregnancy begin to wear off. This is the time to dream and plan ahead. Out of the total weight gain during 40 weeks of pregnancy as 10-12 kg, there is little gain in weight (between 0.7 to 1.25 kg in first 20 weeks). By the end of 20 weeks of pregnancy, there would be a total weight gain of 4 kg. Be careful to watch your weight each time you visit your doctor for monthly check up. If the weight is more than the normal gain coupled with normal blood pressure, it indicates that you are taking excess or wrong kind of food. Consult your doctor if you have raised blood pressure, you may be suffering from Pre-Eclamptic Toxaemia (PET), in which the urine is checked for proteins. In case of a weight loss during this time of pregnancy, consult your doctor, this may effect the growth of your baby in womb.

Do's and don's during second trimester of pregnancy

- Get checked your blood pressure. Normally during pregnancy the blood pressure is slightly lower than pre-pregnancy. In case, it starts rising consult your doctor, this is hazardous for both mother and baby.

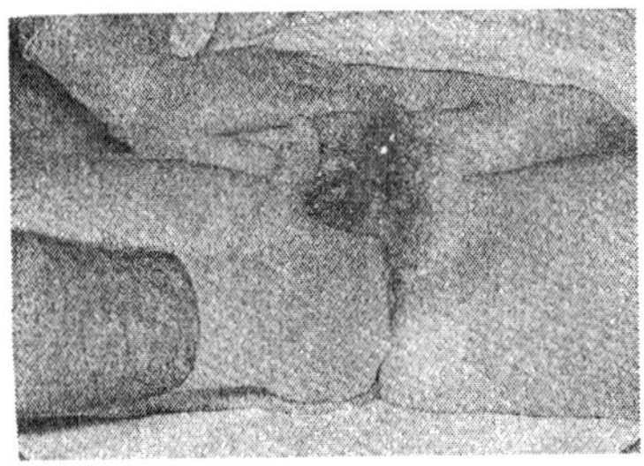

Bimanual Vaginal Examination

- Ask your doctor to assess the development of pregnancy. At twelve weeks, the womb lying deep in the pelvis starts rising out of bony pelvis and can be felt by placing hand on lower abdomen. Your doctor may easily be able to find size of the womb and assess the growth of baby.
- Around 7th week, your doctor may be able to listen to the baby's heartbeat. An ultrasound can pick up the heartbeat. You can hear it around 14th week, when the rate and rhythm of the heartbeat can be observed.
- Go for urine test to find out traces of sugar indicating diabetes and assess functioning of the kidneys.
- Hemoglobin in the blood can be estimated once a month to find if there are signs of anemia; it should be treated immediately.
- If there is swelling on hands, ankles and legs; get yourself examined by your doctor.
- In case of a normal pregnancy, usually between 16th to 20th week, a routine ultrasound scan is advised to find out the proper growth of child and position of placenta. If the position of placenta is near or on the cervical opening, there are chances of severe bleeding. Seek suggestions of your doctor.

- An Alpha Feto Protein (AFP) should be carried out during 15th to 18th week. AFP is a substance produced by the baby, which passes on into the mother's blood stream. In case of abnormally high level, there are chances of a twin delivery or the baby may have congenital defect. Take the matter seriously with your doctor.
- An Amniocentesis is carried during 14th to 18th week or later to detect the abnormality in the baby. If the expecting mother is above 40 and previously she delivered a malformed baby, this test is a must.

Important changes during Second Trimester

- Nausea and vomiting disappears.
- Desire to urinate frequently subsides.

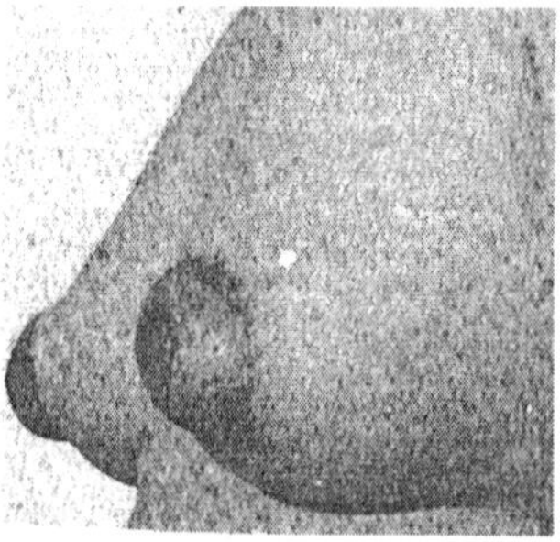

Pigmentation of skin around Nipples

- Gradual increasing bulge in abdomen.
- Enlargement of breasts and its veins become prominent.
- The skin surrounding the breast nipples start darkening.
- Clear water secreting from nipples, which becomes thick and yellowish.
- Feeling of movements of the growing baby in the abdomen at 18 weeks in case of first delivery and 16 weeks in case of subsequent deliveries.
- Small, pink and white streaks become visible on lower abdomen and upper thighs due to the stretching of the skin.
- During this trimester, the appetite returns and mother as well as the baby need nourishing diet.

Do and don't in Second Trimester of Pregnancy

- Normal sex is permissible within the physical constraints imposed by the growing womb.
- Drink plenty of fluid and water (minimum 7-8 glasses of water in a day).
- Avoid excessive intake of sugar, salt and spices.
- Eat well balanced diet to avoid excessive weight gain. Include foods providing fiber in the diet to avoid constipation.
- If you are overweight, there are chances of rise in blood pressure and blood sugar, discomfort on mild exertion, post-operative complications, delayed wound healing, difficult vaginal deliveries, difficulty in shedding extra weight during pregnancy and after the delivery. The average weight gain during pregnancy is 1-12 kg., of this 80% is the womb and its contents.
- Avoid sexual intercourse in cases of previous miscarriages or in case of vaginal bleeding (or spotting). In case your husband understands and respects these restrictions, you can satisfy each other's needs with love and tenderness, omitting sexual intercourse from love- making.
- Do not undertake tiring exercises. To start with exercise for few minutes, gradually increase the duration to 15 minutes everyday.
- Do not exercise if the doctor has suggested bed rest or you are suffering from high blood pressure, heart problem and bleeding (or spotting) during pregnancy. Do not exert to the point where you can get tired. A walk in open in the early morning is the best exercise.
- Stand correctly. Do not exaggerate the hollow of your back. Always stand with your feet apart, distributing the weight of your body evenly on the heels and the back of your feet. Wear low heel shoes.
- Sit in such a posture that the whole length and breadth of your thigh is supported by the seat and the whole of your back is in contact with the back of the chair.

The Third Trimester of Pregnancy

The period from 29th to 40th week of pregnancy is called the third trimester. The expectant mother feels excitement and joy in

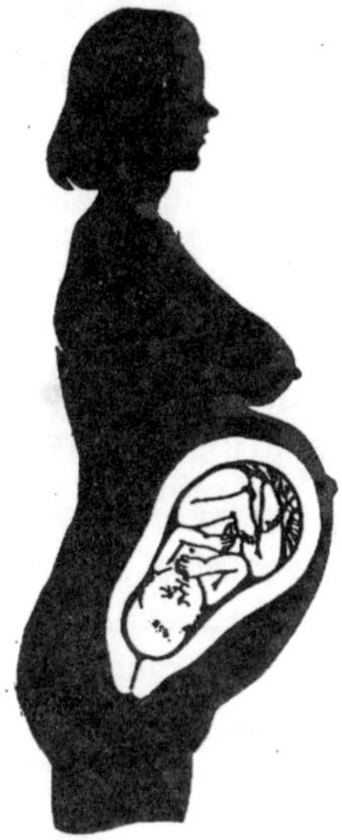

Third Trimester

anticipation of seeing the baby and at the same time the fear of labor and process of painful delivery worries her. During the last month of pregnancy, check the following :

- Fetal movements: There should be three or more movements in one hour. If the movements are less, consult your doctor.
- Blood pressure, urine and swelling of the feet and on other parts of body should be checked and consulted with your doctor in case of any abnormality.
- Abnormality of breasts and nipples : Wear well-fitting bra. In case you find any abnormality in breasts or nipples, report to your doctor. Start a nipple exercise, in case they are small and buried into the breasts.
- Abdominal area : During last month of pregnancy, it is very essential to know the position of the baby, which helps a lot during the process of delivery of child. Abdominal examination gives the information about the size and growth of the baby as regard period of pregnancy, heartbeat of the baby, the amount of fluid in the womb and the position of the baby inside the womb.
- Fatigued and stressed : Some pregnant women feel fatigued and stressed during this period. It is important to relax physically

and mentally. Rest and relaxation are essentially linked with easy and deep breathing, which helps during painful contractions of labor. To relax lie down on your back comfortably, breathe in and out, then gradually tighten the muscles of the different parts of your body in upward direction. You will soon feel relaxed. You can also relax while sitting on a comfortable chair. Lie on your side with a pillow under your head and two under your upper knees.

- Constipation and piles : The bowel movements slow down under the influence of the progesterone hormones of pregnancy, resulting hard and infrequent stool. Avoid laxatives. Better consult a doctor. Constant pressure of baby in womb causes irritation of the blood vessels around the anal opening. This also results in soreness, itching, pain and bleeding while passing stool. Avoid standing for long time and consult with your doctor.
- Thick curdy discharge and itching : However, a clear white vaginal secretion usually increases during this period due to hormonal changes causing such vaginal thrush with a thick discharge and itching in the vaginal area. You may also have burning sensation while urinating. However, avoid soap and nylon undergarments and keep area around vagina dry.
- Breathlessness, discomfort, faint and dizzy and frequent urination : You need rest. This is usually due to low blood pressure and constant weight in the abdomen area. Use an extra pillow to prop yourself up while lying down. Frequent urination during night is due to womb pressing down upon the bladder. You must restrict your fluid intake in the evening. If there is no burning sensation while urinating, there is no need to worry.
- Spotting is an alarming signal. In case of bleeding or heavy leakage of clear watery fluid from vagina, rush to your doctor immediately.
- Contraction of muscles, rashes and swelling : This usually cause suffering from cramps and generally due to calcium deficiency. Painful contraction of muscles is relieved by stretching the legs. Massage the affected calf or foot. After getting a bit relief, walk for some time to tone up blood circulation. If the swelling over the ankles and fingers persists even after sufficient rest, then consult a doctor. This swelling is known as Oedema.

- Burning sensation in the upper abdomen: Heartburn is caused due to valve been relaxed during pregnancy as the enlarged womb presses against the stomach, thus pushing food contents up into the food pipe, resulting in pain and burning sensation in the upper abdomen and below ribs. Actually this valve remains closed in the normal condition and prevents the acidic contents of the stomach from entering back into the food pipe. Do not keep your stomach empty for more than 3 to 4 hours. Avoid spicy and fried food. Have warm milk at night before sleep and take anti-acid tablets.
- Backache : To combat backache, massage the back, starting from shoulders towards the downward **(as shown in the illustrations)**. While massaging use the heel of the hands to make firm circular movement preferably with talcum powder. Holding hot water bottle to the base of spine will help a lot. The male partner should extend this service to his wife.

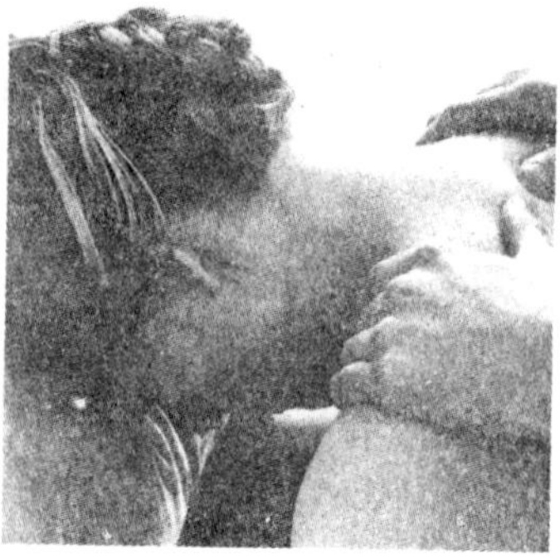

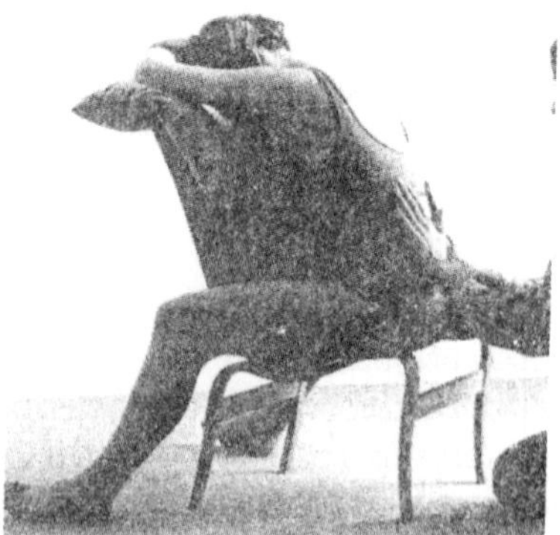

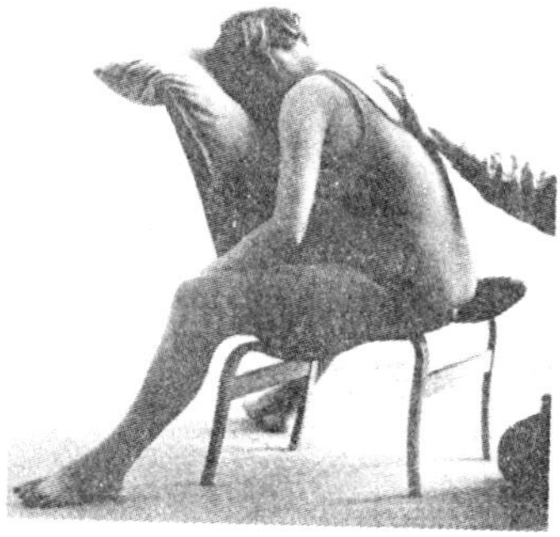

Massaging Abdomen

- To get rid of extra fat on abdomen and breasts : A good time to massage your loose abdomen and breasts is after you shower or bathe. Start with your lower abdomen, making slow, gentle, circular strokes with both hands. Then try some firm strokes, if you like going up and over the bulge, imagining you are lifting the baby back into the pelvis. End the strokes at the top of bulge. Start again at the sides, using the same stroke, but continue up and round your breasts **(as shown in illustrations)**.

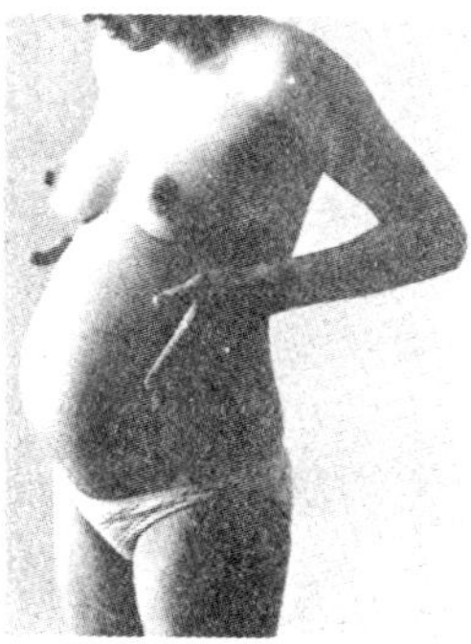

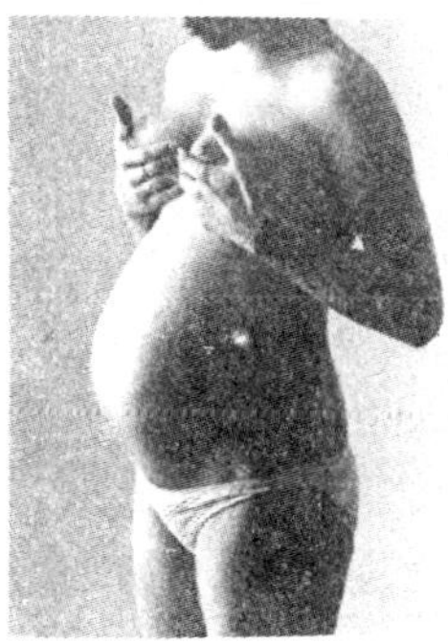

Types of Pregnancy

Radiological Diagnosis of Pregnancy : Main reasons for the employment of radiography are the following :

1. The diagnosis of pregnancy.
2. The demonstration of the fetus in relation to:

   (A) Presentation and position.

(B) Maturity

(C) Structural abnormalities

(D) Multiple pregnancy Intra-uterine death

3. The demonstration of the uterus with reference to:

   (A) Hydramnios

   (B) Placental situation, usually when placenta praevia is suspended

4. Localization of fetal abdomen for the purpose of intra-uterine transfusion.

5. Demonstration of material pelvis and lumber spine including pelvimetry.

6. Fetal cephalometry

Diagnosis of Pregnancy : Radiological method of diagnosis should not be employed before the 28th week and are rarely necessary thereafter to find out the structural abnormalities and in twin pregnancy

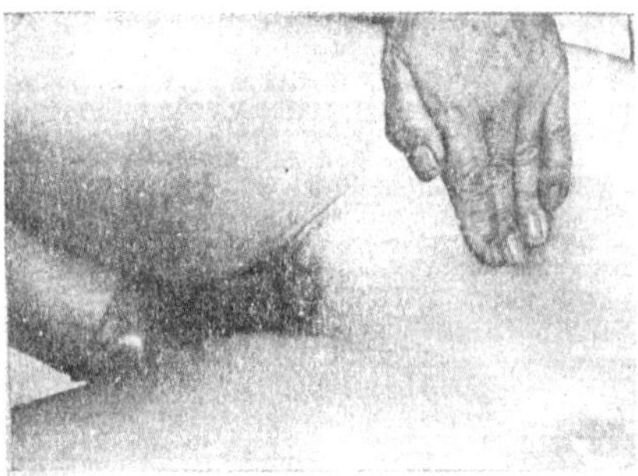

Diagnosis of Pregnancy

when one head is nearer the X-ray tube than other. To find out multiple pregnancy/ the demonstration of the uterus and placental situation, hydramnios and placenta praevia, Tube Shift Method is employed as below :

1. Find out first view of the pelvic inlet demonstrated in contour in the antero-posterior projection. The X-ray tube is centred above the patient's pelvis, so that the central ray of the X-ray beam is directed to pass through a point 3 inches behind the anterior border of symphysis pubis.

2. The radiograph is taken with the patient lying on the left side with a small pilow in between the left loin and the table to keep the lumber spine straight. The thighs are flexed towards the abdomen and knees are flexed 90 degree. The central ray of the X-ray beam is directed through a point just above and behind the great trochauter of the right femur (as shown in the illustration).
3. The radiograph to show the transverse diameter of the outlet and the subpubeic angle is obtained by placing the patient in sitting position (as shown in the illustration). The X-ray beam is directed vertically downwards so that it passes through the mid point of the line joining the two tuberosities clearly defined in the view without distortion.

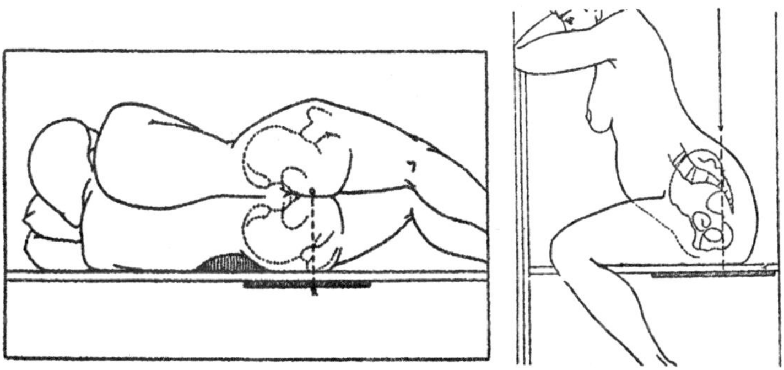

Radiograph of body

The Types of Deliveries : Fertilization is the union of a mature ovum with a sperm. If sexual intercourse takes place within 12 to 24 hours of ovulation, then one of the thousands of sperms deposited in vagina unites with the ovum to fertilize it after traveling uterine cavity and reaching fallopian tube. Once the pregnancy has not established, the production of the hormones estrogen and progesterone continue but there is no shedding- the menstruation stops and a woman is said to have conceived. The fertilized ovum gradually grows into the fetus and it takes about 266 days for a fertilized egg to grow into a fully developed baby. There are various types of deliveries.

Normal Vaginal Delivery

It is aided with a small cut of the vaginal outlet sometimes, the process in known as Episiotomy and has been described in detail in

Chapter 6. **Episiotomy** is done to help quicker delivery and undue downward pressure on uterus and adjoining parts like bladder and rectum.

Suction Delivery : It is a process in which suction is applied to the low descending head of the baby to hasten deliver. It is also called **vacuum method of delivery** and helps the mother to deliver quickly. Anesthesia is not required in most of the cases.

Forceps Delivery

In which baby's head is helped out with the use of forceps e.g. a large pair of tongs, which grasp the baby's head for applying a downward pull. Mild anesthesia is given to the mother to avoid excessive pain.

Essential conditions for the application of Forceps:

1. The cervix must be fully dilated.
2. The head should be in the cavity of pelvis.
3. The head should be in a suitable attitude and a correspondingly suitable position. A forceps delivery must not be attempted until the operator is quite certain of the presentation and position of the head.
4. The membranes must be ruptured.
5. The bladder and rectum should be emptied.

The low forceps operation by traction: **(Refer 14 illustrations)**

1. Introduction of the left blade. Lock the forceps and hold them in the position which they would occupy, if they were in the pelvis of the patient. The left blade has to be applied first.
2. Introduce left blade.
3. Introduce the blade into the hollow of the sacrum.
4. Swing the handle so as to bring the blade gently over the side of the child's head.
5. Bring the left blade in position.
6. Begin to introduce the right blade.
7. Introducing the right blade.
8. Bring the handles into apposition to facilitate locking.

Forceps Delivery

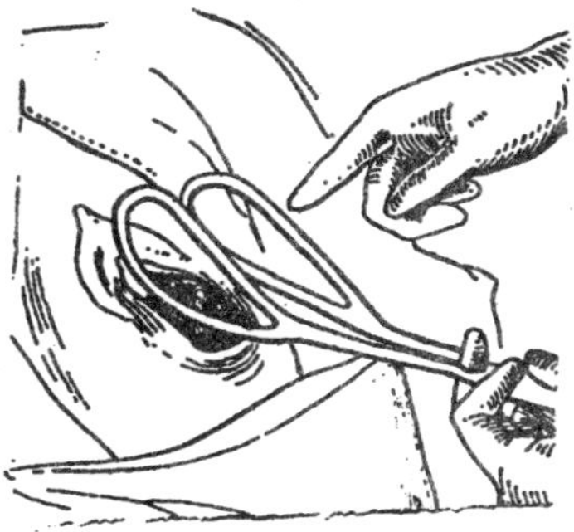

Position 1

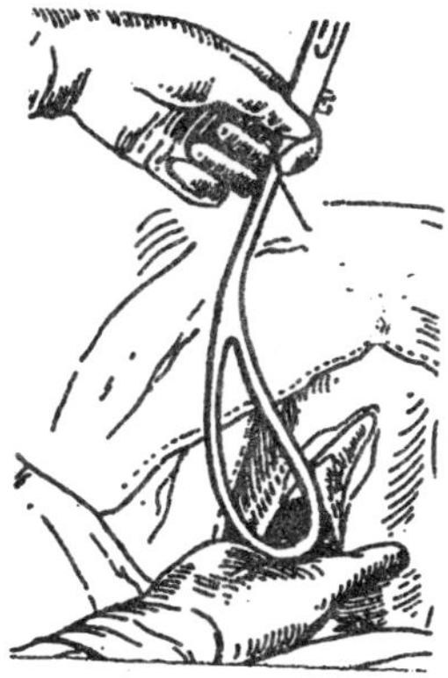

Position 2

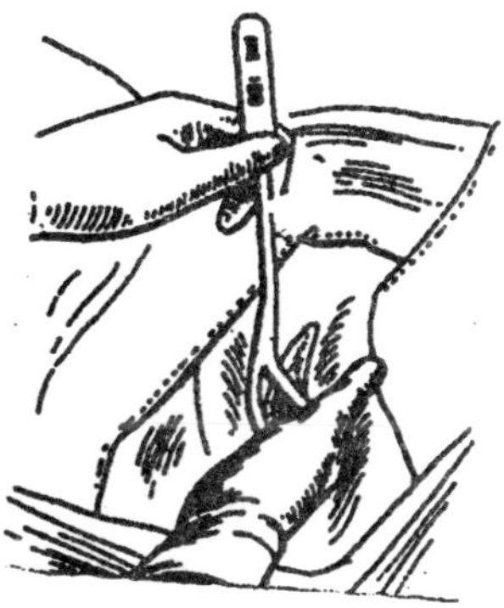

Position 3

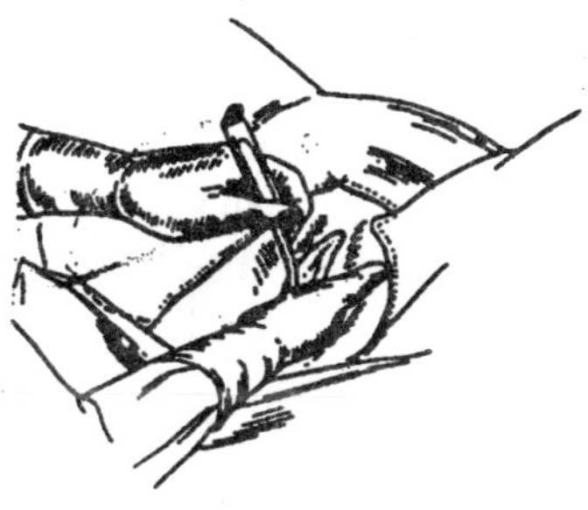

Position 4

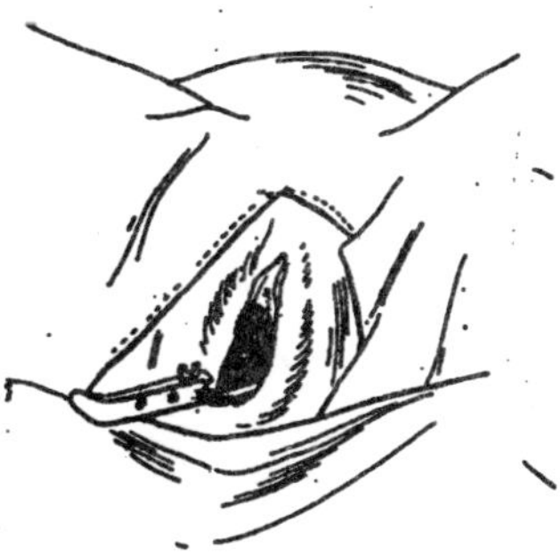

Position 5

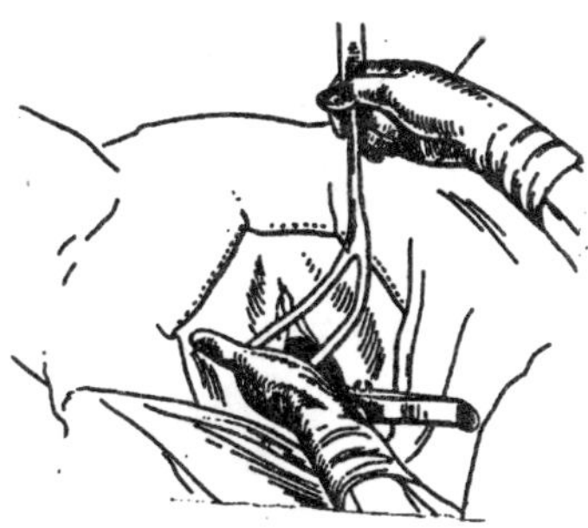

Position 6

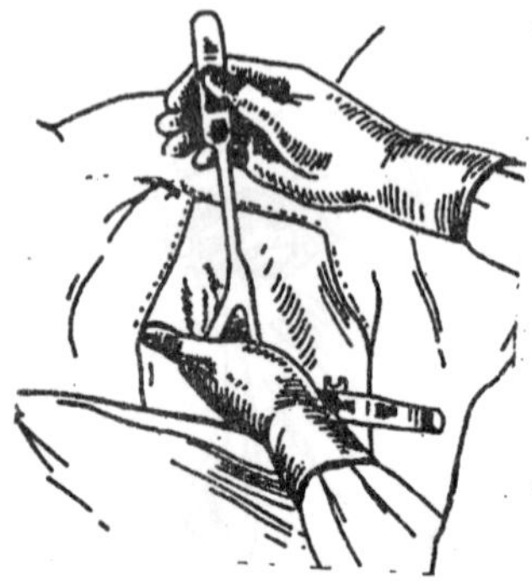

Position 7

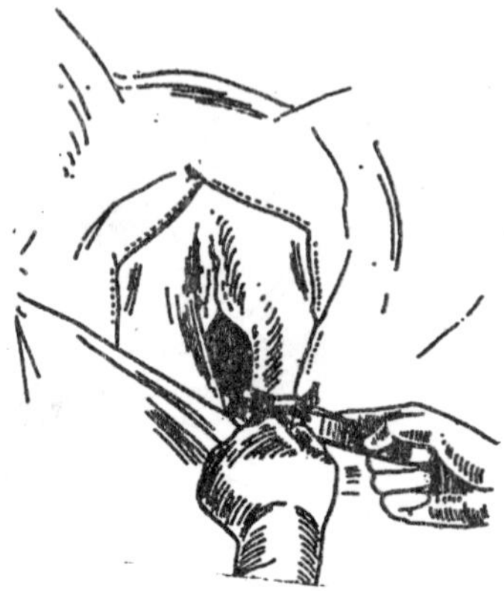

Position 8

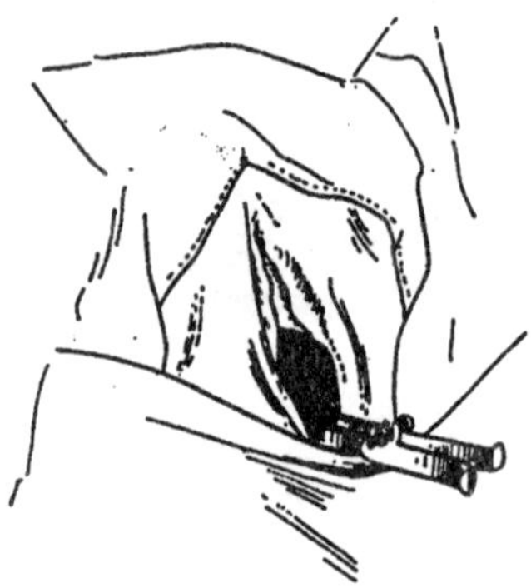

Position 9

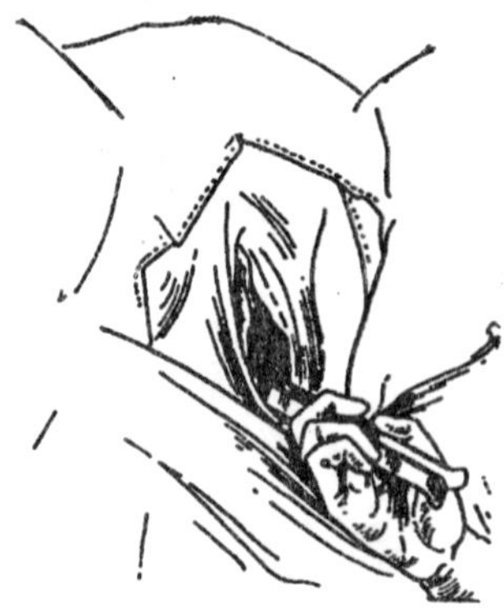

Position 10

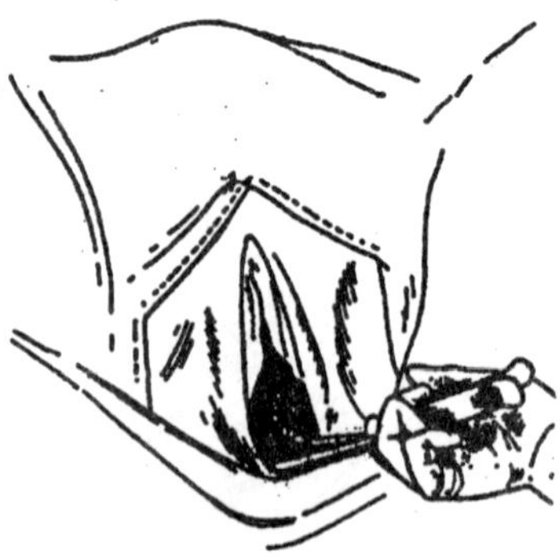

Position 11

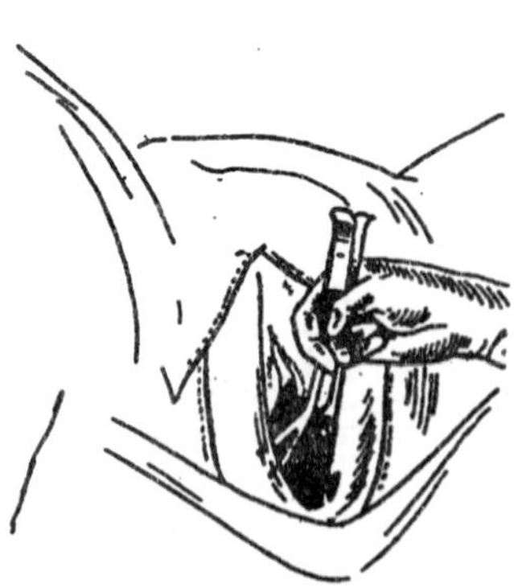

Position 12

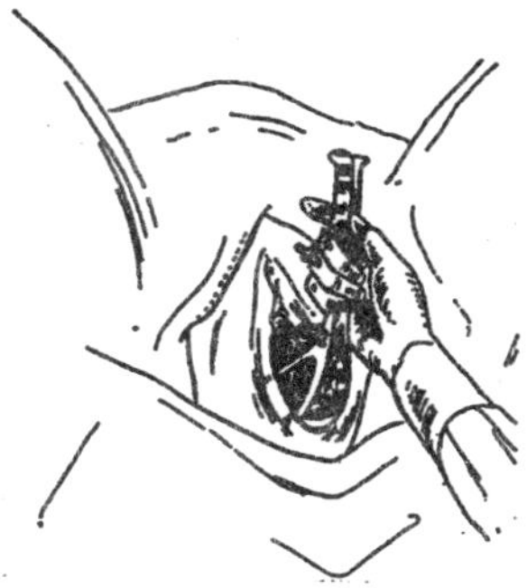

Position 13

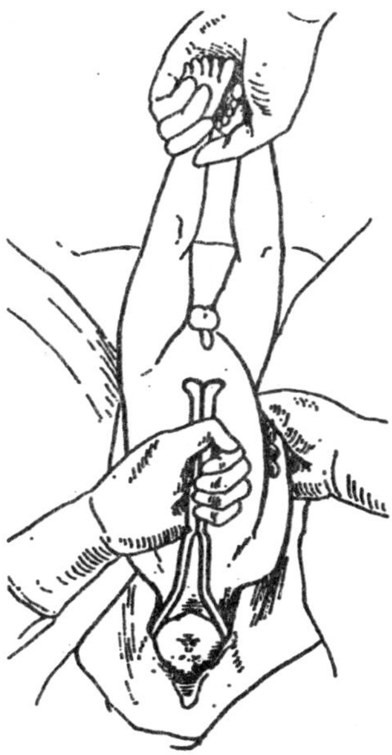

Position 14

9. Locking the handle, fixation of screw gently tightened and ready for traction.
10. Begin traction downwards and backwards.
11. Begin to change the direction of traction as the head begins to emerge.
12. Start traction upward as occiput slips under pubic arch.
13. Traction should be still more upward as flexion of head becomes undone and forehead slips over perineum.
14. Delivery of the child after-coming head by forceps.

Risk of Forceps:

1. Injuries to the soft passages may be caused by carelessness in application of the blades or by too rapid extraction.
2. Hemorrhage may be caused by too rapid extraction.
3. Injuries to the child (e.g. fractures of the skull, intra-cranial hemorrhage, injury to eyes, facial paralysis, sphyxia for compression of head).

Multiple Pregnancy

Do you have any history of multiple births in the family? If yes, then you must watch out and tell your doctor to diagnose seriously. It can be diagnosed by the size of womb or pelvic examination or USC scanning of abdomen. In case of signs of multiple pregnancy, visit your doctor more frequently and have complete rest between 30th to 37th week, to avoid premature delivery. Multiple pregnancy means an extra trouble and sometimes there is a possibility of a caesarean section. Plural births require highly skilled pediatric care. The fetal mortality is much higher; pre-maturity, pro-lapse of the cord and asphyxia of the second twin takes a high toll. Congenital abnormalities in uniovular twins are common. **Locked Twins** is a rare complication, where the first child presents by the breech and the second by the head, the chins being locked during the descent of the first **(as shown in the illustration).**

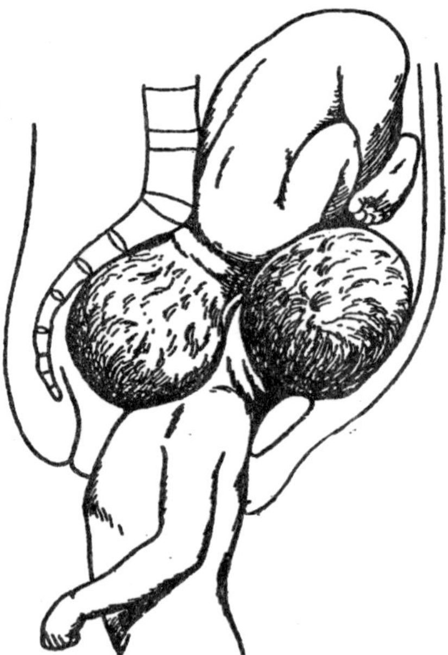

Locked Twins

Delivery of the Head : This is the critical phase, because delay may cause havoc. The reasons for the delay are:

- That when the head passes into the pelvic cavity it is no longer subject to the expulsive power of the uterus.

- That the passage of head is resisted by the ring of vulva outlet. To avoid such risk, episiotomy should always be made in a primigravida when the buttocks are distending the perineum. However, when the child is small and the maternal passages roomy, spontaneous delivery may occur without giving a cut at the outlet of vagina.

The usual method of delivery is to hold the child's body slightly downwards, straddled over the left hand and forearm, and exert gentle suprapubic (nor fundal) pressure on the head as the head enters the pelvic cavity. Gentle traction will deliver the face and head **(as shown in the illustration)**.

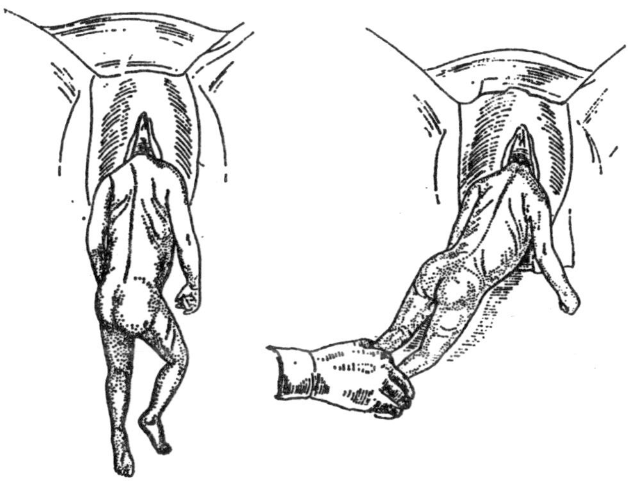

Delivery of the Head

Ectopic or Tubal Delivery

It is a rare complication in which the fertilized ovum or embryo becomes blocked in its passage through the fallopian tube. There the embryo continues to grow as it normally would within the uterus. However, the space between the tube is too small to allow expansion, that may rupture, causing a serious hemorrhage and also intense pain in the pelvis. This may also result acute appendicitis. Consult a doctor for necessary surgery as soon as a tubal pregnancy is suspected before the occurrence of hemorrhage. Ectopic pregnancy remains one of the leading cause of maternal death, the classical triad of pain, abnormal vaginal bleeding and a palpable adnexal mass present in most of the patients with ectopic pregnancy.

Induced Delivery

In this connection, labor is brought on or induced artificially by rupturing the membranes and letting out a little amniotic fluid, which stimulates labor pains. When the pains are too feeble or the delivery is overdue, labor is induced by administrating medicines, which contract the uterus.

Premature Delivery

The termination of pregnancy after the fetus has become viable such as capable of living independently, is called premature birth. And if the fetus is born dead, it is still-birth. Causes which produce abortions can endanger the growth of the fetus resulting in still birth or a premature delivery. Premature delivery is usually the problem with the placenta, the faulty blood supply to the fetus, defective hormone production and effect of injurious toxins and chemicals through the blood to the fetus. The causes of premature delivery are the following:

1. Obliquity of the uterus.
2. Uterus subseptus.
3. Premature fetus.
4. Dead, macerated and flaccid fetus.
5. Hydramnois
6. Placenta praevia.
7. Pelvic tumor.

Breech Delivery

Most babies are born in head-first position instead of feet-first or shoulder first. If the birth canal is adequate and the baby is small, there may not be any serious difficulty because of breech position. If the baby is bulky and the birth outlet small, this could be dangerous to both mother and the baby. Avoid traveling or bulky jerks during the last few days.

Operative Obstetrics

Version: or turning is the artificial alteration of the fetal from one pole to another, or from a transverse to a longitudinal tie. There are three methods of performing version described – External, Internal and combined (Bipolar). Version during labor is an operation which is being carried out much less frequently than in the past. In many cases caesarean section is much safer for the mother and child.

Bipolar Version (combined versions) : This method of version was introduced for the treatment of placenta praevia and was very much in use from the very beginning. Nowadays, this method is much less frequently chosen because of the risks to the child. The patient is placed in lithotomy position, shoulders slightly raised. An anesthesia is necessary, as whole hand may have to be passed into the vagina up to the cervix. The other hand has to be placed on the abdomen over the breech and is moved downwards and to the sides.

The hand is kept in the vagina and one or two fingers are inserted, and are passed into cervix. Press the head upwards and towards the sides. When the head is pressed out of the pelvis, the shoulders will come within the reach of the fingers in the cervix. When the shoulder has been pushed out of the pelvis, the knee is felt, which should be hooked down and thereafter a foot is brought through the cervix to the vulva. Then the head should be pressed into the fundus by the external hand. **(Refer four positions as shown in illustrations)**.

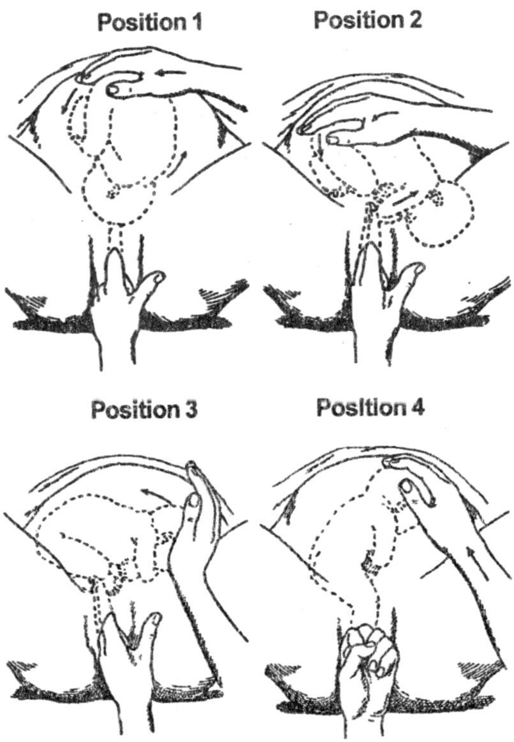

Bipola Version

Internal Version

This operation differs from Bipolar Version only in the fact that the internal hand is introduced inside the uterus. It is indicated in cases where turning of the baby is desirable and necessary conditions are present. Shoulder presentations are the most frequent indication.

Position 1 **Position 2**

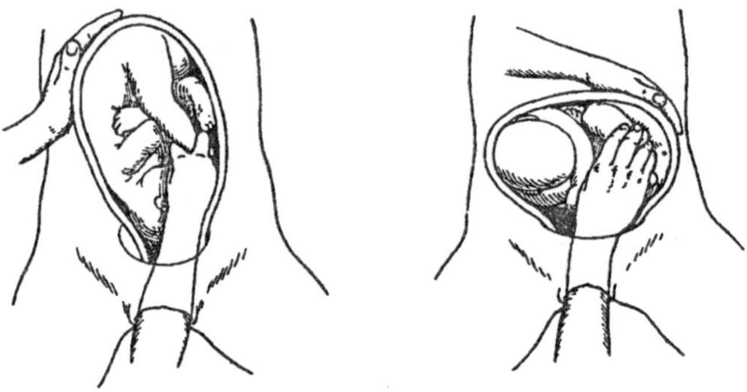

Internal Version

Necessary conditions for doing Internal Version :

1. Membrane intact or not ruptured recently. Avoid internal version in such cases.
2. The abdominal and uterine walls must be relaxed.
3. An anesthesia should always be given.
4. The cervix must be dilated sufficiently to admit the entire hand in uterus.
5. The position of the fetus must have been exactly mapped out by the palpation before the hand is introduced in the uterus.
6. The vulva and the vagina must be thoroughly cleansed.
7. Sterile rubber gloves should be worn.

How to do operation? Pass the hand into the uterus in cone-shape and seize a foot. The patient should be placed on her side or her back. If the knee is felt, the foot or knee should be brought down through the cervix. The head must be pushed up into the fundus of uterus by external hand **(as shown in two illustrations)**.

Vaginal Hysterotomy

This process is artificial dilation of the cervix is conducted by the fingers or by hydrostatic bags in the first stage is an operation, which has nowadays been almost replaced by caesarean section-better and a safer operation.

Under general anesthesia the cervix is exposed by adequate vaginal retraction. With the scissors the cervix is cut at points in clockwise direction. The cut extends to the junction of the cervix and the vaginal wall. Following delivery by the forceps the cut is carefully sutured. The final results of the healing are usually unsatisfactory and lead to reverse hemorrhage sometimes. Incision of the cervix is now very uncommon operation. Attempt to dilate the cervix by the fingers is always almost followed by cervical lacerations and the operation of the incision of the cervix is always to be preferred.

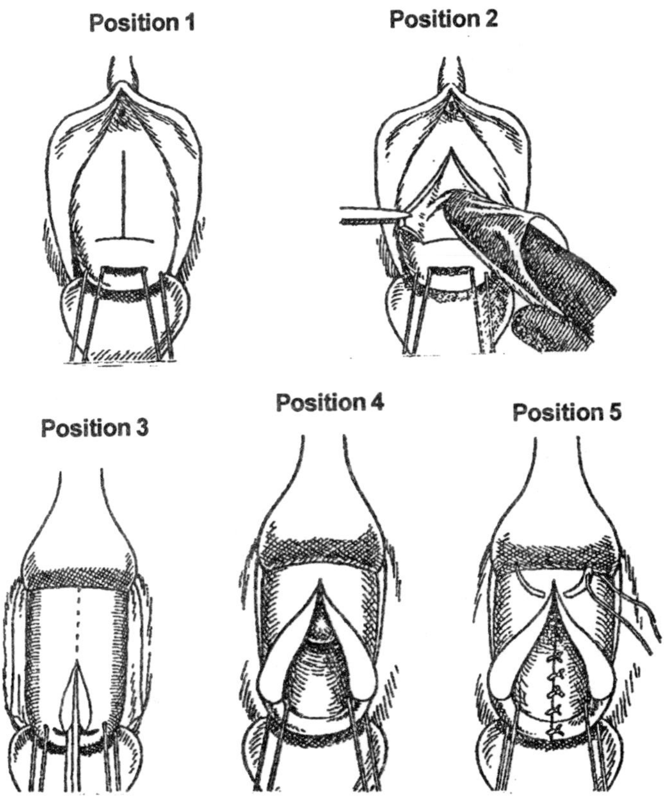

Vaginal Hysterotomy

How to do Vaginal Hysterotomy?

This operation has been almost entirely supplemented by abdominal hysterotomy. The steps of the operation are sufficiently indicated by the illustrations **(Refer five positions)** here as described below:

Position 1. Transverse incisions in anterior vaginal wall.

Position 2. Dissecting bladder from uterus and vagina.

Position 3. Bladder and vaginal wall drawn up.

Position 4. Bulging down the membranes.

Position 5. Suturing anterior incision.

Displacement and Abnormalities of Uterus

There are serious displacements of uterus usually during pregnancy. Generally, they occur together, but occasionally simple retro-version is found. The cause in majority of cases of uterus displacement has existed before pregnancy ensued and merely persists after the uterus begins to enlarge. There are four possible terminations :

1. Spontaneous rectifications
2. Abortion
3. Sacculation of the uterus
4. Incarceration

Diagnosis and causes of displacement of uterus : It may be diagnosed by :

- Increase in backward displacement.
- Pain on micturition occurs, passing into retention if incarceration occurs.
- Undue enlargement of abdomen (distended bladder).

Generally, the enlargement of uterus and abdomen occurs due to pregnancy plus large tumor, hydramnnios, multiple pregnancy or even a mere mistake as to the date of conception. The bladder must be carefully emptied by catheter before examination.

How to treat displacement and abnormalities of uterus?

1. If by12th week the uterus is still retroverted, then a large ring pessary (made of plastic) is inserted into the vagina.

2. The patient is instructed to adopt the semi-prone position and remain in bed for a couple of days in the **Sim's Position (as shown in the illustration).** It is found after 24 to 48 hours the fundus can be felt in the abdomen. The pessary should be left in vagina until after the 16th week of pregnancy (under doctor's supervision).

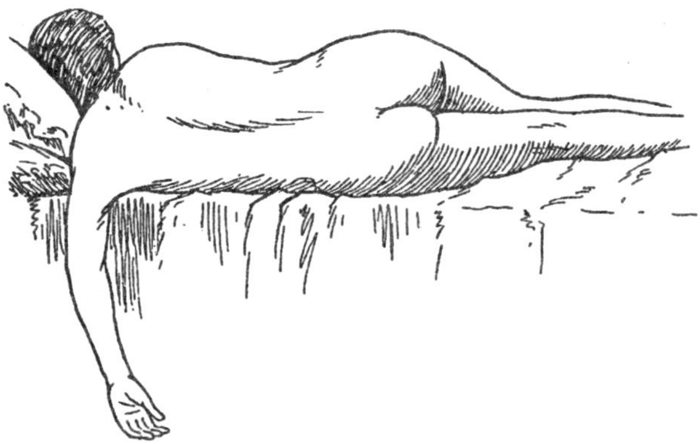

The Sim's position

3. If the uterus remains retroverted after 48 hours, then manual reposition of the uterus may be undertaken. Simple manual reposition is done by inserting two fingers in the posterior fornix and pushing the fundus upwards and forwards, manoeuvring it past the side of the sacral promontory; the cervix is then caught backwards by one finger and the other hand on the abdomen catches the fundus and depresses it into its ordinary position. After the uterus has been replaced a large ring pessary should be inserted and not removed until after the 16th week of pregnancy.

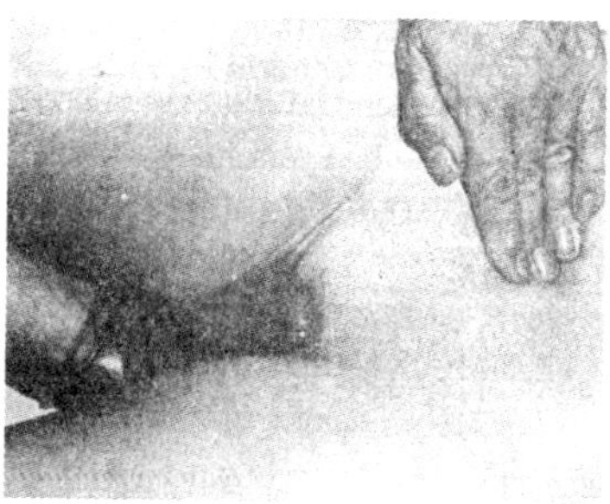

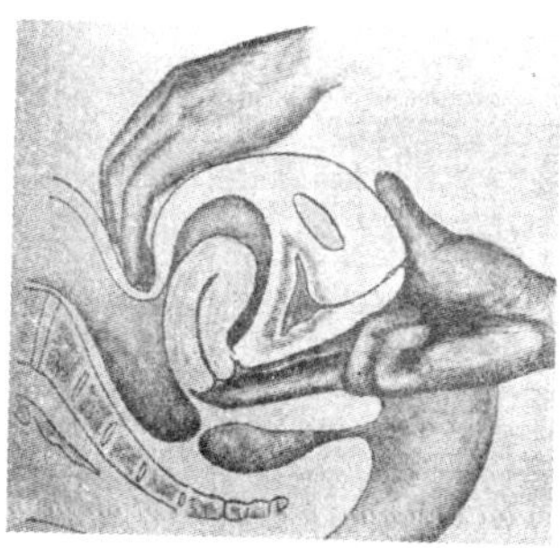

4. In case of patient with a history of preveous abortions, a laparotomy should not be delayed.

Abnormalities of Uterus: The malformations of the uterus are usually the result of incomplete fusion of two Mullerian ducts or of incomplete absorption of the septum between them. The complications recorded include a high incidence of abortion and premature labor, of inertia during labor, retained placenta, of transverse lies and breech presentations. There are eight types of major developmental abnormalities of the uterus **(as shown in the illustration)** as below:

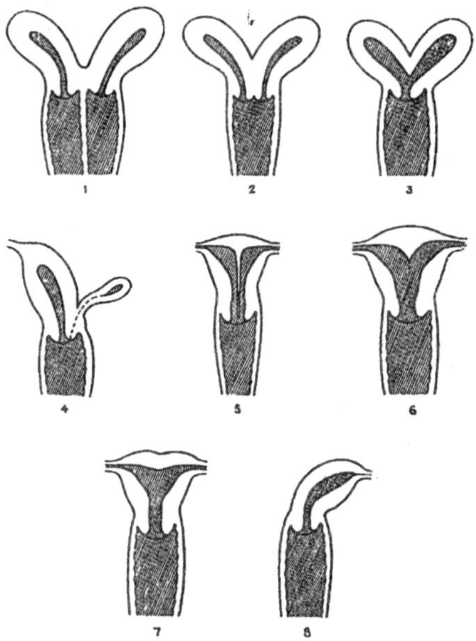

Abnormal Uteruses

1. Uterus didelphys (complete duplication of uterus, cervix and vagina)
2. Uterus bicornis bicollis
3. Uterus bicornis unicollis
4 Uterus bicornis unicollis (with one horn rudimentar)
5. Uterus septus
6. Uterus subseptus
7. Uterus arcuatus
8. Uterus unicornis.

List of Contents required in Doctor's Maternity Bag

Items for Examining Patient:

Fetal stethoscope

Finger cots

Disposable gloves

Disposable paper masks

Anesthetics

Trilene inhaler

Trilene 6 ml. (5 amps.)

Antiseptics, etc.

Antiseptic liquid

Hibitane obstetric cream

Sterile swabs or cotton wool balls

Two sterile maternity pads

Soap and nail brush

Razor and blades

Two large gallipots

Two small gallipots

Two kidney dishes (8" size)

Instruments

One needle-holder

Two pairs Spencer Wells forceps

One pair pointed scissors

One pair episiotomy scissors

One pair toothed dissecting forceps

Two no. 3 round pointed ½ inch circle needles

Two no. 11 triangular cutting ½ inch circle needles

Sterile cord ligatures or clips

Two tubes catgut (size 2/0)

Two tubes catgut (size 2/0) with cutting needle attached

Black silk or soft braided nylon

Two disposable sterile catheters

Two disposable sterile mucus extractors

One pair (Wrigley's) forceps

One pair (Kocher's) forceps

One pair vulval retractors

One metal sterilizer

One lithotomy webbing sling

One infant tracheal tube

One infant laryngoscope

Oxygen spark-let infant resuscitator

Syringes and necessary drugs

Two disposable 20 ml. Syringes with two 6 inches needles

Six 2 ml. Syringes with needle (21G x 1-1/2 inch and 25 G x 5/8 inch)

Injection Lignocaine ½ % (in 50 ml bottle)

2 amps. Pethilorfan100 mgs.

2 amps. Pethidine100 mgs.

Injection Lethidrone10 mg (In 1 ml)

6 amps. Syntometrine 0.5 mg (in 1 c.c.)

6 amps. Ergometrine 0.5 mg (in 1 c.c.)

3 amps Synkavit 1 mg (in 1 ml)

Miscellaneous items

Plastic apron

Gown and cap

Sterile disposable gloves

Urine testing equipment

Large torch or headlamp

Two sterile test tubes for cord blood

Sterile disposable towel

Low-grade thermometer

When the delivery has to be conducted in the patients' place

The following precautions are required:

1. The room for the confinement should be large enough to allow for free working space. It should be well ventilated and should have maximum amount of light. The room should be very close to a bathroom. The place/house should be located where the living conditions are satisfactory and most hygienic.
2. The patient should lie on a hard bed, which doesn't sag. To prevent this an hard thick board may be inserted under the mattress. At the onset of labor, a supply of hot water should be available in/adjoining the room.
3. Ensure that a reliable person has been engaged to attend to the patient during the pregnancy and postnatal period.
4. Care should be taken that no member of the family is a source of infection to the mother and the baby.
5. Domestic animals should not be allowed to enter the room.

Requisites for the confinement for the mother

1. Two polythene sheets.
2. Strong clean brown paper to protect the mattress.
3. Two sets of clean sheets and pillow-covers.
4. Three old but clean sheets.
5. Two old night dresses for labor.
6. Three night dresses with an opening in the front for breastfeeding.
7. Two firm brassieres to support the breast.
8. Sanitary belt.
9. Safety pins.
10. Two bath towels.
11. Two hand towels.
12. Two face cloths.
13. Soap in a soap case.
14. Hot water bottle.

Requirement for delivery

1. One wash basin.
2. Two jugs

3. One bucket.
4. Plenty of newspapers.

Requirements for the baby

1. One cot or basket complete with mattress.
2. Sufficient sheets and blankets.
3. Four night gowns.
4. Four vests.
5. Three dozen napkins.
6. One 4 inches crepe bandage for binder.
7. Four pairs bootees.
8. Two woolen caps (in winter).
9. Two shawls (in winter).
10. Five or six bibs of polythene or any soft material.
11. One bath or large basin.
12. One bathing apron.
13. Two bath towels.
14. Two face cloths.
15. Baby soap in a soap dish.
16. Needle and thread, safety pins.
17. Zinc and castor oil cream.
18. Small basket or tray to carry baby's things.
19. 24 sterilized maternity pads.
20. ½ kg. sterilized cotton.
21. Three cord ligatures.
22. Six cord dressings.
23. Sterilized cord powder.

Birth Control and Abortion

Birth control, also known as contraception refers, to the prevention of fertilization-the union of the sperms and egg produced by ovaries. Most of the newly married couples want to know about the family planning techniques. Birth control is very important in the following cases:

- In case a woman is in poor health. She should try to control until she is healthy enough to face pregnancy and childbirth.
- Couples have a desire for children but want to space them out.
- There have been previous Cesarean section deliveries a couple of times.

Following are the various most widely used methods of birth control:

- Abstinence: A truly safe method of birth control. The semen is ejaculated near the entrance of vagina without having had actual intercourse. In certain cases the ejaculated semen may come into contact with a virginal hymen and gain access to the vagina until it reaches to the uterus. Some marriages were able to survive with this method.
- Rhythm method: There is certain time each month when a woman is not likely to become pregnant. Usually a woman in childbearing age sheds an egg from her ovary every month on about fourteen day after the onset of her menstruation (with a regular 28 day interval) between the menstrual periods. She might ovulate between 12th to 16th days. The sperm can live for at least two days within the Fallopian tubes, the place at which fertilization takes place. Thus a woman is more likely to become pregnant in case of sexual contact during this period. This method is about 85-90% effective.
- Coitus interruptus: This is one of the oldest technique for birth control if the male partner has proper control over the withdrawal of his organ and the other partner has no objection to this practice, as some women reach a climax when their male partner ejaculates. It is not a 100% safe method of birth control, as in few cases part of the semen ejaculated from male partner may remain deposited on the female organ. Males who suffer from premature ejaculation usually have poor control over ejaculation. This method of birth control is not recommended as a regular practice as a man has a great need for completing the sexual act once he has started.
- Condom: A thin latex sheath placed on the male organ to accommodate ejaculation of the semen. This is a frequently used safe method for birth control. The condom is discarded and thrown after single use. Most of the couples complain of lack of enjoyment during sex act when a condom is used and is less preferred due to the following reasons:

- 1. Decrease sensation when used.
  2. Interrupt lovemaking when put on.
  3. It may break while in use.
  4. It may leak due to manufacturing defect.
  5. Sometimes, it may burst when in use or slip off after orgasm before removing. In case of leakage, the woman should immediately place one or two contraceptive suppositories or contraceptive jelly or foam deep into her vaginal canal. Avoid douching.
- Douches: It is cleansing of vaginal canal by use of a syringe and stream of water. It is one of the poorest methods because it is not possible to flush out completely by douching and some of the sperms in the folds of the vagina may penetrate into the cervix.
- Diaphragm: Diaphragm is a circular rubber device that lifts tightly in the vagina and completely covers the cervix. A gynecologist may suggest the correct size of diaphragm after examination. The diaphragm can be inserted while standing or while lying on the back or in sitting position as one sits for toilet by inserting fingers. The front end of the diaphragm will be tucked in back of the pubic bone. The diaphragm is removed the next morning or about five hours after termination of relations.
- Contraceptive jellies, foams and creams: They are commercial, highly effective products in destroying sperm within the vagina, which are inserted into the vagina an hours before the intercourse. You may follow the instructions mentioned on the wrapper before use.
- Intrauterine devices (IUDs): A plastic or plastic-metal object inserted by the gynecologist into the uterine cavity. It is 98% effective device. The cervix is dilated, usually during a menstrual period and the device is pushed into the uterine cavity. However, women feel mild discomfort. The device blocks the entrance of the sperm into the Fallopian tube, where fertilization usually takes place. The device is usually changed after three years. The IUD should not be inserted or removed if inserted in case of the following conditions:
  1. If the woman has heavy menstrual periods or bleeding in between the periods.
  2. The woman has fibroid tumors.

3. In case of extremely painful menstruation.
4. If the woman suffers from lower abdominal cramps.
5. There is cervical infection.

However, a woman who has not borne any children should avoid wearing an IUD as an infection may result in future fertility. In case of a uterine infection, it should be treated with antibiotics. The device should be removed promptly in case the woman is pregnant.

- Oral contraceptives (Birth control pills): The pills are taken orally. They inhibit ovulation or formation of egg as without ovulation pregnancy is not possible regardless of how many sperm reach the Fallopian tubes. Each tablet contains two female hormones: one estrogen and another progesterone. These pills are 100% effective and should be taken strictly according to the advice of your doctor. It eliminates any disagreeable contraceptive odor. Sometimes, complications as below may arise while taking the birth control pills:
    1. A feeling of headaches and nausea.
    2. A bloated feeling with some weight gain due to fluid retention. Prolonged use of pills is not advised.
    3. Swelling and tenderness in the breasts may develop in some women.
    4. Inflammation of the veins in the legs (plebitis).

Avoid using oral contraceptives in the following cases:

1. Obese women.
2. Woman having chronically high blood pressure.
3. If suffering from liver disorder.
4. In case of heavy smokers and older women.
5. If suffering from varicose veins or phlebitis.
6. In case of heavy smokers.
7. In older women.
8. Women suffering from fibroids of the uterus.
9. Women having breast tumor or have cystic disease of the breasts and family history of breast disorders.

- Surgical birth control : An incision is made in the lower abdomen, the tubes are grasped with a forceps and tied or cut in their middle portion or are cauterized with an electric cautery. A laparoscope (metal instrument) is inserted through a incision in the navel through which the gynecologist looks in the abdomen and applies the cautery to the Fallopian tubes. It is a 100% effective method for birth control.

- Vasectomy : It is technique for cutting the vas deferens, thereby making the male infertile. In case the couple has many children and the husband wishes to spare the wife the discomfort of surgery. However, cutting the vas in no way interferes with a man's potency or ability to have or enjoy sex.

Some signs of confirmed pregnancy

- Stoppage of Menstruation (monthly bleeding known as periods).
- Laziness, heavy feeling, irritability and presence of physical disturbances.
- Morning sickness and vomiting from second month onwards, which usually stops in the fourth month, or in some cases continues throughout pregenancy period.
- Heaviness in breasts.
- Breast nipples get prominent and areola starts turning darker from pinkish.
- Tightening of abdomen after about four months.
- Frequency in micturation due to pressure of the pregnant uterus on the urinary bladder.
- Genitals feel warmer due to more blood and congestion.
- Vagina remains excessive moist.
- The fetal movement starts usually in the fifth month onward.
- Vagina is usually hot and moist.
- Uterus rises above the pelvis when the pregnancy is advanced.
- The movement of the fetus increases, feeling the limbs, head and neck of the fetus.

The effect of drugs or chemicals

Name of drug/chemicals	*Teratogenic effect*
Alcohol	Growth retardation, cardiac, limb and facial anomalies.
Androgens	Cleft lip-plate and masculinization.
Chlorambucil	Malformaions and fetal loss.
Dicumarol	Bleeding and fetal death.

Diphenylhydontoin	Facial, cardiac and limb anomalies.
Excessive smoking	Growth retardation.
Gentamycin	Eighth nerve damage.
Heroine	Intrauterine death, low birth weight of baby and sudden infant death.
Indomethacin	Low birth weight and platelet dysfunction.
Iodides	Hypothyroidism and goiter.
Lithium carbonate	Goiter.
Methotrexate	Congenital malformation and abortion.
Oral contraceptives	Cardiac, limb and visceral anomalies.
Quinine	Deafnes and thrombacytopenia.
Radiation	Mental retardation.
Streptomycin	Eighth nerve deafness.
Tetracycline	Staining of teeth and enamel hypoplasia, inhibition of bone growth and congenital cataracts.
Tolbutamide	Fetal death and thrombocytopenia.
Heavy dose of Vitamin D	Mental retardation.

Abortion

Loss or failure of early pregnancy in several forms: complete, incomplete, inevitable, missed, septic and threatened is known as Abortion.

- **Complete Abortion:** is the termination of a pregnancy before the age of viability almost in 50% cases. It occurs at less than 20 weeks from the first day of the last normal menstrual period or involving a fetus of weight less than 500 gm.
- **Incomplete Abortion:** is the spontaneous passage of some (not all) of the products of conception associated with uniform pregnancy loss.
- **Inevitable Abortion:** is a pregnancy in which rupture of the membranes and/or cervical dilation takes place during the first half of the pregnancy period.
- **Missed Abortion:** is the retention of a failed intrauterine pregnancy, which can be detected by an ultrasound.
- **Septic Abortion:** is a variant of an incomplete abortion due to infection.

- **Threatened Abortion:** is a pregnancy in which vaginal bleeding or uterine cramping occurs. 50-60% such pregnancies come in the category of complete abortion.

Causes of Abortion: There are several causes for an abortion. Some of the prominent causes are the following:

- Endocrine abnormalities (in 25-50% cases).
- Genetic factors (in 10-70% cases).
- Trisomy (in 40-50% cases).
- Monosomy (in 15-25% cases).
- Reproductive tract abnormalities (in 6-12% cases).
- Tripoidy and tetraploidy (in 5-15% cases).
- Abnormality of placentation.
- Effect of venereal diseases.
- Chronic cardiovascular disease and chronic renal disease.
- Diabetes mellitus.
- Environmental factors such as alcohol, anesthetic gases, effect of drugs, radiation, smoking and toxins.
- Other factors such as advanced maternal age, delayed fertilization, short interval between pregnancies.

Signs and symptoms : These include the following :

- Vaginal bleeding (bright red to dark colored).
- Abdominal cramping. (generally rhythmic accompanied by pelvic or low back pressure).
- Cervical dilation with tissue visible at the cervical openings.
- Severe vaginal hemorrhage.
- Cervical polyps and cervicitis.
- Urinary tract infection and lower abdominal discomfort.
- Loss of early symptoms such as fullness of breasts or morning sickness.
- Disseminated intra-vascular coagulopathy can occur when an intrauterine fetal demise in the second trimester has been retained beyond six weeks after the death of the fetus.

Specific measures : are the following :

- Rh-negative mothers should be treated with Rh immune globulin after completion of the abortion, because ovulation may occur as early as two weeks after an abortion.

- After an abortion, control the bleeding, prevent infection and relieve pain.
- Ensure that all the products of the conception have been expelled from the uterus. If retained tissues are present and cannot be ruled out, curettage must be performed immediately.
- Septic abortion requires urgent and aggressive management. Antibiotics, fluid therapy and prompt evacuation of the uterus are indicated.
- If significant pain or bleeding persist, especially bleeding leading to hemodynamic alterations, evacuation of the uterus should be conducted.

Maternal disorders and their effect on the fetus

Disorder	*Adverse effect*
Toxemia of pregnancy	Infra-uterine growth retardation, respiratory depression of the fetus due to use of sedatives and need for curtailment of pregnancy.
Antepartum hemorrhage	Fetal and birth asphyxia, premature labor and anemia.
Polyhydramnios	Anencephaly, high intestinal obstruction and ectopia vesicae.
Oligohydramnios	Bilateral renal agencies or hypoplasia obstructive, obstructive uropathy, deformed limbs or face.
Rupture of membrances	High risk of pneumonia in the baby.
Malnutrition	Intrauterine growth retardation, anemia and deficiency of iron.
Thyrotoxicosis	Neonatal thyrotoxicosis and goiter.
Maternal diabeties	Premature delivery, often by cesarean section, intrauterine death, early asymptomatic or symptomatic hypoglycemia.

Thrombocytopenic purpura	Transient neonatal thrombocytopenia due to transplacental transfer or antiplatelet antibody.
Maternal infection	Abortion, intrauterine death, fetal growth retardation, multisystem involvement such as hepatitis, meningoencephalitis, anemia, thrombocytopenia, microcephaly or hydrocephalay, congenital malformation with viral infections during the first trimester of pregnancy.

If the mother is diabetic?

The following complications may arise in case of a diabetic mother:

- Fetus may suddenly die during last trimester of pregnancy.
- Pre-term delivery may have to be induced to avoid third trimester fetal death.
- Neonatal respiratory distress.
- Hypoglycemia, hypocalcemia and hyperbilirubinemia.
- Polycythemia and increased viscosity of blood.
- Higher risk of congenital anomalies.
- Cardiomyopathy and persistent pulmonary hypertension.
- Macrosomia or large size of the body and its risks during delivery such as birth trauma, asphyxia and increased possibilities of cesarean section.
- Intrauterine growth retardation.

Effects on fetus in case of intrauterine infection?

A variety of maternal infections may be transmitted to the fetus during pregnancy by various modes, such as hematogeneous through the placenta, direct infection of placenta, ascending infection from the vagina resulting in amnionitis and during passage through the birth canal. Such infections may be the following:

- Viral infections (cytomegalovirus, herpes simplex, hepatitis, cox-sackie, rubella, mumps etc.)
- Protozoal infections (toxoplasma gondi and malaria).

- Spirochetal infections (treponema pallidum).
- Bacterial infections (listeria and monocytogenes).

Effects of a deformed pelvis?

The birth of the baby in case of a deformed and contracted pelvis become very difficult and result in:

- The head of the baby may not get fixed up in the true pelvis.
- The baby might get struck up at the lower end.
- Perenium might get torn giving rise to bladder and rectal complications.
- The uterus might burst.
- Baby or the mother and sometimes both may lose their lives.

Under such circumstances the only way to save the mother and the baby is surgery by cutting through the wall of abdomen. The operation is called cesarean section. Remember, this operation can only be repeated twice or at the most three times on one woman and she has to completely adopt scientific method of birth control.

5
External and Internal Genitals

Every woman on way to become a mother should know about her body thoroughly. There are several women, some of them going to be married or are expectant mother but they know least about the organs of their body. Most of the teenagers feel hesitant to question about male or female genitals though their knowledge is essential for every one to make married life and pregnancy more enjoyable and also allay fears and misconception.

The Uterus: The womb is the compartment of female body in which a baby forms and grows till birth. It is also termed as uterus, a pear-shaped hollow thick walled muscular organ situated deep in the lower abdomen, placed between the bladder in front and the rectum behind. The uterus is usually of size 3″x2″x1″ when in non-

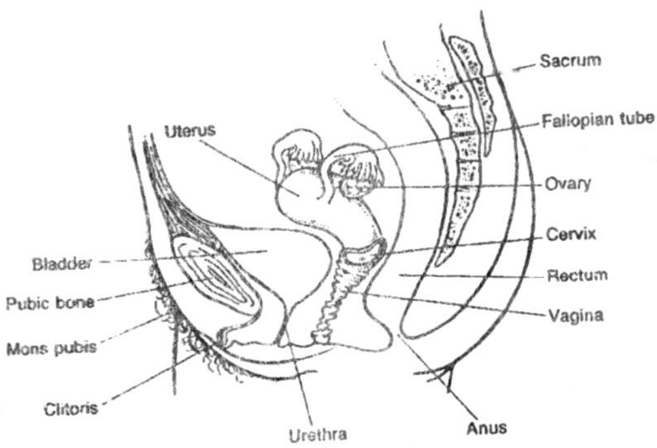

Internal Organs

pregnant state and it stretches gradually in size to accommodate a fully formed baby. The lower part of the uterus is narrow and is called the cervix with an opening in its tip. The cervix projects into the vagina, creating the space between the vaginal walls and surface of the cervix called vaginal fornix.

The upper broad end of the uterus opens on either side into two long tubes, called the fallopian tubes varying from 7 to 12 cm. in length, each ending in a funnel-shaped opening guarded by five finger-like projections called fimbria. The funnel-shaped opening lies close to the ovary on either side. The cavity of the uterus is a potential space only, the anterior and posterior walls being normally in contact. The cavity of the body is triangular in shape 1″ wide at the fundus and 1.5″ long. The cavity of cervix is 1″ long, and is spindle-shaped. The whole length of the uterine cavity is thus 2.5″. The virgin uterus weighs about 42 gm. The measurement and the weight of uterus of a pregnant woman is slightly more than a virgin uterus.

During pregnancy the uterus enlarges in order to contain the rapidly growing ovum inside it. At the beginning of pregnancy it is an organ measuring 3 by 2 by 1 inches. At the end of pregnancy it measures about 12 by 9 by 8 inches and its weight also increases from45 to about 1000 gm. All the component tissues of the uterus share in this growth – the serous, muscular, mucous layers, the blood vessels, nerves and lymphatics.

External Genital-Vagina: The external organs of generation are generally spoken of as the vulva. The illustration below gives the name and relative position of female external genital organs:

(a) Prepuce of the clitoris

(b) Vestibule (anterior part)

(c) Orifice of the vagina

(d) Vestbular fossa

(e) Glans clitoridis

(f) Frenulum

(g) Labium majus

(h) Labium minus

(j) Orifice of the urethra

(m) Posterior commissure

(p) Anus

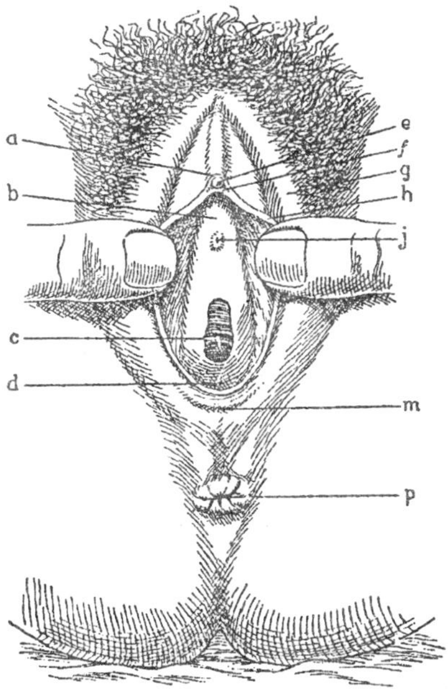

Female external genital organs

The Mons Pubis: Which is the only part of the genital organs visible when the woman is in the upright posture, is a cushion of fat in front of the pubic symphysis, covered after puberty with more or less short curly hair.

Labia Majora: The mons pubis is continued in a backward direction into the two outer lips of the vulva – the labia majora. Each labium majus has a lateral and a medial surface. The lateral is covered with the same short crisp hair that covers the mons. The medial surfaces, which are usually in opposition, are smoother and are devoid hair. Posteriorly the fat disappears from the labia, and they are just two folds of the skin that meet at the posterior commissure.

Labia Minora: Between the labia majora, and in the case of most virgins visible only on drawing them apart, are two triangular folds of soft, smooth, moist skin. These are the labia minora or nymphae. In front they meet as the prepuce of the clitoris; posteriorly they are joined by a fine fold called the frenulum labiorum or fourchette. They have no hair, are well supplied with sebaceous and sweat glands.

The Vestibule: is the smooth, almond-shaped area bounded by the labia minor on the both side. At its apex is the clitoris, and in the center it is perforated by the urethra and the vagina. The vestibular fossa is the portion of vestibule behind the vaginal orifice and in front of the frenulum labiorum.

The Clitoris: is the homologue of the penis in the male. The small glans is rich in nerve endings, and is exquisitely sensitive. The whole organ is highly erectile, and is regarded as seat of the voluptuous sensations experienced by the female during coitus.

Vaginal Orifice: This lies just behind the orifice of the urethra. Behind and at the sides it is usually bounded by the hymen. In the virgin it is more or less closed by the hymen, and is completely hidden by the labia minora. In parous women the hymen is absent, and the orifice is frequently exposed by the gaping of the labia.

Hymen: This is a crescentic or circular fold of connective tissue covered with skin – like that of the vagina. It closes in the orifice of the vagina in the virgin, leaving an aperture varying in size, but usually large enough to admit one finger. The hymen is usually ruptured at the first coitus, when there may be slight bleeding. At the first labor it is almost invariably completely torn up.

The Vagina: The vagina is the canal, which unites the uterus and the vulva. Its direction is approximately parallel to the plane of the pelvic brim. It has a faint sigmoid curve, its lower and the upper portions being directed more directly upwards and the middle portion more backwards. It joins the uterus at an angle, which is nearly a right angle. The anterior and posterior walls are in contact so that on section it forms a transverse slit in the pelvic diaphragm. From below upward it is in relation anteriorly to the urethra and the base of the bladder; posterioly to the perineal body, the rectum and the recto-uterine peritoneal pouch. It is wider above than below. The vagina has four coats as below:

1. The cavity is lined by a modified skin covered with stratified epithelium.
2. Below the epithelial layer is another layer of connective tissue, which passes towards the surface in the form of papillae, just as in the subcuticular layer of the skin.
3. Next comes the muscular layer, with its subdivision into an inner circular and outer longitudinal layer.

4. The outermost coat is the connective tissue sheath, which contains a large plexus of veins and very free blood supply.

Abnormalities of the cervix and vagina: Cervical abnormalities are diagnosed clinically. Retention cysts of the cervix varying in size from a few millimeters to 4 cm., single or multiple are commonly diagnosed during routine sonography. Multiple cysts may be a cause of benign enlargement of the cervix. Cervical carcinoma is usually diagnosed clinically. The vagina, having four inches length runs anteriorly and caudally from the cervix between the bladder and rectum. Garner's duct cysts most common cystic lesions of the vagina are mesonephric duct remnants that form single or multiple cysts along the lateral wall of the vagina. Solid masses of the vagina are rare but common congenital abnormalities of the female genitract. As in carcinoma of cervix, sonography is not used for diagnosis of the caranoma of the vagina.

The Penis: Penis is the male genital organ that serves a dual function of erection and as a route of excretion of urine and semen.

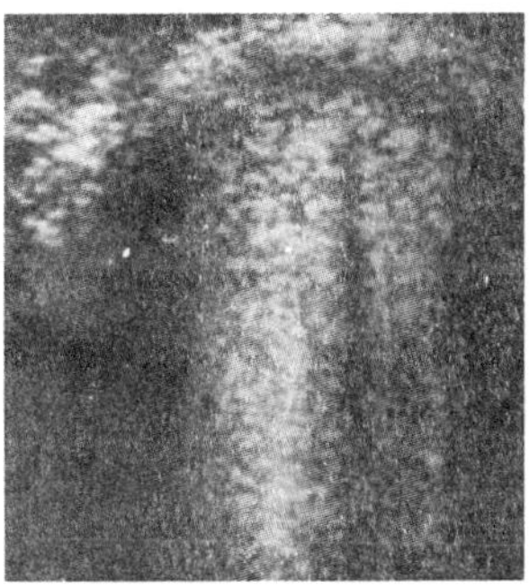

Sonogram of Penis

It is composed of three cylindric structures of cavernous – the two corpora cavernosa are the main erectile structures. The blood supply to the penis is primarily via the right and left internal pudendal arteries, which enter the base of the penis (as shown in the illustration) primarily supply of blood to the skin and glans of the penis. Until recently, it was felt that psychologic factor accounted for most cases are cause of impotence. However, studies using nocturnal penile tumescence have revealed that a majority of the cases of impotence have organic causes. Subsequent studies have shown that vasculogenic impotence is one of the most frequent causes for erectile failure. Vasculogenic impotence may be due to poor arterial inflow into the penis (arteriogenic impoptence) or excessive venous leakage of blood from penis (venogenic impotence) or both. The frequency of various causes of the impotence are:

Vasculogenic	**37.5%**
Diabetes mellitus	**20%**
Psychogenic	**11.7%**
Neurogenic	**6.7%**
Malegnancy	**5.8%**
Testoterone and Trauma	**3.3%**
Other causes	**11.7%**

Ovary: Ovary having 1.5 inch length, 0.75 inch breadth and thickness resembles the egg of a pigeon in appearance are almond-shaped flattened bodies, connected with the base of the uterus by

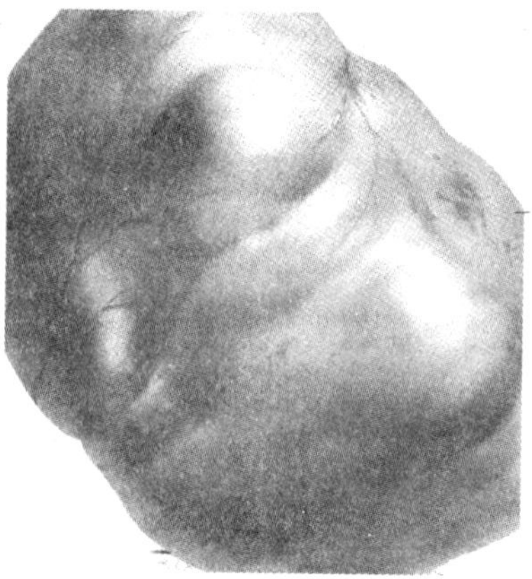

Ovary cyst

means of ligament tightly attached to the fallopian tubes. Polycystic ovary disease is a complex endocrine disturbance resulting from chronic anovulation. The most common symptoms are amenorrhea, hirsutism (accumulation of excess superfluous hair on the body), obesity and infertility. Polycystic ovarian diseases, Functional cysts, Follicular cyst, Corpus-luted cyst, Theca-luteal cysts, Ovarian Remnant Syndrome (causing pelvic inflammatory disease or tumor), Parovarian cysts, Post menopausal Adnexal cysts, Endometriosis (presence of functioning endometrial tissue outside the uterus), Torsion of the ovary associated with cysts or tumors and ovary cancer.

Epithelial tumors are harmful Nonneoplastic lesions, which need immediate treatment. Pelvic inflammatory disease is a common condition that is increasing in frequency. It is usually bilateral and caused by sexually transmitted diseases with the patient presenting with pain, fever and vaginal discharge. Method of ultrasound transvesical retrieval with laproscopy is a popular method to detect ovarian disorders.

Abdomen and Liver: Abdomen is the seat of the functioning of all body organs. The liver is the largest organ in the human body weighing approximately 1500 gm. in the adult. The liver lies in the right upper quardrant of the abdomen, suspended from the right hemidiaphragm. It can be divided into three lobes-the right, left and candate lobes. The right lobe of the liver is separated from left by the main lobar fissure. The left intersegmental fissure divides the left lobe into medical and lateral segments. The candate lobe is situated on the posterior aspect of the liver. Your liver has many important functions to perform, for it is great chemical laboratory of your body. The liver can be affected by a number of serious disorders such as virus infections, parasites, disturbance of the circulation, stone formation in the bile duct, injuries due to poisonous substance and various kinds of tumors. Most of the foods we eat are stored in the liver; after having been digested and absorbed from the gastro-intestinal tract.

A vast network of tiny blood vessels arises from stomach, small bowel and spleen which in turn flows into the liver. Food materials from the digestive tract are able to reach the liver cells, where they are chemically changed and stored. These energy foods and vitamins stored in the liver are stock piled, which are needed by muscles, bones, nerve and other tissues. The various abnormalities of liver are liver cyst, jaundice, hepatitis, infections, serum, toxic, fatty liver, cirrhosis of the liver and cancer of the liver. Jaundice is a disease marred by a yellow discoloration in the skin or in the whitest of the eyes. To treat jaundice, one must first find the cause of the jaundice. If the trouble is due to some parasite such as malaria parasite, proper medication may bring the condition under control. If the jaundice is due to presence of a stone or other obstruction, surgery will be needed for relief and cure. Hepatitis is an acute inflammation of liner caused by infectious or tonic agent. The skin may be discolored and the whites of the eye turn yellow. Various substances and organisms may be responsible for hepatitis, including germs, viruses, toxic agents and many other substances. Infectious hepatitis often occurs in the epidemis due to certain viruses spread mainly by contaminated food or water. Fatty liver is due to excessive amount of fat being deposited in the liver cells, which occur most frequently in overweight persons or due to excessive intake of food, particularly fat. Cancer may arise in almost any organ of the body. When it begins in stomach or large bowel, the liver may soon be involved.

The Gall Bladder and Pancreatitis: The Gall Bladder is a small, pear-shaped, muscular organ closely attached to the under surface of the liver. The size and shape of normal gall-bladder (usually its transverse diameter exceeds 5 cm. vary widely in individual patients. The disorders of gall bladder include signs and symptoms of acute or chronic cholecystitis and jaundice. Cancer sometimes occurs in gall bladder. In as much as a person can live quite well without the gall bladder, it is wise to have diseased organ removed to avoid the risk of serious complications. Pancreas is an important gland situated below the liver, which produces strong digestive juices necessary for assimilation of food. Pancreatitis means inflammation of the organs – which may be mild or very severe. The treatments vary according to the seriousness of the condition. Avoid taking alcohol in any form, for this may only aggravate the condition. Avoid stress as far as possible.

The Urinary Tract: The human body is a living engine, which burns fuel – the food, and requires a constant supply of oxygen as

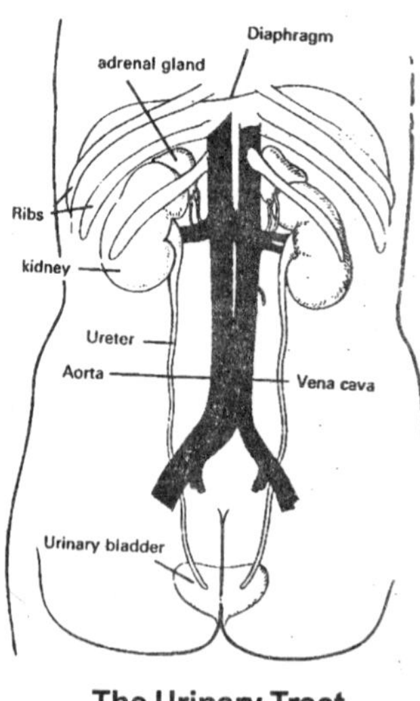

The Urinary Tract

well as water and various chemical substances, which provide energy to the organs of the body. For repairing the damaged tissues constantly, keeping check on all these living cells and chemicals there are two remarkable organs – Kidneys.

Normally, the body filters about 300 liters of fluid each day leaving approximately one liter of urine to be excreted from the body. As the urine flows down the tiny tubules towards the center of kidney, it is finally collected in the renal pelvis, from there it finds its way down through the uterus to the bladder, where it remains until it is eliminated from the body. The common disorders of the urinary tract are kidney stones, polycystic disease (which begins before birth), Bright's disease (Nephritis), cancer of the urinary tract, hydronephrosis, kidney infection, prostate gland, tuberculosis of kidney, urethritis (inflammation) and uraemia (toxic condition associated with kidney failure).

6
Pregnancy and Childbirth

Duration of Pregnancy: When a woman becomes pregnant the period between the beginning of her last menstruation and the birth of the child is approximately 280 days. This is the 'menstruation-delivery interval' and upon it is based the usual method of calculating the probable date of confinement. But it does not represent the actual duration of pregnancy. Pregnancy begins at the moment of conception when the ovum is fertilized by spermatozoon and we have no means of knowing exactly when that occurs, so we have no precise knowledge of the actual duration of pregnancy.

How to calculate probable date of confinement?: The nearest approach to an accurate estimate of the probable date of confinement in women who have been menstruating normally is the method of counting 280 days from the beginning of the last menstrual period. The first day of the last period is taken because it is usually the date best remembered by the patient. The actual date, 280 days on, is estimated roughly by adding seven days and counting forwards nine calendar months. For example, supposing a woman began her last menstrual period on 3rd of September, add to that seven days and count forwards nine months .The date of probable confinement would be the 10th of June.

There is another method of calculation for estimating the date of confinement. It has been suggested that the duration of pregnancy coincides with the length of ten menstrual cycles, but the evidence is inconclusive, and the calculations of the date of confinement on such a basis are not more accurate than those reached by the ordinary methods.

Causes of the Onset of labor: Why labor should be in the great majority of cases after the lapse of forty two weeks of gestation is a question which is still unanswered. Following are some of the important views in this regard:

1. The heightened reflex irritability of the uterus during pregnancy. This grows progressively greater as pregnancy advances. It was assumed that ultimately the irritability, which is shown by increasing frequency and strength of the intermittent contractions, led to the strong contractions characteristic of labor.
2. The distension of the uterus at term may be enough to determine reflexly the onset of the labor pains. Cases in which the uterus is unduly enlarged tend to premature labor, as in case of twin pregnancy or excess of liquor amnii (hydramnios)
3. References have been made to the fact that the irritability of the uterus is greatest at the time, which correspond to the suppressed menstrual periods.
4. It has been observed that possibly the prolonged pressure of the fetus may eventuate in the dilatation of the cervix. However, sometimes the cervix is partially open for sometime before labor begins.
5. Children born at the 40th week of gestation have the best chances of survival.

Physical Examination: The doctor often asks certain questions regarding the previous pregnancy such as difficulty in previous delivery, abortions or miscarriages (if any) in past, the birth of premature or

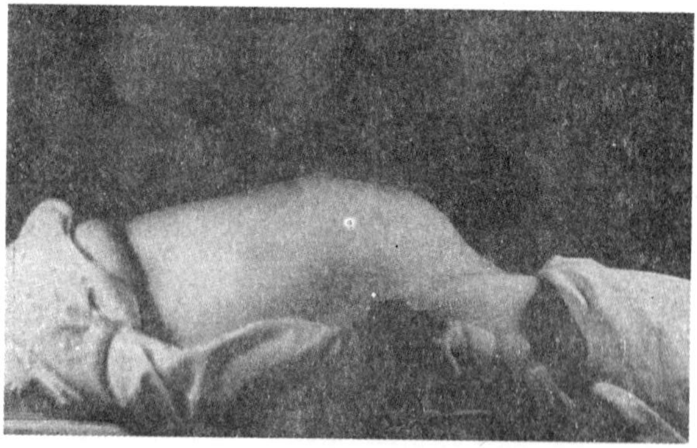

Physical Examination of Pregnant

macerated fetuses or death of children occurring in early infancy (if any), the blood of both parents should be examined and the patient should be questioned about her present health, existence of cardiac or pulmonary disease or toxaemia, for example breathlessness, palpitation, cough, excessive vomiting, persistent headaches, swelling of the hands or face, diminished amount of urine, dimness of vision, condition of the bowels, the presence of vaginal discharges and their nature, swelling of the feet or legs, presence of haemorrhoids or varicose veins etc. should be enquired into.

After preliminary questioning is finished, the patient is asked to undress and lie upon an examination couch. Firstly, a general survey of circulatory, respiratory and digestive system is made. See that the doctor inspects the breast noting their development, the condition of nipples, areola (the darkish part around nipples) and the presence and the amount of secretion from them (if any). The mouth should always be examined for septic teeth, gums and tonsils. The blood pressure should then be estimated by sphygmomano meter. It is important to test the blood group of expectant mother for the investigation of the:

1. Haemoglobin
2. Rh group
3. Blood group
4. Wassermann reaction.

The patient's height is recorded and it may be worthwhile to mention that women of short stature (five feet or below) are more likely to have small pelvis than taller women. The patient's weight is noted and a check on weight gain is made during the pregnancy.

Abdominal Examination: In early pregnancy, note the size of uterus and exclude any morbid abdominal conditions. Prior to the 26th week of pregnancy abdominal diagnosis of presentation and position is often inaccurate. The level of the fundus, the presence of uterine soufflé, hearing the heart-beat should be examined. At the 38th week, a final review is carried out and relationship of the fetal head to the maternal pelvis determined. A study is be made to determine the size of the head related to the pelvis brim. It is important that in a primigravida, the head should normally become engaged in the pelvis during the last two or three weeks. It may be still movable during the last fortnight of pregnancy due to pelvic contraction, an abnormally large head, a posterior position of the occiput, placenta praevia, a pelvic tumor or simply due to faecal accumulation in the pelvic colon and rectum. **A thorough examination of abdominal region should be conducted by the doctor to find out if the head is able to enter the pelvis.**

Pelvic Examination: The objects are twofold- to investigate the condition of the pelvic organs and to estimate the size and shape of the pelvic canal. **It is necessary to measure the pelvis by your doctor by means of a bimanual examination (as shown in the illustration).** The diagnosis of pregnancy is confirmed and the presence or absence of pelvic swellings such as uterine fibroids or ovarian cysts can be determined. If the fundus of the uterus can be palpated abdominally there is no need to carry out the pelvic examination at the first visit and can be postponed until need arises.

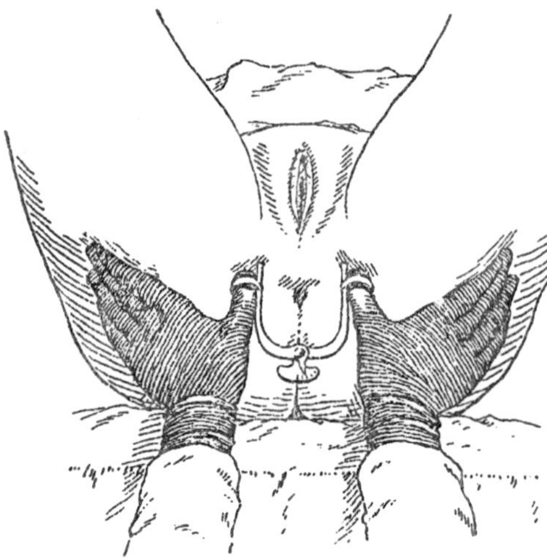

Pelvic Examination

There are three methods of pelvic examination as below :

1. External Examination: **The measurements are made with a pair of calipers (as shown in illustration)** to find out any deformity to be recognized at once.
2. Internal Examination: Interspinous diameter is measured with calipers. The two, anterior-superior spines are located, where the points of caliper are placed on their outer lips and the measurement read off. Normally, it is 9-1/2 to 10 inches (24 – 25 cm.). The Intercristal diameter is also measured at the points

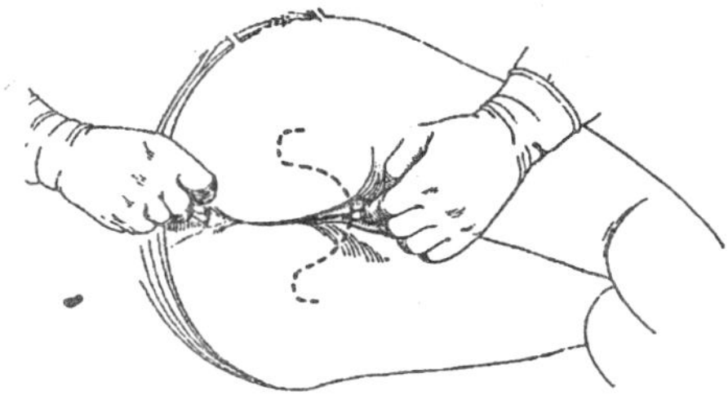

Position 1

Position 2

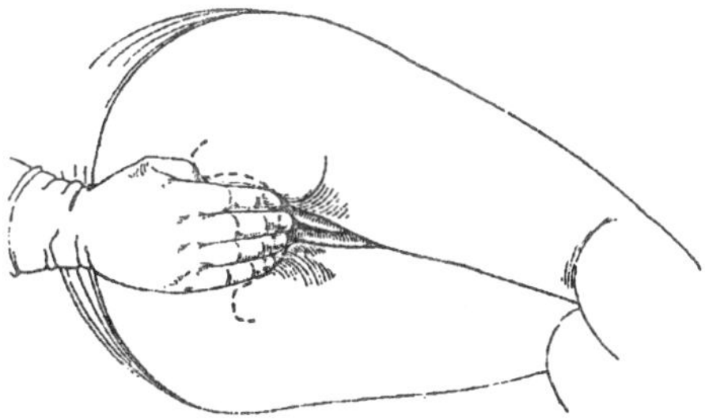

Position 3

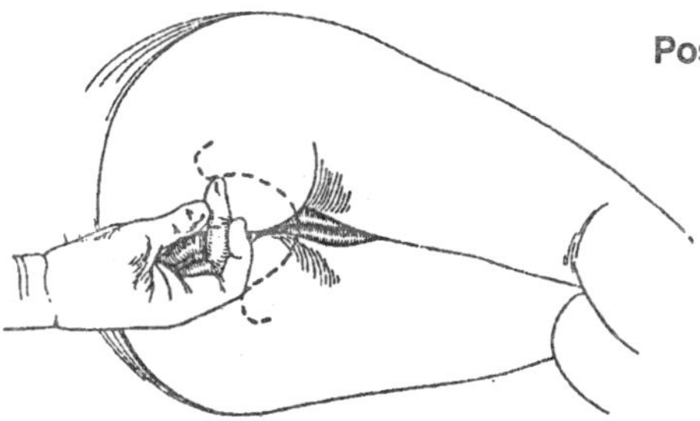

Measuring Pubic Area

passed slowly round the iliac cresta until the points of greatest separation are found when the measurement is read Normally, it is 10-1/2 to 11 inches (26-27 cm.).

3. By X-rays: The size of the pelvis and the fetal head can be assessed by X-ray.

This process is known as Radiographic Pelvimetry.

The illustration 1 shows how to measure transverse diameter of the outlet by measuring the anterior-posterior diameter of the outlet with the pelvimeter. The illustrations 1 and 3, show measuring the sub-pubic arch and anterior segment of the outlet by simple methods of estimating the

shape and the capacity of the sub pubic arch and the transverse diameter of the outlet.

Blood Pressure: The blood pressure of the patient should be ascertained at each antenatal visit. During pregnancy the blood pressure should not rise above 140/90. If after a suitable period of rest, the pressure remains above this figure, then hypertension is said to exist. During the middle trimester of pregnancy the blood pressure is often low and the reading of 110/70 may be recorded. This physiological drop is of great interest and is called the 'mid pregnancy drop' in blood pressure.

Urine and Hemoglobin: Usually, the patient is asked to pass urine before she undresses for the physical examination. Examination of urine is most important throughout pregnancy. The possible presence of albumin is most important point to attend to, besides checking the presence of sugar, pus and other abnormalities. Urine should be examined once a month in the first six months, thereafter more frequently as pregnancy advances. If the albumin is present in the urine along with a vaginal discharge, a mid-stream specimen of urine should be obtained and a doctor should be consulted.

The hemoglobin should be checked throughout pregnancy. It should be estimated as routine in all pregnant women at the 30th week. If you are suffering from anemia, there is plenty of time to correct this. All Rh negative patients have their blood examined for the presence of antibodies at regular intervals.

Weight: Be carefully when the weight increases during pregnancy, since fluid retention in the tissues along with the increase in weight, is the earliest signs of toxaemia. In normal pregnancy, the increase in weight begins with the 4th month and continues at an average rate of about 2 kg per month till about the 39th week, the total weight being about 12 kg. Any abnormal gain in weight should determine a careful investigation.

The Last Four Months of Pregnancy: Special attention should always be paid to the following examinations every month:

1. Urine
2. Blood Pressure
3. Checking the position of fetus
4. Fetal heart-sounds (regularly in last six weeks)

5. Checking the relative sizes of head and pelvis (regularly in last four weeks)
6. The mobility or engagement of the head.

Exercise, Rest, Sleep and Diet: Labor is a great muscular feat and must be prepared for by adequate exercise (with the consultation of your doctor). Avoid long journeys during the last trimester of pregnancy. An afternoon rest should be taken daily. It is essential during the later months-either in bed or a couch with the feet up and all clothing loosened. At least eight hours sleep should be obtained every night. Women engaged in an industry or at a place where labor work is involved should cease such work for at least eleven weeks before labor is due.

In case of healthy women no special diet is necessary, but the food must be adequate in quantity and simple and nutritious in quality. Overfeeding should be discouraged. Reduce intake of salt after mid-pregnancy. 100 gm of protein are required daily and of this 50 gm should be absorbed through milk, eggs and lean meat. All good mixed diets contain enough carbohydrate and fat. Fresh fruits and green vegetables should be taken in plenty. Drink at least 6 to 8 glasses of water daily. Constipation must be strictly avoided. A daily motion should be secured.

Clothing: It should be the aim in regard to clothing during pregnancy to avoid any pressure on the breasts, and any constriction at the waist or round the lower limbs. High heel shoes should be replaced with those with low or medium heels in the later months.

The Fetus

The child in womb becomes theoretically capable of living a separate individual existence about the 28th week of pregnancy. It is important to know the age of a fetus or embryo both for clinical and medico reasons.

- At the end of 4th week: The embryo is much curved, head and tail being close together. It measures from 2.5 to 4 mm. The brain and cord are enclosed, eye and ear vesicles are visible. The heart is prominent and is beginning to divide in four chambers.
- At he end of 8th week: The embryo is about an inch (25 mm.) long in measurement. The head has a human shape, whereas

the tail has nearly disappeared. The hands and feet begin to appear. Eyes, nose and ears are recognizable. The external genitals are visible, but sex is not distinguishable. The embryo now becomes the fetus.

- At the end of 12th week: The fetus is about 3-1/2 to 4 inches long weighing about 50 gm. The intestines are enclosed in the abdomen and umbilical cord is beginning to show spiral turns. Sex can be determined by the presence or absence of the uterus. Most of the bones begin to emerge.
- At the end of 16th week: The fetus is about six inches (15 cm.) long and weighs about 190 gm. Sex is clearly defined at this stage. The fine downy hair starts appearing on the skin.
- At the end of 20th week: The fetus is about 7 to 8 inches (18-20 cm.) long and weigh about 450 gm. The head is still relatively large. The cord is about 12 inches long.
- At the end of 24th week: The fetus is about 9 inches (23 cm.) long and weighs about 930 gm. Fat begins to deposit under the skin. Hair appears on the head.
- At the end of 28th week: The fetus is about eleven inches (28 cm.) long weighing about 1300 gm. The eyelids are now open and the papillary membrane starts disappearing. The body is now covered with fine hair (lanugo). The intestines contain a dark green tarry matter known as meconium. A child born at this time very seldom survives.
- At the end of 32nd week: The fetus is nearly 12 inches long weighing about 2075 gm. The hair on the scalp is thicker.
- At the end of 36th week: The length of fetus is nearly 14 inches weighing about 2500 gm. The subcutaneous fat increases, the face is less wrinkled and the body more round. A child born at this time has a very fair chance of survival.
- At the 40th week: The total length reaches 20 inches weighing about 3200 gm. The fingers have complete nail, the skin is pink and smooth. The diameter of the head becomes normal. In the male the testicles are in the scrotum.

Position of the fetus: The position of fetus is in its relation to the pelvis of the mother. There are four commonest positions of a vertex presentation as follows:

1. Left occipito-anterior (L.O.A.)

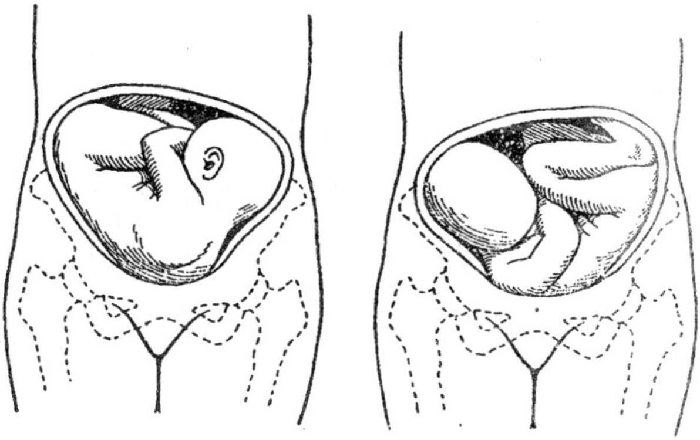

Position of Fetus in Relation to Pelvis

2. Right occipito-anterior (R.O.A.)
3. Right occipito-posterior (R.O.P.)
4. Left occipito-posterior (L.O.P.)

Diagnosis of Presentation and Position of the abdominal examination: The patient should lie on her back, the shoulders slightly raised and the knees drawn up to relax abdominal muscles. The clothes must be so arranged as to allow free exposure of the abdomen. Abdominal palpation is carried in four steps.

Sketch 1

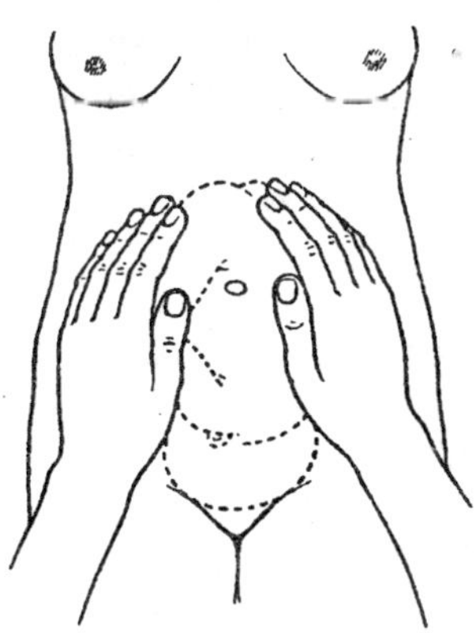

Sketch 2

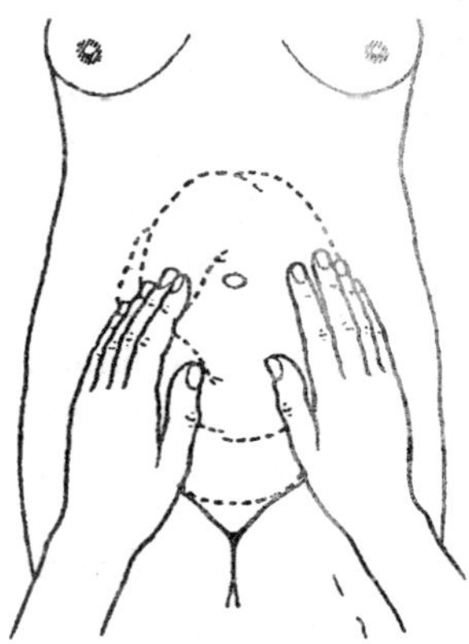

Position 1

Sketch 3

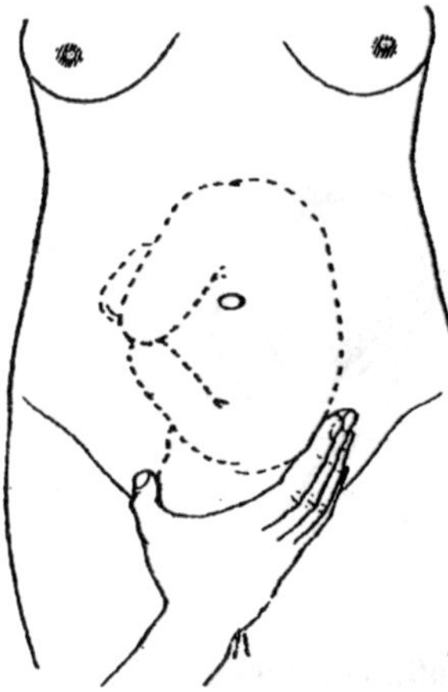

Sketch 4

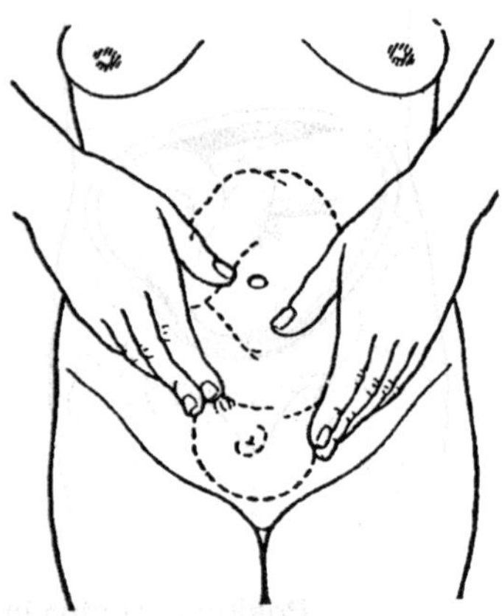

Position 2

Abdominal Examination

1. First Step: Palpate the fundus with both hands **as shown in Sketch 1**.
2. Second Step: Palpate with both hands on sides **as shown in Sketch 2**.
3. Third Step: Slip the hands down and palpate the sides of uterus **as shown in Sketch 3**.
4. Palpate the lower pole of the uterus **as shown in Sketch 4**

Vaginal Examination: Where necessary, this must be done as seldom as possible to avoid risk of a septic. The strict precautions should be observed in making vaginal examination, especially in the last days of pregnancy or in labor. The patient's external genitals should be carefully prepared and washed. The labia are then separated and examining fingers are passed into the vagina without coming into contact with them.

Radiological Examination: In cases in which obesity or undue rigidity makes abdominal examination difficult or unsatisfactory, examination by X-rays is most helpful.

The Clinical Course of Normal Labor

Labor is the process by which the products of conception, such as the fetus, liquor amnii, placenta, and membranes are separated and expelled from the uterus. There ate two groups as below into which all labors may be divided:

1. Eutocia: normal or physiological labor, in which here is no complication and the delivery is completed within 24 hours by natural unaided efforts of the mother.
2. Dystocia: abnormal or pathological labor. In this case two or three weeks before the onset of labor the patient experiences a feeling of 'lightening'. The uterus sinks lower in the abdomen with the result that the waist becomes lowered. During the last few days there is a marked increase in the secretions of the genital tract and the vulva becomes moist and succulent.

Three Stages of Labor

Labor is divided into three stages as described below. The first stage lasts about 12-15 hours, the second stage about two hours and the third stage takes 20 minutes to half an hour. In the patients belonging to working class, the average time is considerably shorter. The first stage occupies 8-10 hours, the second stage one hour or less and the third stage 20 minutes to half an hour. These are average figures and labor class women usually complete their labor in a much shorter time.

Stage of Dilation (The First Stage of Labor): which extends from the onset of true pains to the full dilation of the cervix. The occurrence includes periodic pain due to contraction of the uterus and therefore synchronous with a hardening of that organ, which can be felt by hands are placed on abdomen. There is continuous discharge from vagina (Cervical mucosa), also known as 'show'. As the pain becomes more frequent and severe, the patient begins to cry out and feels relief by sitting bent forward. A gentle massage on the back from shoulder to lower back is also helpful for the patient to relieve tension. It takes 12 to 15 hours to complete the first stage. At the end of it there is usually a sudden gush of fluid indicating that the fetal membrane have ruptured.

Stage of Expulsion (The Second Stage of Labor): This is a stage of expulsion and extends from the complete dilation of the cervix to the expulsion of the child. The pains often stop for few minutes after the rupture, and then begin again with greater frequency. These gradually become more expulsive or 'down bearing' in character. The patient usually braces herself by holding on to some solid object or pressing her feet against the foot of the bed. The

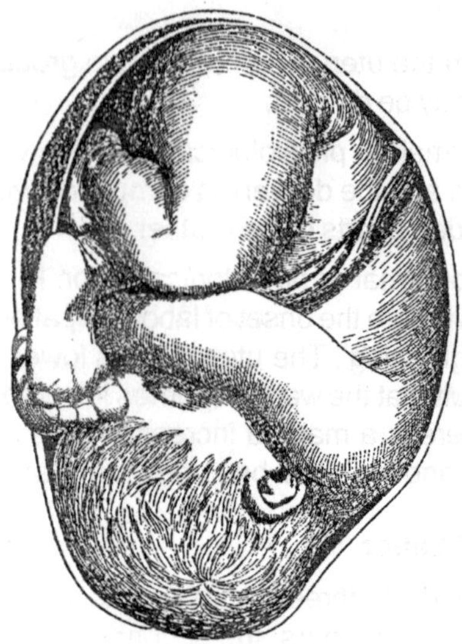

Normal Fetus

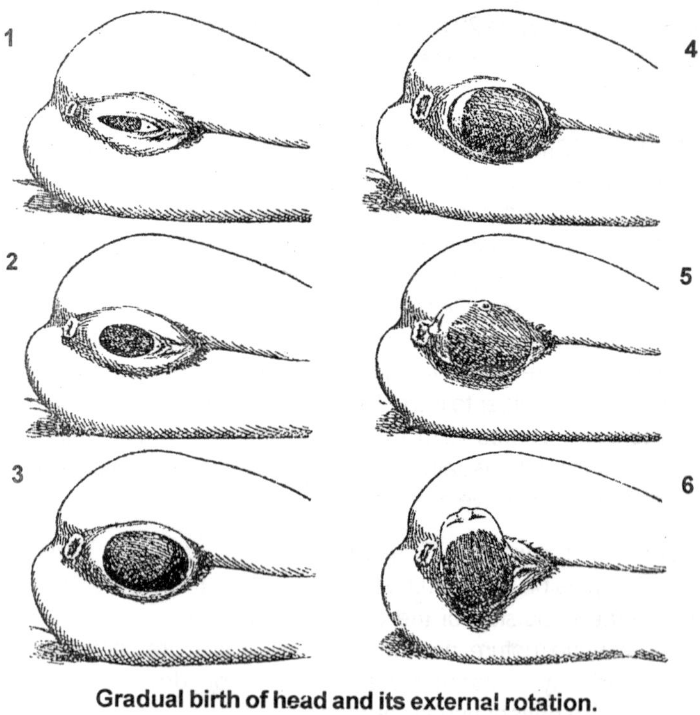

Gradual birth of head and its external rotation.

diaphragm is thus fixed and the intra-abdominal pressure brought to bear on the expulsion of the child. The patient perspires freely. The effect of these pains is to drive the head through the cavity of the pelvis. It presses upon the rectum and on the perineum, which begins to bulge a little during the pains. The vulva also begins to gape more. Gradually, the pains become longer and more frequent, the head recedes a little, but with each succeeding pain it is driven a little farther down. The perineum bulges more and more, the vulva too gapes more and more and the scalp of the baby is seen when the head is forced down during a pain. Larger and larger area of the head comes to lie in the vulva opening during successive pains. The opening becomes transformed from a slightly gaping slit to an oval and ultimately an almost circular opening. The perineum meantime has been so pressed that it becomes stretched out and thinned. Gradual birth of head and its external rotation have been shown in the sketches.

After the head is born, there is a short pause during which the face of the child becomes congested. After the head, the shoulders, followed by the trunk and lower limbs are pushed out, and then comes a gush of the remainder of the liquor amnii. After the end of the second stage the retracted uterus may be felt as a firm tumor extending up to just below the umbilicus.

Stage of Delivery (The Third Stage of Labor): This is stage of delivery of child and extends from the birth of the child to the birth of the placenta. There is usually a short cessation of pains with a corresponding relief to the patient. Ultimately, the uterus begins to contract again, and may be felt by the hand to grow more hard and solid. Sometimes, there are little gushes of blood during the pains, indicating the separation of the placenta. Many times there is no bleeding. In the end, the placenta is expelled by a strong pain into the vagina. The third stage may take a few minutes to an hour or even more. The average time is about 20 minutes.

Separation of Placenta: The resumption of pains after the birth of child indicates still further contraction and retraction of the upper segment. This brings about such a disproportion between the placental site and the placenta when the attachment between the two are torn through. The placental site may be reduced in area 4-1/2 by 4 inches (11 by 10 cm.) without separation taking place. There are two methods of expulsion of placenta:

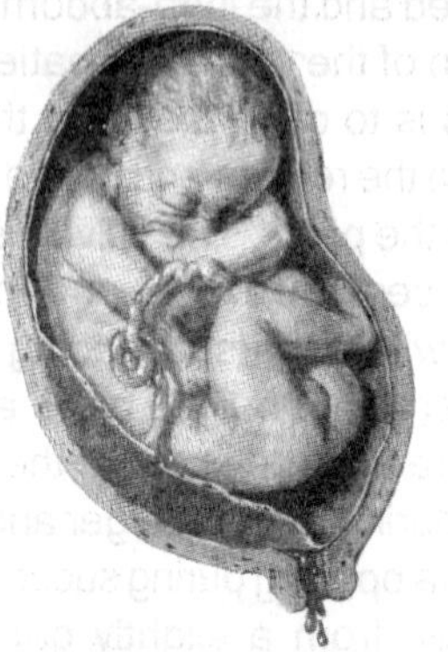

Partial placenta pervia

Schultze's Method: In which the placenta is expelled like an inverted umbrella when the fetal surface comes first and the membrane trailing behind)

Dubcan's Mechanism: Its also known as Matthews Duncan. The lower edge of the placenta is first extruded, and the whole organ slides down folded longitudinally upon itself. This method is more common.

Control of Hemorrhage: As the placenta is separated from the wall of the uterus, the blood vessels passing from the one to the other are torn across, and many of the large sinuses in the uterine wall thus laid open. Bleeding is, however, prevented by the retraction of the uterus, which causes the separation. If owing to exhaustion of the uterus, retraction fails to occur after the separation of the placenta, then free and alarming bleeding may take place – post partum hemorrhage.

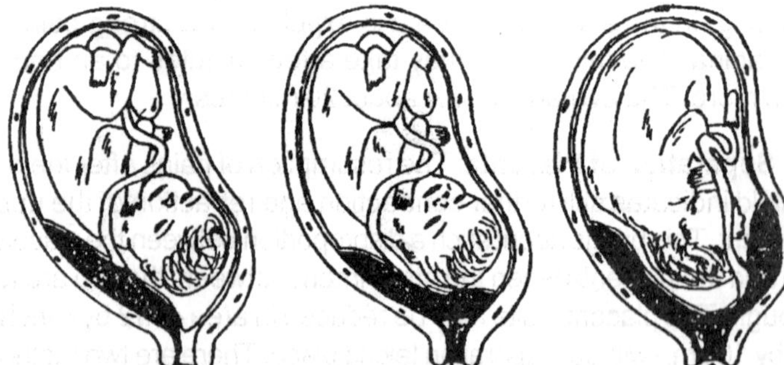

Position 1 Position 2 Position 3

Hemorrhage

Vaginal secretion: The vaginal secretion in a healthy pregnancy differs only in its increased quantity from that of a healthy non-pregnant woman. It is whitish in color, containing epithelial cells, leucocytes and mucus. It also contains numerous large 'vaginal bacilli'. It has been observed that the acidity of the vaginal secretion is inimical to the life of other organism than the 'vaginal bacillus', followed by the appearance of organism in the vagina. Thus during the puerperium the lochia (discharge from the uterus after labor) is alkaline, which contain many organisms, mostly saprophytic are found.

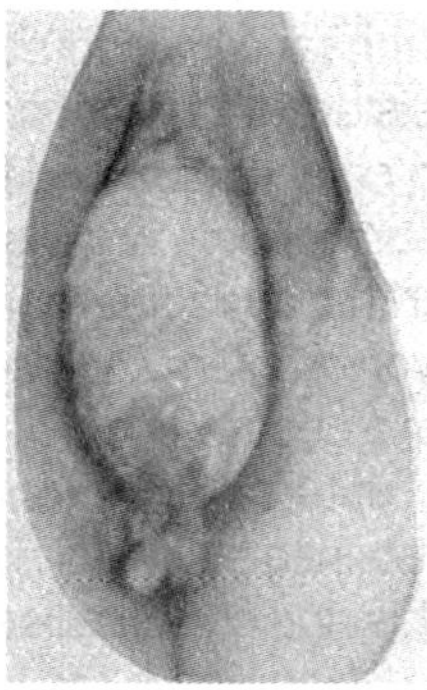

Method of cleaning genitals after labor: Nature follows the principles of antisepsis in labor. The birth canal can be divided into three parts:

1. The vulva, including the entrance to vagina. This area swarms with organism of various sorts. It may therefore be designated the Septic Tract.
2. The vagina, containing the vaginal bacilli with their acid secretion, a few fungi, and some leucocytes. This is Antiseptic Tract.
3. The cavity of the uterus, separated by the plug of mucus from the vagina, is entirely devoid of any form of organism. It is therefore the Aseptic Tract.

Cleansing of vulva: Wherever possible the patient should have a complete bath at the very commencement of labor, and the nurse should see that the rectum and bladder are emptied. It is usually suggested that the patient should be given an enema in every case, irrespective of whether the bowels have acted naturally or not, unless the patient is in strong labor when the nurse arrives. The nurse should then pay special attention to the genitals. The hair should be shaved.

Before a vaginal examination is made the vulva is swabbed with a antiseptic solution. The labia minora must be separated and wiped with pledgets of wool soaked in an antiseptic solution. The pledget must always be drawn from being backwards to prevent carrying forward any septic matter from near the anus. Pledget must not be used for more than one wipe.

Puerperal Infection: The term puerperal infection can be used to describe any infection during or after labor. It generally applies to infection of the uterus and surrounding tissues after delivery. This can vary from mild to life threatening in severity. Some of the most severe infections may appear within hours of the delivery. Vigilance and aggressive diagnosis and treatment are required. The puerperal infection causes due to colonization and infection of the tissues of uterus, peritoneum or surrounding organs. Abscesses thus formed usually contain both aerobic and anaerobic bacteria. Nearly 50% of the uterine infections involve Chlamydia trachomatis. The risk factors of this infection includes a cesarean delivery, unhygienic procedure during labor, prolonged rupture of the membranes, prolonged labor, multiple examinations, retained placental fragments, urinary catheter, low socioeconomic status and chronic diseases including diabetes.

The signs and symptoms of the infection are fever and tachycardia often developing rapidly after delivery, uterine tenderness, signs of septic or cardiovascular shock, hypertension, anxiety, disorientation, prostration, impaired renal function, hemolysis or hemoconcentration. The infection can be diagnosed by the following:

1. Urinary tract infection (including Pyelonephritis).
2. Wound infection.
3. Infection in intravenous line (due to contaminated fluids).
4. Disturbed abscess.
5. Septic thrombophlebitis.
6. Necrotizing fascitis.
7. Transfusion reaction.
8. Amniotic fluid or pulmonary embolism.
9. Cardiogenic shock.
10. Toxic shock syndrome.
11. Mastitis.
12. Afelectasis.

Possible associated conditions include septic shock, adult respiratory distress syndrome, acute renal failure and disseminated intra-vascular coagulation.

Vaginal Examination: The use of abdominal palpation instead of this method of examination in normal cases has already been recommended. Where a vaginal examination is necessary it must be done with scrupulous care. The patient should be on her back rather than on her side, so as to diminish the risk of the hand coming into contact with the anus. Cleanse the hands and vulva before conducting the examination. The labia minora are held apart by the fingers of the left hand, and the fingers of right hand introduced without coming into contact with the vulva at all, or at least only the inner surfaces of the labia minora which have also been cleansed.

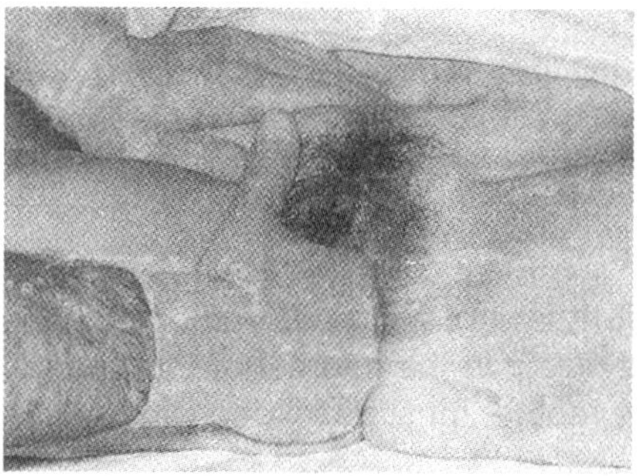

In case, the patient is passing through the stage of labor, it is well to introduce the fingers into the vagina during a pain and prolong the examination until it has passed off, so that one can learn the state of matters both during and between pains. Ascertain the following points:

1. State of labor; how far advanced it is?
2. Presentation and position?
3. Are the membranes ruptured? If not, be careful not to rupture the same.
4. State of vagina and perineum as to distensibility or rigidity, moistness or dryness.
5. Is pelvis normal?
6. Is cord prolapsed?

Symphysiotomy

Symphysiotomy is an operation, which is rarely performed nowadays owing to improved results of caesarean section. The object of this operation is to enlarge the pelvic capacity during labor by dividing the ligaments of the symphasis pubis. This division is followed by a separation of pubis bones because the weight of the limbs rotate the hip bones outwards and downwards. The result of the movement is to provide an immediate increase in the dimensions of the pelvis. The following conditions are necessary for conducting an operation:

1. The child in the uterus must be alive.
2. The disproportion between the head and pelvis must not be too large.
3. The soft passages must be well dilated or readily dilatable. The operation is followed by extraction of the child and therefore should not be performed unless the cervix is fully open, and vaginal canal and vulva both are large enough to allow rapid extraction.
4. The canal must not be grossly infected. The operation is performed solely in the interest of the unborn child, and all risks to the mother must be fully considered.

A strict aseptic and antiseptic technique is essential while conducting surgery. The anaesthetized patient is placed in the lithotomy position. Ensure that the ends of pubic bone do not spring apart too far when the joint is cut open. Hemorrhage may be an alarming factor during surgery, usually due to torn veins in the region of the neck of the bladder so every care should be taken to minimize injury to the bladder and urethra. About ten days rest is required by the patient after symphysiotomy operation.

Episiotomy: This means the deliberate incision of the perineum in order tp prevent excessive stretching of the pelvic floor or to avoid an extensive tear where this appears inevitable. Episiotomy is best performed when the perineum is bulging and about 4-5 cm. of scalp is showing. If it is performed too early there may be excessive bleeding and in case of too late damage may have already been sustained by the pelvic floor. Local anesthesia is employed, in which two fingers are inserted into the vagina and with a pair of blunt-pointed scissors an incision is made from the mid point of perineum in a post-lateral direction. The length of the depth of incision must be such that it doesn't hurt the head. The vaginal edges are united with chromic catgut interrupted stitches. The sutures should be tied very gently on this delicate area. Occasionally, due to infection, the whole wound breaks down and requires secondary suture after healthy granulation tissue has been established. The following illustrations should be referred for symphysiotomy-episiotomy operation and application of local anesthesia.

Illustration 1: Position ready for the surgery.

Illustration 2: Introducing the local anesthetic.

Illustration 3: Pudendal nerve block.

Illustration 4: Cutting the perineum.

Illustration 5: Stitching the deeper tissues.

Illustration 6: Episiotomy completed.

Position 1

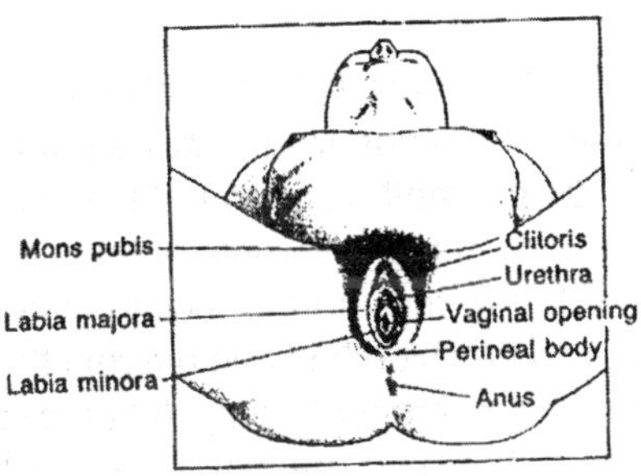

Position 2

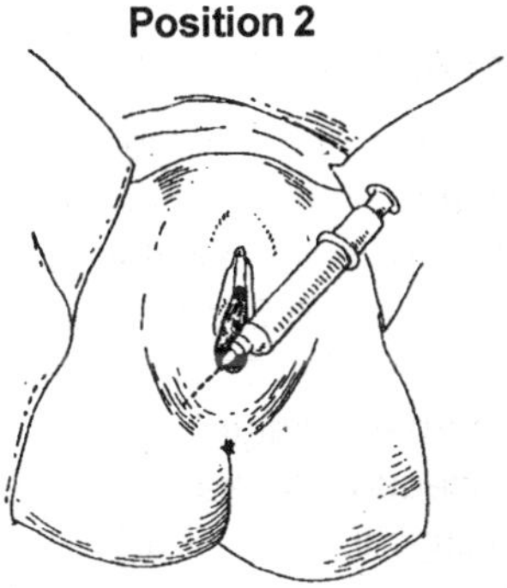

Position 3

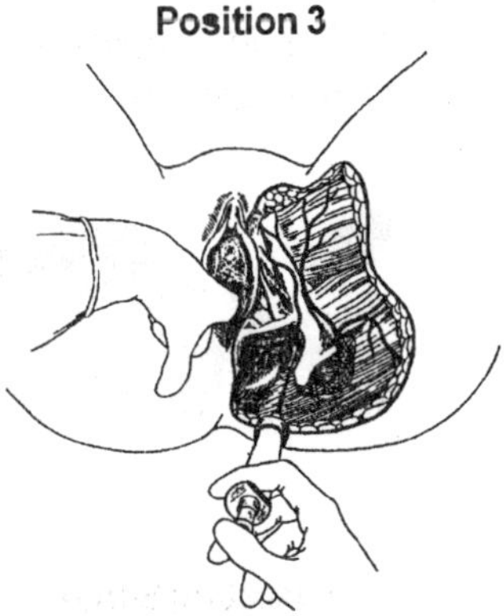

Position 4

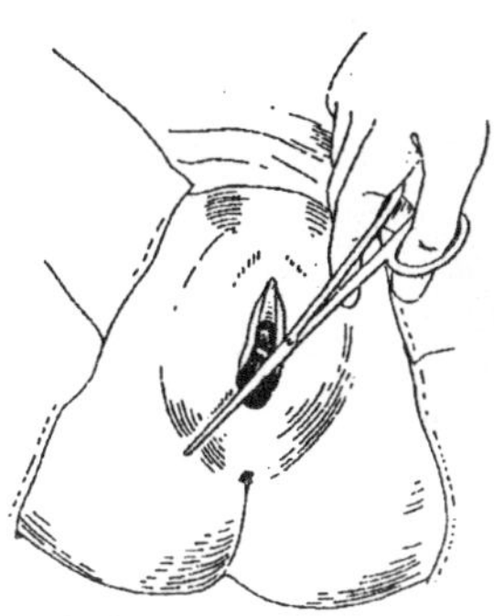

Position 5

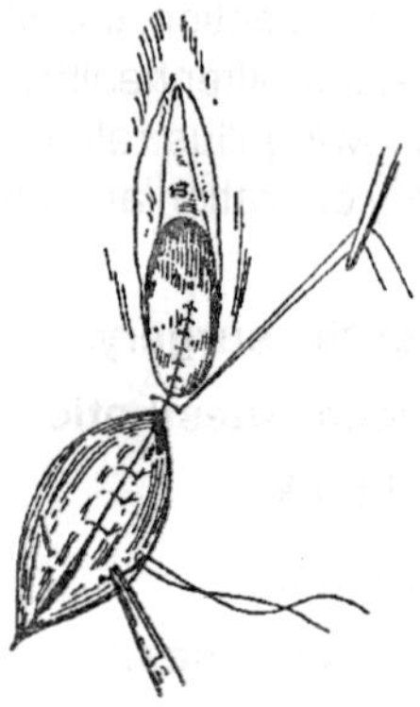

Position 6

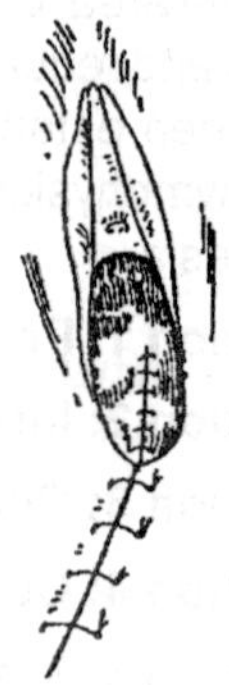

Episiotomy

CAESAREAN SECTION

It is a major surgery in which the delivery of child is made cutting through both the abdominal wall and the uterine wall. This surgery was, however, introduced in 1876 by the method of amputating the uterus. In 1882, new developments changed the whole outlook on the operation by innovation of suturing the uterine incision with absorbable catgut in such a way to control bleeding and prevent the subsequent leakage of 'lochia' into the peritoneal cavity. Advances in surgical methods and asepsis since then have made this operation safe when performed under proper conditions.

The circumstances, which make caesarean section desirable are varied in nature and may be assessed by individual obstetricians. But the more common conditions fall within the following:

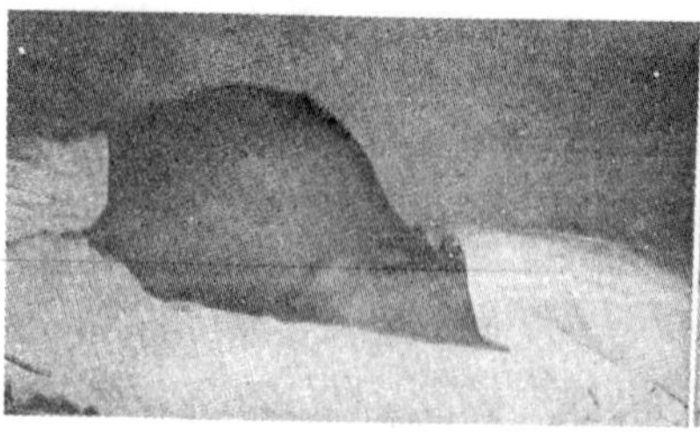

Ready for Delivery

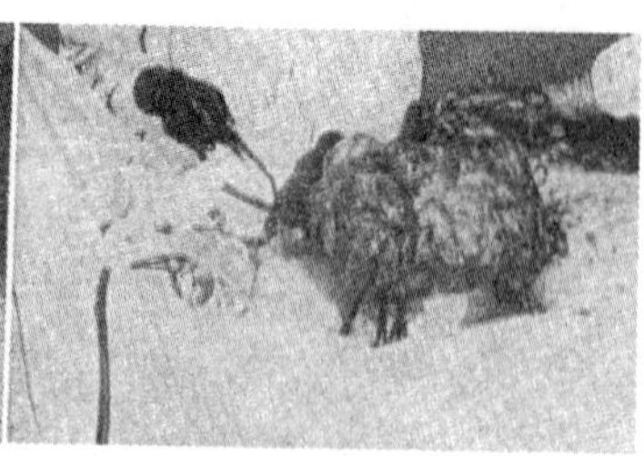

Conducting Surgery

1. Cephalo-pelvic disproportion and contracted pelvis.
2. Disordered uterine action.
3. Fetal distress.
4. Placenta praevia.
5. Previous caesarean section or hysterotomy.
6. Pre-eclampsia.
7. Diabetes mellitus.
8. Elderly primigravity.
9. Bad obstetric history.
10. Prolapse or presentation of cord.
11. Breech presentation in a primigravida in some cases.
12. Brow presentation.
13. Transverse lie.
14. In a newly dead woman with a living fetus and un-dilated cervix. A healthy fetus may remain alive in uterus for 10-15 minutes after mother's death.

A caesarean section is not recommended in the following conditions :

1. Where the child is dead or in such danger that it is unlikely to survive.
2. When the maternal passages are believed to be grossly infected, usually as a result of much handling.
3. The operation is not one to be attempted in bad surroundings, by the inexperienced operator or without proper assistance.

In this technique the abdomen is opened by an incision between umbilicus and pubes. The operation is carried in the following process as shown in the illustrations below:

Illustration 1: After opening the abdomen, pick up the utero vesicle fold of peritoneum prior to incising.

Illustration 2: Pushing the bladder off the lower segment.

Illustration 3: Enlarging the opening in the lower segment.

Illustration 4: Delivering the fetal head.

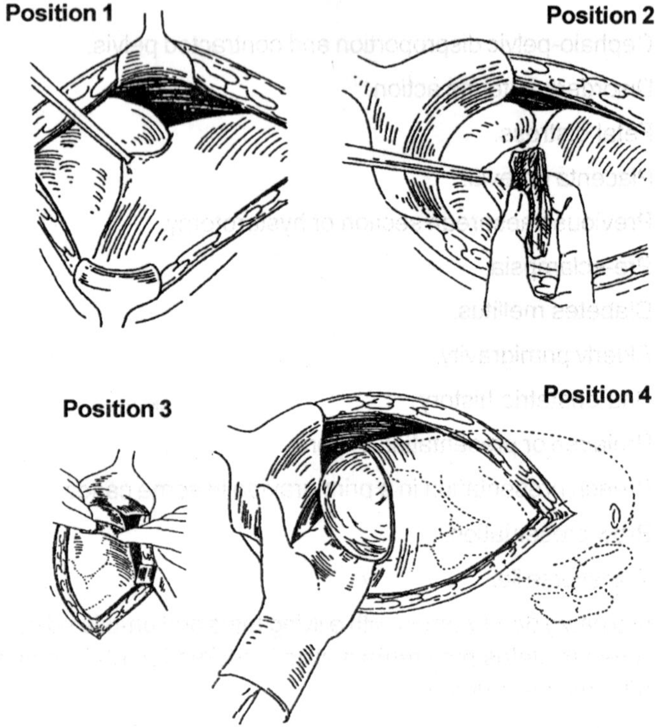

Caesarean Section

The results of Caesarean section to mother and child can never be considered apart from the proper indications for the operation, which all are such as would involve serious risk to both patients if vaginal delivery were chosen – such as contracted pelvis, serious pre-eclamptic toxaemia, accidental hemorrhage, placenta praevia, cardiac disease, etc.

The physiology and management of the puerperium :

The pueperium is the period immediately following labor, during which the maternal organs return to their normal condition. It takes six to eight weeks. It may be noted that the 'return to normal' is incomplete in certain respects such as the striae on the skin remain as permanent scars, the vulva remains slightly enlarged and the structure of the uterine wall remains permanently altered in some degree. The uterus and other generative organs become reduced to their normal condition by a series of processes that are known collectively as involution. The involution of the uterus is the most striking and one of the most important phenomena in the puerperium. At the beginning of pregnancy the uterus is measuring externally 3 by 2 by 1 inches whereas at the end of pregnancy, it measures about 12 by 9 by 8 inches. At the close of labor the uterus is about six inches long by 4-1/2 inches broad and 3-1/2 inches thick.

7
Breast Care and Breastfeeding

Glossary of terms for Breastfeeding

Afterpains	Contraction of uterus during breastfeeding in the first few days after childbirth, due to oxytocin released.
Allergy	Symptoms when fed even a small amount of a particular food.
Alveoli	Small sacs of milk secreting cells in the breast.
Amenorrhoea	Absence of menstruation.
Antibodies	Proteins in the blood and breast milk, which fight infection.
Areola	Dark skin surrounding the nipple.
Artificial feeds	Any kind of milk/ other liquid given instead of breastfeeding.
Artificially fed	Receiving artificial feeds only, and no breast milk.
Attachment	The way a baby takes the breast into mouth. A baby may be well attached or poorly attached to the breasts.
Bedding in	A baby sleeping in bed with mother instead of in a separate cot.
Breast abscess	Presence of painful, red swelling on the breast. The presence of pus caused by infection.

Blocked duct	A milk duct in the breast becoming blocked with thickened milk, so that the milk in that part of the breast doesn't flow out.
Bonding	Mother and baby developing a close loving relationship.
Breast Pump	Device for expressing milk.
Breast refusal	Baby not wanting to suckle from mother's breast.
Breastfeed history	All relevant information about mother and the baby in past and their present breastfeeding situation developed.
Breastfeeding supplementer	A tube through which a baby can drink artificial milk or expressed breast milk while suckling.
Breastfeeding support	A group of mothers who help each other to breastfeed.
Breast shell	Also known as breast shield and are used when nipples are flat.
Breast milk Substitutes	Any food or drink, which is used to replace breast milk
Barbiturates	These are drugs, which are used to make people sleepy or for control of fits. These may make you addictive to them if taken frequently. This medicine gets secreted into breast milk and therefore may affect the baby.
Bromocryptine	This is a medicine, which may be sometimes used to suppress breast milk production. Its use is harmful for the baby.
Calories	Kilocalories to measure the energy available in food.
Casein	Protein in milk which forms curds.
Colic	Regular crying, sometimes with signs suggesting abdominal pain by the baby after feeding.
Cold compress	Clothes soaked in cold water to put on the breast.

Colostrum	The special breast milk that women produce in the first few days after delivery. It is yellowish or clear in color.
Complementary food	Solid food given from the age of 4 to 6.
Calmpose	A medicine which is used to calm the nerves and for inducing sleep. Sometimes, it is used for control of fits. The medicine if taken by the mother may produce jaundice, sleepiness or loss of weight in the newborn baby.
Calomel	A drug used as a purgative. It affects the baby in about 50% cases.
Cascara	A laxative made from the bark of a tropical tree It is secreted in the breast-milk and it affects about 50% of the babies causing diarrhea.
Chloral hydrate	A chemical compound which is sometimes used to make a person sleep. It also reduces blood pressure. This medicine is used in women who have toxaemia of pregnancy. The medicine is secreted in the breast milk and may harm the baby.
Choking	This can occur sometimes while eating or drinking breast milk, food or liquid taken into the windpipe instead of food pipe. The baby develops sudden difficulty in breathing and it coughs violently and may soon turn blue. Choking is more common amongst low birth weight and weak babies in comparison to normal birth weight and strong babies.
Cracked nipple	When the skin of the nipple has a split (break) because of excessive dryness or rash.
Cold compress	Cloths soaked in cold water to put on the breast.
Contaminated	Containing harmful bacteria or other harmful substances.
Dehydration	Lack of water in the body, generally due to diarrohea in children.

Demand feeding	It means that the baby should be given feeds whenever he demands them or when the baby appears to be hungry.
Discharge	It refers to the secretion of liquid from an opening. Normally, this discharge is in the form of a greasy material, which is secreted from around the areola of breasts. This discharge is good as it kills the germs on the skin.
Drainage	Sometimes, the abscess in breast does not get better with antibiotic treatment. The pus inside the abscess can be drained by making an incision. Once the pus is drained tension is relieved and the mother feels comfortable.
Ducts	Small tubes which lead milk to the nipple.
Dummy	Artificial nipple for a baby to suck.
Early contact	A mother holding her baby during the breast feeding.
Effective suckling	Suckling in a way which removes the milk efficiently from the breast.
Engorgement	Swollen with breast milk, blood and tissue fluid. Engorgement breasts are often painful and oedematous , and the milk doesn't flow well.
Eructation	The curdled milk baby brings out. During feeding, the baby may swallow some air which can come out as a 'burp' (breaking the wind) This is called eructation (belching). Sometimes, baby brings out some fresh milk along with curdled milk. Do not worry.
Express	To squeeze and press out milk.
Expressed milk	Milk, which has been pressed out of the breasts.
Engorged breasts	Breast engorgement occurs when these are not emptied properly and frequently, as a result the milk builds up in the milk tubes which makes the breasts swollen, lumpy,

	hard, painful and hot. It is not only because of excess of milk production but is also caused by leakage of fluid from vessels blocked by increased pressure in the breasts. A mother with engorged breasts feels hot, sweats a lot and may feel thirsty.
Ergot Alkaloids	Used for the treatment of migraine. They can suppress breast milk production and cause other harmful effects on the baby.
Fissure in nipple	Break or crack on the skin, usually appear in breast nipples and areola. It is very painful and sometimes blood oozes out from it. This may also get infected.
Flat nipples	Nipples which do not protrude out from the areola at any time are flat nipples (the nipple which sticks out less than average). The baby may have a lot of difficulty in suckling them.
Foremilk	The watery breast milk that is produced early in a feed.
Formulae	Artificial milk for babies made out of a variety of products, including sugar, animal milk, soy bean and vegetable oils. They are usually in powder forms, to mix with water.
Full breasts	Breasts which are full of milk, hot, heavy and hard from which milk flows.
Follicle	It is a small cavity or recess in the skin or some other part of the body from where secretion takes place.
Growth factors	Substances in the breast milk, which promotes growth and development of the intestine and helps the intestine to recover after an attack of diarrhoea.
Growth spurt	Sudden increased hunger for some time.
Hind milk	Fat-rich breast milk produced in a feed. In fact, during breastfeeding the baby gets the milk in two phases. In the first phase it gets fore milk – that is milk, which is already present in the milk tubes. This is weak

because of low-fat contents. Hind milk is the major part of breast feed, which the baby gets only after the 'let down' reflex begins to work. Usually, the gap between fore milk and hind milk is small, but sometimes it may be up to two to three minutes. Do not discontinue feeding if the milk doesn't seem to come out after the initial phase. You will not give the complete feed to the baby if you stop feeding before 'let down' reflex has started to work.

Hormones — Chemical messengers in the body. They are substances produced in one part of the body the endocrine glands, and are carried to another part of the body by the blood stream where they produce their effects. If the mother is taking hormones, these can be passed to the baby and can cause ill effect. Some hormones may also suppress breast milk.

Heroin — It is a narcotic drug available in the form of a white powder derived from morphine. This medicine causes addiction. It is secreted in breast milk and can cause sleepiness in the baby and produces constipation. Sometimes, it may cause serious breathing problem.

Hygiene — It means being clean and keeping healthy conditions. Hygienic conditions are must while breastfeeding the child.

Immune system — Those parts of the body and blood, including lymph glands and white blood cells, which fight infection.

Ineffective suckling — Suckling in a way which removes milk from the breast inefficiently or not at all.

Infection — When germs enter the body and multiply. If caused by certain germs (bacteria), infection should be treated by antibiotics in consultation with a doctor. Some infections can be prevented by

	immunizations or preventive measures. Infective conditions are harmful for both mother and the child.
Inflammation	This means having become red and swollen as a reaction to an infection or injury.
Inverted nipple	If the nipple is buried inside the areola of the breast, it is inverted. The condition is rare. Before considering the nipple to be inverted, try to hold the nipple between the thumb and the finger and try to pull it out. If the nipple comes out, it is not inverted.
Jaundice	A yellow discoloration of the white portion of the eyes and the skin is seen in case of Jaundice. It is very common in newly born babies after two days age. If the palms and soles of the feet are yellow, you should consult a doctor immediately.
Lactation	It refers to the period during which a woman is breastfeeding the baby.
Lead	A harmful substance. Some ointments applied to the breasts may contain lead. Some breast shields may also contain lead. These can cause several bad effects including damage to the brain.
Let down reflex	This is a reflex which enables pushing the milk from the full milk glands to the ducts and then to the nipples. It is stimulated by suckling, but it can also occur even while preparing to breastfeed the baby, e.g. sight and sound of the baby. While in some women the let down reflex is very prompt, in other it may be 2-3 minutes after the baby suckle. In the latter situation the mother should wait until the milk begins to flow freely. Let down reflex is smooth if the baby is put to breast within half an hour of the birth. If the first feed is delayed, let down reflex may be slower in getting established. Positive attitudes, avoiding tensions and natural breastfeeding all help in maintaining the let down reflex.

Lithium	A medicine which is used for treatment of some psychiatric disorders. This can be secreted into the breast milk and harm the baby. A woman who is on lithium should consult a doctor regarding continuation of medicine or breastfeeding.
Low birth weight	A new born baby who weighs less than 2500 gm. Such babies need special care. It is suggested to seek doctor's advice.
Lump in breast	A localized swelling in the breast, which is painful to touch. This can occur in any part of the breast and at times more than one lump is present in the breast. Sometimes, it is accompanied with fever and chills. The lump can increase or decrease during a feed. Better consult a doctor.
Mastitis	An infection of the breasts caused by poor or delayed emptying of the blocked duct. As a result of blockage the milk leaks out into the breast tissue and causes infection. The breast feels hot, painful, swollen with a shiny skin. Fever may also be present. Besides treatment, continue to breastfeed to prevent formation of abscess.
Milk glands	These are located inside breasts and help in producing and secreting milk. The milk glands swell up before the feed time, since at this time they are filled with milk. Immediately after a feed, these milk glands are empty.
Montgomery's Tubercles	Prominences around areola of the breast. They become prominent during pregnancy and secrete oily material, which provides natural lubrication. It kills germs on the skin, and keeps nipples and breast supple. Do not try to remove the secretion.
Natural feeding	Natural breastfeeding means giving your baby breast feeds whenever he/she is crying or seems to be hungry. It also includes feeding the baby when your

	breasts are full or leaking or when you wish to feed the baby. This approach meets the needs of the baby as well as the mother.
Protractile Nipples	Means that the nipples stick out from the breast. Protractility helps the baby to draw the nipple and areola further into the mouth. When the baby suckles, he is able to empty the breasts easily and completely.
Radioactive	Breastfeeding is avoided after exposure to radioactivity. Consult a doctor before any procedures are undertaken on a woman who is breastfeeding her baby. Radioactive substances leave harmful effects on feeding mothers.
Supplimentation of Breast Milk	Milk which is given in addition to the four months of age supplementation may be advised. If the mother is very sick or the baby is not able to take breast milk. After four to six months age supplementation with milk and food is advised, since breast milk alone may not be sufficient to meet the increasing demand of baby.
Weaning	The process by which breastfeeding is initially supplemented and ultimately replaced by artificial milk and/or semisolids. Weaning should start by about four to six months and should not be delayed.

Breastfeeding and Disorders of Breasts

If possible plan to feed your baby yourself. There are many fine formulas in the market, but human milk is best for human babies. If you nurse him yourself, he will probably have fewer stomach upsets, less diarrhea, and almost no constipation. He will also have less skin troubles. It is beneficial for the mother too. You will feel better yourself, your pelvic organs will return to normal more quickly, and your skin will improve. This is one of the nature's ways to keep a woman young and beautiful.

Diet of a feeding mother : The mother should be sure to take sufficient fluids every day, particularly milk. The calcium in the milk is needed for baby's bones and teeth and also to protect her own system. She should take milk in the form of milk products, soups and drinks. She should also contain a liberal amount of vegetables and some extra protein in the form of beans, peas, eggs and cheese.

How often to feed your baby? : Feed your baby as much as he desires, certainly at least every three or four hours. The more milk he gets from the breast, the more you will have, provided your fuel intake is sufficient. To find that the baby is getting enough feed here is a simple way. Weigh him just before you feed him, and again right after the feeding. The difference in the weight will let you know how much the breast milk he is getting at each feeding. If he fails to show weight gain each week, you may need to give him one or two bottles of formula each day. This should only be done after he has nursed his full time at the breast.

What to do in case of swollen breasts and sore nipples? : If your breasts become swollen and painful, apply warm, moist packs two to three times a day. Take care not to burn the skin. Gentle heat will relieve any congestion in the breast. If the nipples become sore, carefully sponge them with rubbing a lubrication oil, and then rinse with clean water.

Lifted breasts and breastfeeding : No other part of a woman's body is so attractive and enjoy the supreme position as her breast, in the overall beauty, charm and grace of a woman. Lifted, well-rounded, shapely and stiff bust of a woman gives her an added attraction and such a bust symbolizes the youthful beauty of a woman. Shapeless, small, sluggish or over-developed breasts rob the attraction of a streamlined figure. With the passing of youth the busts get drooped, but if this occurs in youthful days (which usually happens with the majority of women due to their sheer negligence) early attention should be paid to avoid these defects. Breast care is very important. If woman's breasts get drooped and flabby at an early age, it will fail to give necessary sexual perception. It is rightly said by a scholar that, **'what is the use of breasts which are neither useful to the husband, nor to the child.'**

Lactation (Breastfeeding) : There is no other nourishment to a child than mother's milk. Breast milk is normally available within 60 to 72 hours after delivery. An infant should be allowed to suckle 12 hours after the delivery, which helps for the normal flow of the milk. The first flow that comes out of the breast is known as colostrums. Its sucking helps the child in its excretion of faeces. With the flow of milk the breast becomes stiff and warm. The woman feels exhausted,

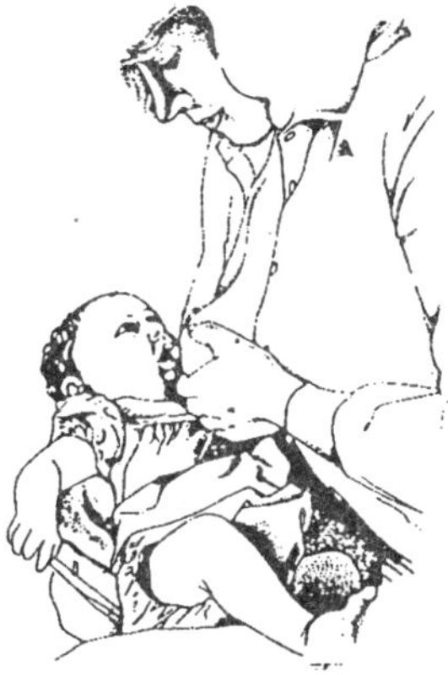

Position of breast-feeding

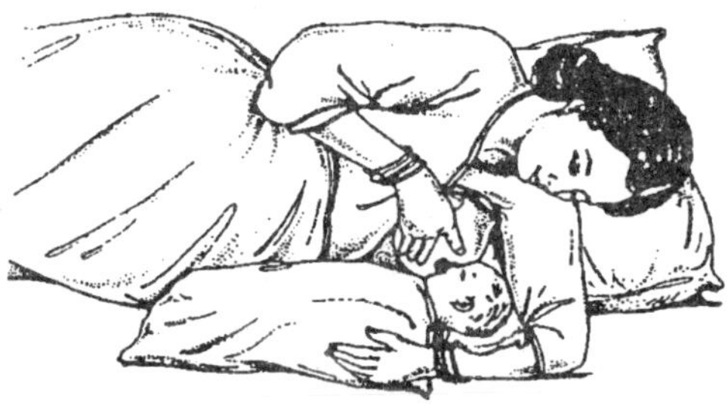

Position of breast-feeding while lying down

gets some headache and sometimes there is some fever as well. This fever is known as breast fever. During this fever a woman feels pulsation in breast and sometimes pain in the armpits. Fomentation with ice subsides this pain within 24 hours. Even fomentation with the pods of poppy gives much relief. To relieve a woman from breast pain extra milk should be sucked out with Breast Pump.

Some important facts about human milk : Before a child takes up to breast milk, it is necessary to examine mother's milk to avoid complications. Milk, which either floats or sinks in water, which gives soar taste, or is thick, gives different smell, or appears black, yellow or red should be considered impure. If the breast milk is defective and impure the following herbal treatment helps supply of pure milk :

Mix very minute quantity of each spice (available from a good herbal store): Patol Patra, Neem Patra, Vijasar, Devdaru, Padh,

Murva, Giloya, Kutki and dry ginger in ¼ cup water and prepare a docoction. When the water will be reduced to fifty percent, get it filtered and give it to the mother twice a day (in the morning and evening). Make sure that the mother should include wheat bread, kidney bean, ghee and milk in her diet.

Remember, if the busts are heavy, it doesn't mean that there is plentiful supply of milk. A calm, cheerful and a slim woman has more milk than a resentful and peevish woman. For plentiful supply of milk the following home remedies should be adopted :

1. Cumin seed (aromatic seed) to be steeped in the milk and allowed to dry. Give it to the feeding mother followed by some milk.
2. Cook white cumin seed and paddy rice in milk and give it to the feeding mother.

Sometimes, there is excess supply of milk in the breast, which remain leaking all the time. Necessary care should be taken to keep the breast clean or there is danger of nipples being cracked or sore. The nipples should be washed often, particularly after feeding the baby. If there is pain in the breast, maul the roots of 'Indrayan' (an herb available from a herbal store or a good 'pansari' shop) and apply the lotion on the busts.

Advantages of breastfeeding for the baby? : There are many advantages of breastfeeding for the baby. Moreover, breastfeeding strengthens the bond of love and affection between a mother and her baby. Few important advantages are the following :

- It is the most perfectly balanced food, containing everything that your baby needs for the first four months of life, and many may be even longer. It helps in the optimum growth of the baby without making him overweight.
- It contains special protective substances, which help in the prevention of many illnesses, infections and allergies. Diarrhea, respiratory infections, ear infections, eczema and asthma are less common in breast-fed babies than in bottle-fed ones.

Advantages of breastfeeding for the mother? : There are several advantages of breastfeeding for the mother also. Above all, breastfeeding the baby gives the mother a sense of fulfilment and satisfaction. Some of the advantages are following :

- If the baby is breast-fed immediately after birth, it helps in controlling the bleeding the mother has after delivering the baby.

- Breastfeeding helps the womb return to its normal size.
- Breastfeeding helps the mother to get back into proper shape by helping her to shed excessive weight that has gained during the pregnancy.
- Breastfeeding is useful for prevention of cancer.
- Exclusive breastfeeding helps in spacing children. However, this is not foolproof and some contraceptive may be required. Better consult your doctor.
- Breastfeeding is very convenient since you do not require to carry around feeding bottles, sugar, the milk powder, arranging for warming up of feed and cleaning the feeding bottle or utensils etc. especially when you are out or during journey.
- Breastfeeding is not expensive than giving artificial milk.
- You do not have to get up in the middle of the night to prepare the feed or warm up the milk.

Breastfeeding vs. Artificial feeding : Many illnesses and obesity in older age are more common in artificially fed babies than breast fed ones. A chubby appearance of an artificially fed baby cannot be considered better than a slim but healthy appearance of a breast-fed baby. Remember, the appetite of your baby will depend on the fat content of the milk. The composition of artificial milk remains same throughout, whereas in case of breastfeeding the later part of breast milk contains the higher amount of fat than the earlier part. A bottle-fed baby ends up drinking larger amount of milk in order to satisfy his need. It is easy to overfeed the baby on artificial milk, it is almost impossible to overfeed breast milk.

Breast milk is more easily digestible than the cow's milk. Proteins in the milk curdle in the stomach as soon as it reaches the stomach. The proteins in cow's milk is more than that formed by the breast milk. The curds formed by cow's milk are more and much thicker than breast milk curds. Thus breast milk is more easily digested than cow's milk. The baby who is given artificial milk may remains full up to four hours after the feed, but breast-fed baby will get hungry earlier, i.e. in two to three hours after the feed. The proteins from cow's milk pass out in the faeces and urine in larger quantities than breast milk proteins. Therefore, there is much less wastage of breast milk proteins than cow milk proteins. Thus a baby fed on cow's milk drinks more milk than a breast milk fed baby and may become fat, which is not healthy.

What is colostrums? : Colostrum is the first milk after child-birth, which is yellow in color and thick in consistency. It comes out of the breasts during the first few days after the baby's birth. Many women throw away colostrum and regard it as accumulated milk of pregnancy and therefore unfit for the baby. Others are worried because of its yellow color and thick consistency. Few people believe that it is too difficult for the baby to digest such a thick milk and therefore unsuitable for the baby. Colostrum must definitely be given to the newly born baby. It is very rich in proteins, cells, minerals and vitamins. At the same time it is low in fat and carbohydrates (sugar). A newly born baby given colostrums have has five times the vitamins than an artificial fed baby has. The antibodies in colostrum protect the new born's intestine from absorption of whole proteins and therefore relieve from allergies.

Anatomy of the Breast : The breast contains many tiny glands whose function is to produce milk. The milk thus produced is conveyed to nipple through ducts that terminate there. The contour of the breast is determined not only by the amount of glandular tissue but by the amount of fatty tissues that is present. Women generally want to know about the characteristics and functioning of breasts.

Size of breasts : Both the breasts are not always equal in size. In many women, one breast is slightly larger than the other. In most of the cases, the size and shape of the breasts tend to follow a familiar pattern. There is tendency for the girls to develop the same kind of breasts as their mother has.

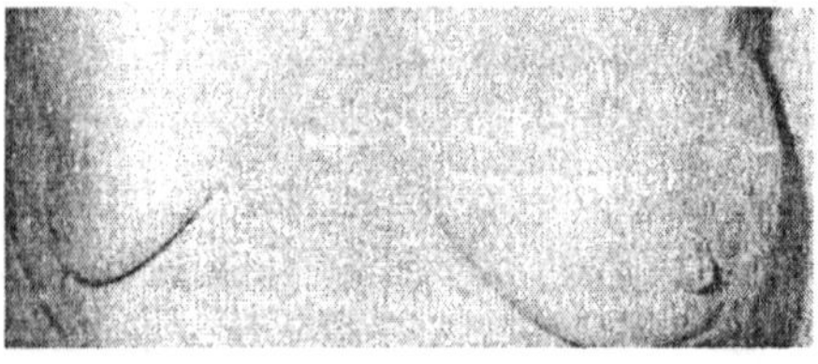

Unequal Breast

How to exercise and maintain the youthful contours of breasts? : Breasts are body's characteristic not affected by exercise. To maintain the youthful contour of breasts, wear a good uplift brassiere and also avoid marked fluctuations in weight, which tend to weaken the ligaments supporting the breasts. Do not press too strongly on one portion of the breast. Any metal supports in the brassiere are harmful to the breasts. Women are generally worried about the shape of breasts during pregnancy and after childbirth. But it doesn't necessarily lead to disfigurement. Many women discover that their breasts are improved by pregnancy and nursing. Much can be done to maintain a youthful figure as one enters the forties and fifties. Avoidance of overweight and the wearing of a proper breast support will help greatly.

Can small breasts be made larger? : In most adolescents, underdeveloped breasts may be associated with slow development of the rest of the body and low production of female hormones. If this is the case, the breasts will enlarge spontaneously as the child matures. In recent years, good results have been obtained by inserting a Silastic bag containing either saline or silicone gel beneath the breast to give it appearance of being larger. Breast surgery is one of the most successful procedure to give breast larger appearance, but it is very costly treatment and uncommon in India.

Medications to ensure increased milk production and breasts to dry up : No medication is necessary, as only a small percentage of women will be unable to produce sufficient milk. The breasts are dried up when a mother wishes to stop nursing. There are several efficient drugs that cause the breasts to stop secreting.

What is inverted nipples and how it can be cured? : Nipples that are folded in upon themselves instead of protruding out from the surface of the body are inverted nipples. If they are treated from the earliest youth, it is possible to prevent a certain amount of inversion. This involves daily treatment by everting and massaging them. It is important to do this during pregnancy if nursing is to be attempted.

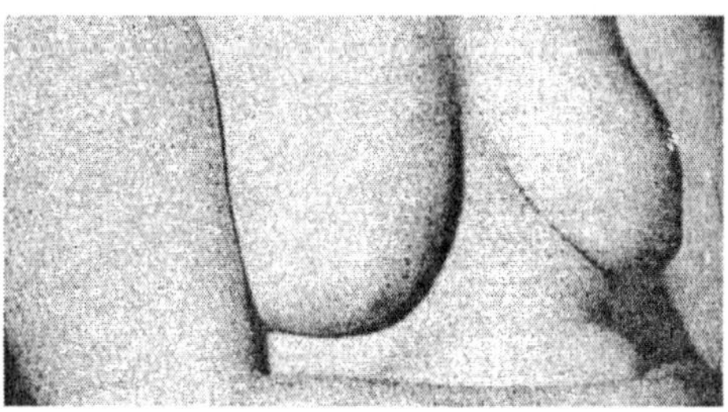

Breast without nipples

Effect of menstrual periods on breasts : In many women tenderness and engorgement of the breasts take place for a few days before periods and subside on the first or second day of the period. In some patients in whom the sensitivity and tenderness is extreme; this condition can be relieved somewhat by restricting salt and fluid intake for few days before menstruation and by giving large doses of Vitamin B complex. In the rare case, hormone therapy may be indicated. Breast sensitivity and enlargement are essential significance before a menstrual period. This is a normal cycle phenomenon related to hormone secretions.

How often should a woman have her breast self-examine?: Every woman should have her breast examined at least once a year or if she should feel something unusual or develop pain in breast, she should seek medical attention. Here is an easy method of self-examination of the breasts:

1. Lie flat in the bed face up. Place a small pillow under the right shoulder and back of your chest. This prevents the breast from sagging to the side of the body, thus permitting a more satisfied examination.
2. Place your right arm on top of your head.
3. Place the fingers of your left hand together in a straight position and gently draw the flat portion of the fingers, not the tips, over the inner half of the breast, starting at the top and working down towards the bottom of the breast. It is easier to feel a lump. The fingers are moistened with a little mineral or baby oil or soap. This allows the fingers to glide smoothly over the breast.
4. Lower your right arm and place it at your side.
5. Again, take the flat portion of the fingers of your left hand and glide them over the outer half of the breast toward the nipple. Start this at the top of the breast and work down toward the bottom of the breast.
6. Repeat the above process in reverse, for examination of the left breast.
7. Milk each nipple gently but firmly to note any discharge. Normally there is no discharge.
8. After completing the above, stand in front of a mirror in a good light and inspect your breasts carefully. Look particularly for the following abnormalities :
   - A sore or ulceration of the nipple.
   - A change in the size of a breast.
   - A change in the level of one of the nipples.

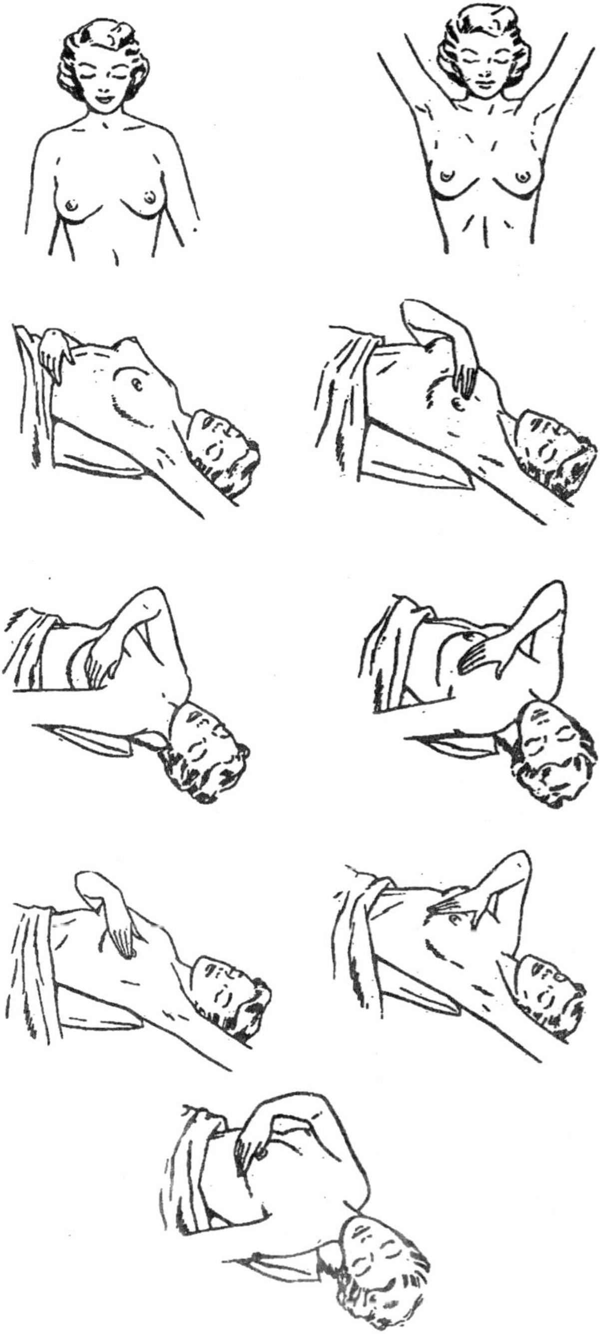

- A change in the appearance of the skin overlying the breast, especially a dimpling or indentation in its contours
- The presence of a lump or a protrusion of any part of the breast.

Breast Infections : Breast infections in all nursing mothers who have recently gone through pregnancy are usually common. In most of the cases in case of breast inflamed or developing an abscess, nursing can be continued (preferably consult your doctor) without harming the child and the mother. In case of a breast abscess, the following treatment is suggested :

- Apply warm compresses to the inflamed area.
- Doctors usually prescribe large doses of an antibiotic medicine.
- Incision and drainage of the breast if and when the abscess localized.
- Discontinue nursing if it becomes too painful to the mother or if the breast requires surgery.
- Small abscesses can be drained by an registered medical practitioner. But large ones must be opened under general anesthesia in the hospital.
- After drainage of breast abscess, the breastfeeding can be continued in the opposite breast, but it is usually necessary to discontinue nursing in the infected breast. Occasionally, breast abscesses will form spontaneously in women who have not been pregnant. Such infections can be treated in the manner outlined above. Rarely, a breast becomes involved in an infection caused by tuberculosis or syphilis (V.D.).

Breast Tumors and Cysts

1. Cysts occur most often in women between the ages of 30 and 45. They appear as single small, rounded masses no larger than a pea, or they may grow to the size of a lemon or orange. Cysts tend to be multiple.
2. Adenomas, fibro-adenomas, or cystadenomas are seen frequently as non-tender, non-painful lumps in young women between the ages of 18 and 35. They too can be as small as a pea or grow to the size of an orange.

3. Milk cysts (also known as galactocele) are cysts caused by blockage of a milk duct in women who have had children.
4. Intractal papilomas tumors are warty growths within a breast duct and the first recognized because of a yellowish, greenish or bloody discharge from the nipple. They may be so small that they cannot be felt when examining. They tend to occur most frequently in women between the age 30 to 40.
5. Fat necrosis and hematoma are conditions as a result of an injury to the breast. They lead either to destruction of some fat tissue within the breast. The lump caused by fat necorosis can occasionally resemble the lump produced by the breast cancer.
6. Cancer lesions first evidence themselves between small, painless, hard lumps, which can occur anywhere in the breast. Women between the age group 40 and 50 are most prone to develop breast cancer, although the disease is also seen in young women in their 20 and 30s, and in older women between the age 60 to 70.

Surgery of the breasts

The safest procedure is to remove every localized lump from every breast and in this way many early malignancies will be discovered at the earliest possible time. In some cases in which solitary cyst is present, needling of the cyst to drain it may be done instead of a surgery. In case of chronic cystic mastitis, where one has lumpy breasts containing innumerable areas of the lumpy masses, surgery is not always performed and a careful examination of the patient is conducted before surgery. A microscopic diagnosis can be made. In many cases, presence of a lump can be diagnosed by X-ray. The procedure is called **'Mammography'**. Remember, a negative mammogram is not proof that the breast is free from tumor as about 10% of the breast cancers sometimes will not show on mammography. The modern medical techniques have reduced the amount of radiation greatly. Mammography is usually recommended in case a woman has a family history of breast cancer, or she herself had a previous breast tumor or cancer etc. If there are symptoms of a breast cancer, a mammography should be performed within a period of two to three weeks.

In case of a lump in the breast?

An incision between one and two inches long is made over the lump and the entire lump is removed and submitted to microscopic examination to determine whether or not removal of the entire breast is necessary. A biopsy (the removal of the isolated lump) is usually recommended. The lump is submitted to immediate microscopic examination while the patient is still under anesthesia (A technique of preparing the tissue by freezing it before cutting and staining it, which is often induced by intravenous related drug). A microscopic examination usually gives positive information in almost hundred percent of cases. A woman generally feels discomfort for a few days following breast removal. The technique of removal of breast is known as **'Mastectomy'.** Remember, an early detection of the breast tumors by periodic examination will often prevent a breast tumor from reaching an incurable stage. Removal of the breast with or without its underlying muscles and the lymph glands that drain are the procedures usually advocated by the surgeon, as some surgeons remove only the breast leaving the glands intact, depending upon the condition. Blood transfusions are sometimes given when the entire breast has to be removed.

After the breast has been removed

An operation for removal of a breast is not dangerous if conducted by an experienced surgeon and a patient gets out of bed usually the very next day. This operation, in no way, does alter the activities of a woman. It is not certain that most non-cancerous lumps sometimes turn cancerous. It is not possible to tell positively before surgery whether the lump is actually benign or malignant. A woman may allow herself to become pregnant if the lump is found to be a benign one. If it is detected as hundred percent positive cancer, it is advisable for her to avoid pregnancy. A breast removal surgery should in no way alter the activities of a female and return to the normal living. **'Chemotherapy'** is helpful in the incidence of recurrence of cancer after surgery, as this process helps to reduce recurrence rates markedly. Chemotherapy must be continued anywhere from one to three years after breast removal. The examination should be followed up twice a year. There is no proof that tumors of the breast are inherited, but there are families, have a tendency towards greater tumor formation. It is permissible to have breast operation during menstrual period.

Plastic Surgery of the breasts

Following are the indications for plastic surgery upon the breast :

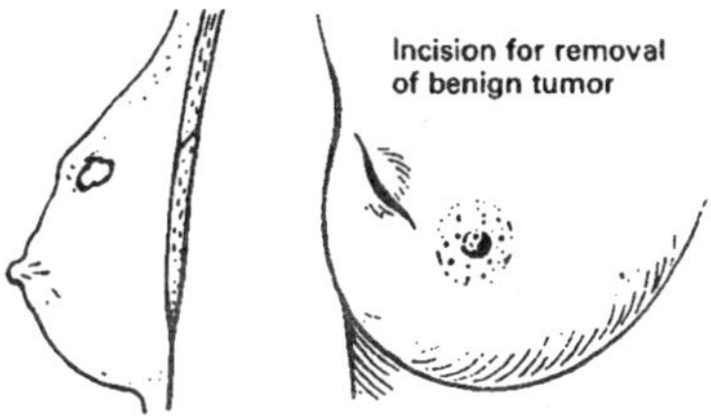

Benign tumor of breast

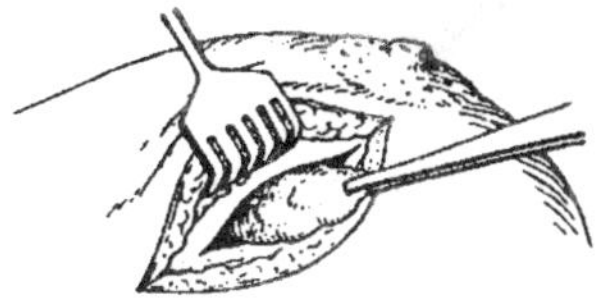

Tumor is removed

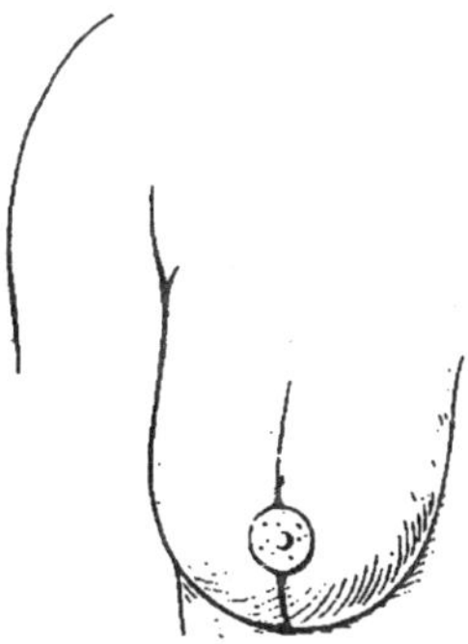

Incision around nipple

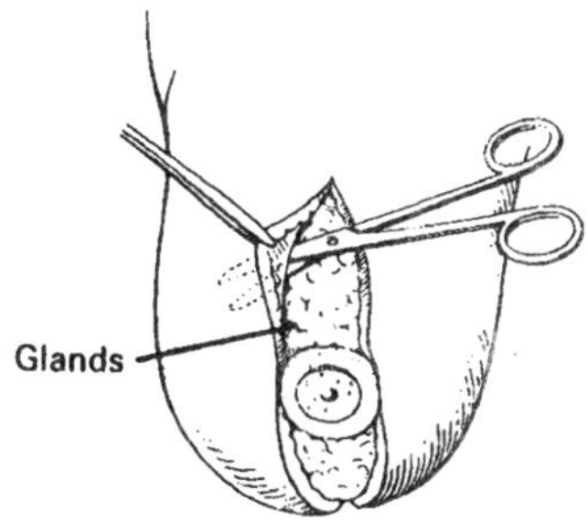

Breast tissue uncovered

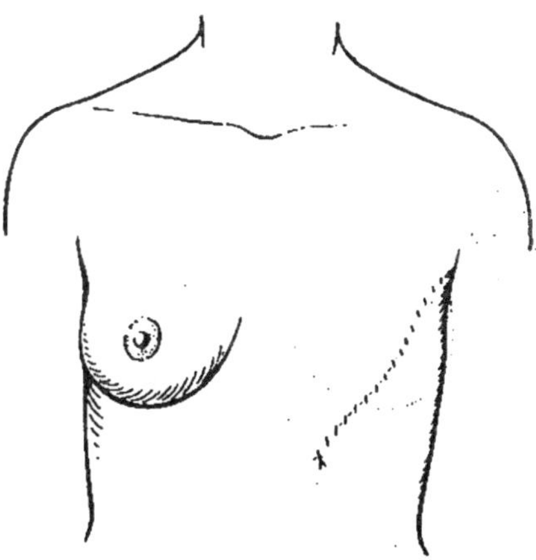

Appearance of incision
after breast removal
for malignant tumor

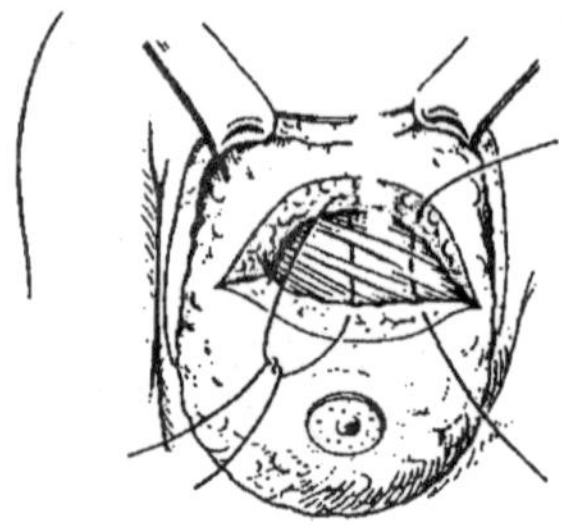

Section of breast removed

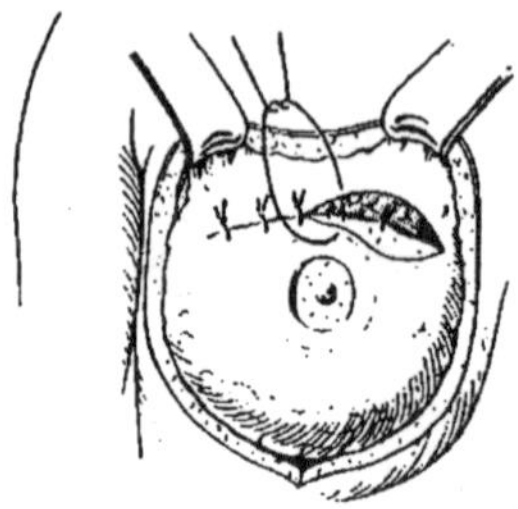

Deep and superficial sutures

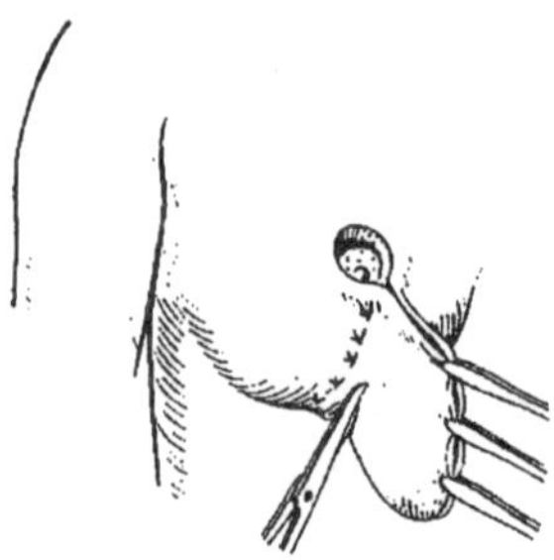

Excess skin removed

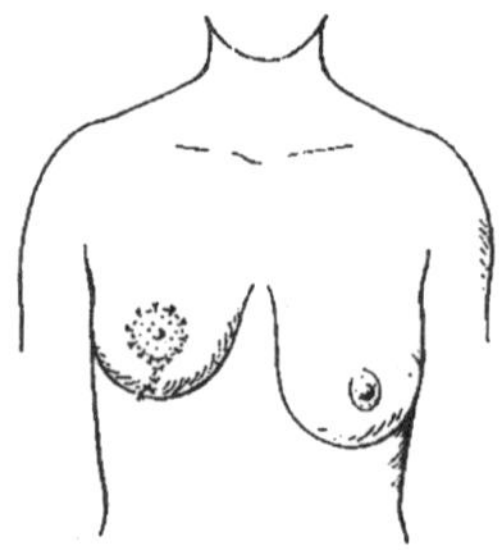

Finished suture

1. Marked enlargement or under-development.
2. Marked sagging (known as pendulous breasts).
3. Marked psychological disturbances caused by the feeling that one's breasts are ugly and that they interfere with one's happiness.
4. Breast reconstruction following mastectomy.

A sac composed of a plastic material can be placed beneath the tissues of the breast. The sac is then filled either with a salt solution or a silicone gel. The sac may be inserted either through an incision made below the breast or around the nipple. Make sure that a lapse of a year or more should exist between mastectomy and breast reconstruction. And breast reconstructed after mastectomy will not experience erotic sensations. Generally, a woman can develop a normal pregnancy after having plastic operation upon her breasts, but usually it is not possible to nurse a child successfully. Remember, this operation should not be embarked upon lightly; this is a major surgical procedure to be performed only by an expert in the field. The ideal time to undergo plastic surgery would be after a woman has finished childbearing. However, many young women wish to have breast surgery performed; this is feasible as soon as maturity has been reached.

After a breastplasty

It takes two hours to perform a breastplasty. Women often ask, if new nipples can be reconstructed. In some cases a rim of tissue around the opposite nipple is removed and is used as a free graft on the newly constructed breast. After a breast surgery, the breast can give the outward appearance of a real breast. However, not always, a certain amount of asymmetry may result. To reconstruct a breast, if the major pectoral muscle has been left in place during a mastectomy operation, an implant is placed beneath it. This will produce a mould on the chest wall giving it the appearance of a breast. If the pectoral muscle has been removed along with the breast, a flap of skin and muscle from the back of the chest or from the flank is brought onto the chest wall. This is done in a series of procedures using the principle of a pedicle graft. The results of a plastic surgery are usually permanent. Most scars are placed beneath the breasts and appear only as thin white lines, without exhibiting the signs of ugly or disfiguring. Soon after surgery upon the breast one can do the following :

- Bathe : After ten days.
- Walking : As soon as one leaves the hospital.
- Walking up and down stairs: As soon as one leaves the hospital.
- Perform household duties: After three to four weeks.
- Drive a car : After four weeks.
- Resume sexual relations : After four weeks.
- Return to work : After four to six weeks.

Link between Bras and Breast cancer

A study has revealed a causative factor for breast cancer that can increase your risk of getting the disease by hundred percent. A woman who wears a bra 24 hours a day is 113 times more likely to get breast cancer than a woman who wears a bra less than 12 hours a day. A woman who never wears a bra is 21 times less likely to get breast cancer than a woman in the general population. The straps, side panel, under-wires and other structure of the garments cut off drainage from the lymphatic. Look for the garments, which helps remove toxins and waste products from the cells of the body.

The longer you wear the bra, the more hours those toxins remain trapped in your breasts. The end result after years of bra use, can be a breast tumor or a cancer. According to medical reports, the cause of breast cancer has been regarded as biochemical and genetic. Bras and other tight clothing can contribute to the development of breast cancer as a result of cutting off lymphatic drainage so that toxic chemicals are trapped in the breast. So the take-home message to women from medical experts for a risk-free, cost-free life style experiment is : **Wear bras as little a possible.**

Selecting and wearing a bra : Select a bra that's not too tight. When you try it on, slide two fingers under the shoulder straps and the side panels. If the bra fits properly, your fingers should slide easily. The bra should also not leave marks or dents on your skin. If it doesn't, it is too tight. Women need to realize that wearing bras is a cultural phenomenon, not a natural one.

Massage-the most soothing relief for breasts : A gentle massage can help to improve circulation to the breasts and decrease pain. With your fingertips, make small, gentle, circular motions over the entire surface of the breasts. When you feel a cyst or a lump, massage gently around it, but never so hard that you irritate the tissue or cause any pain.

A castor oil pack applied to your breasts decrease inflammation and eliminate pain.

Disorders of Breast

Relieve Engorgement and blocked duct : Expressing milk is very useful to relieve such conditions. There are many situations in which expressing breast milk is useful and important to enable a mother to initiate or continue breastfeeding. Expressing of milk is very useful in the following cases :

- Keep up the supply of breast milk, prevent leakage of breast milk.
- Prevent the nipple and areola from becoming dry and sore.

The most useful way for a mother to express milk is by hand. It needs no appliance, so she can do it anywhere and at any time. It is easy to hand express when the breasts are soft. It is more difficult when the breasts are engorged or tender. The oxytocin reflex may not work as well when a mother express, as it does when a baby suckles. A mother needs to know how to help her oxytocin reflex, or she may find it difficult to express her milk.

How to express milk by hand? : To express breast milk by hand, the following steps are required :

1. Wash your hands thoroughly.
2. Sit or stand comfortably and hold the container near your breast.
3. Put your thumb on the breast above the nipple and areola, and your first fingers on the breast below the nipple and areola, opposite the thumb.
4. Now press your thumb and first finger slightly inwards towards the chest wall. Avoid pressing too hard; that can block the milk ducts.
5. Press your breast behind the nipple and areola between your fingers and thumb.
6. You must press on the lactiferous sinuses beneath the areola.
7. Press and release, press and release. This should not hurt or you feel uncomfortable. If it hurts, or you feel uncomfortable; the technique is wrong.
8. At first, milk will not secrete, but after pressing a few times milk starts to drop out. It will start flowing in streams if the oxytocin reflex is active. Press the areola in the same way for the sides to make sure that the milk is expressed from all segments of the breasts.
9. Avoid rubbing or sliding your fingers along the skin. The fingers should be more like rolling. Avoid squeezing the nipple. Remember, pulling or pressing the nipples will not generate flow of milk. Express one breast at least for three to five minutes until the milk flow is slow. Then express the other side and finally repeat both sides.

Expressing breast milk with Breast Pump

If hand expression is difficult, a feeding mother can use a breast pump. Rubber bulb pump is also used for expressing milk, but it is not very efficient, especially when the breasts are soft. They are suitable for collecting milk to feed a baby. The milk collected in a breast pump is often contaminated. Breast pump is useful mainly to relieve engorgement or when hand expression is difficult. Syringe pumps are more efficient than rubber bulb pumps. They are easier to clean and sterilize.

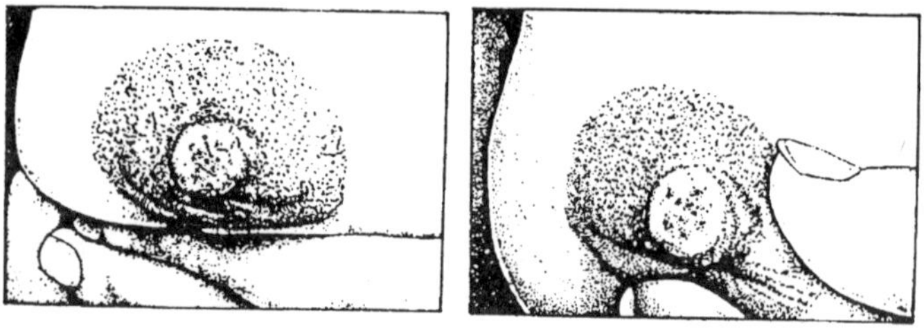

Expressing with a Syringe Pump

To use a syringe pump, put the plunger inside the outer cylinder. Now put the funnel over the nipple. Make sure that it touches the skin all round to make an airtight seal. Pull the outer cylinder down, the nipple is sucked into the funnel. Pull and push a few times, after a minute or two, milk starts to flow and collects in the outer cylinder.

Warm Bottle Expressing

This method is used to relieve severe engorgement when the breasts are tender, the nipple is tight and hand expression is very difficult. Take a glass bottle (minimum 700 ml size) with a wide neck (at least 2 to 4 cm. diameter) that the nipple can fit into it easily. Boil water in a pan. Pour hot water in the bottle to start warming it up. Then almost fill the bottle with hot water. Wrap the bottle in the cloth and pour hot water back into the pan. Put the neck of the bottle over the nipple, touching the skin all round to make an airtight seal. Hold the bottle steady till it cools down and makes gentle suction, which pulls the nipple into the neck of the bottle. Repeat the process again and again. In fact, the warmth helps the oxytocin reflex. Keep the bottle attached to the skin as long as the milk starts flowing drop by drop. Pour out the breast milk and repeat on the other breast. After some time, pain if any will subside and hand expression or suckling may become possible.

When to start expressing breast milk?

The mother should start to express milk on the first day within six hours of the delivery if possible, which helps to :

- Establish lactation.

- To feed a low-birth-weight (LBW) baby.
- To feed sick newborn.
- To keep up her milk supply.
- To build up milk supply if it seems to be decreasing.
- To leave milk in store for the baby when she is out (when mother is working).
- Relieve symptoms such as engorgement or leakage of milk.
- Keep skin of the nipples healthy (Express a small drop to rub on her nipples after a bath or shower.

The mother may only express a few drops of colostrums at first that helps breast milk production to begin. She should try to express milk as much as she can. In this way, the baby starts suckling soon after delivery. This should be repeated after every three hours, including during the night.

Flat and Inverted Nipples

This problem is rare (hardly 4-5% mothers). But if the nipples are flat or inverted, this can however make it difficult for the baby to feed. If the problem is noticed, hold the areola of the breast between the thumb and the first finger. If the nipples protrude out, then baby will be able to feed the child without any problem. In most of the cases, the nipples improve at the times of or soon after the delivery when baby starts breastfeeding (without any treatment). Her breasts will improve and become softer in a week or so after delivery. Suckling by the baby helps to pull breast nipples out.

Remember, a baby should suckle from the breast, not from the nipple. Baby needs to take a large mouthful of breast. Mother should have plenty of skin-to-skin contact with the baby and to let the baby explore mother's breasts. If the baby doesn't attach well by himself, help to position him so that he may attach better. Help mother to try different positions to hold the baby in the first day before her breast milk comes in and breasts are full. Sometimes, putting baby to the breast in a different position makes it easier for the baby to attach. The following techniques prove helpful for better breastfeeding :

1. The lactating mother should try to make her nipples stand out more before a feed. This will help the baby to attach and start feeding himself. The mother needs to use a breast pump if the nipples do not protrude out as desired.

2. Many times shaping the breast makes it easier for the baby to attach well and feed properly. To shape the breast, mother should support it from underneath with her fingers and press the top of breast gently with her thumb.
3. Mother should be careful not to hold her breast too near the nipples. If baby cannot suckle effectively in the first week or two, help mother to express her milk and feed the baby in a cup.
4. Try to express breast milk directly in the mouth of baby, so that it is easier for the baby to attach to the breasts and he may be more willing to suckle himself.
5. If it is acceptable to both partners, the husband can suck on her wife's breasts a few times to pull out the nipples.

Engorgement of the Breasts

The engorgement of the breast results because of accumulation of milk in the breast, which cause pain and tenderness. The following are the main causes of engorgement :

1. Plenty of milk accumulating in the breast.
2. Delay in starting the breastfeeding
3. Not expressing milk soon after a breastfeeding.
4. Infrequent removal of milk from breasts.

The following preventions are recommended when having breast engorgement :

1. Poor attachment to breast.
2. Ensure good attachment soon after the delivery.
3. Encourage unrestricted feeding.

Mastitis

If you are having pain and swelling in some portion of the breast, you are perhaps suffering from Mastitis. The other prominent causes of mastitis are the following :

- Blocked duct occurs when the milk is not removed from part of the breast.
- The duct is blocked by thickened milk with the symptoms like lumps, which is tender and sometimes redness of the skin over the lump.

- Inflammation of breast tissue (which is called non-infective mastitis).
- Many times, the breasts get infected due to bacteria (which is called infective mastitis).
- Poor drainage and infrequent breastfeeding by the mother.
- Insufficient suckling due to poor attachment of baby.
- Pressure from the fingers during feeding the baby.
- Wearing tight bra and clothes.

The following steps should be adopted to cure mastitis :

- Frequent breastfeeding.
- Expressing milk from the breasts after feeding the child.
- Avoid stress and over work.
- Reduce frequency and length of the feed.
- Gentle massage towards the nipple.
- Warm compresses.
- Lift the lower part of breast to help the baby to feed or drain better.
- Trauma to breasts, which damage tissues and nipple fissure, which allows bacteria to enter.

Why and when the baby is crying too much?

When the baby cries too much, do not assume that he is hungry or the mother doesn't have enough milk in her breasts to feed the baby. When a baby cries a lot, it creates much tension in mother-child relationship and among other members of the family. The mother should find out the reason of baby's crying. There may be various causes for this due to :

1. Discomfort due to hot or cold weather.
2. A tiredness, illness or pain in the stomach.
3. Hunger for not getting enough milk.
4. Effect of drugs taken by the mother.
5. Baby may be allergic to the protein in some foods in mother's diet. Some of such foods include cow's milk, soy products, eggs, peanuts, caffeine in coffee, tea, colas etc. which may pass into the breast milk and sometimes upset the baby.

Over-supply of milk may occur if the mother takes her baby off the first breast and start feeding him from the second breast. The baby may get too much foremilk and not enough hind-milk. Such babies may have loose green stools and a poor weight gain. In case of colic, the babies cries and pulls his legs as if he has abdominal pain. When giving the baby milk, hold him upright in a sitting position or against shoulder.

Sore Nipples

In case of sore nipples look for the cause, check attachment and examine breasts as below to find out :

- Engorgement and fissures in the breast.
- Check baby for candida infection and tongue-tie.
- Baby's bottom for candida rash.

Adopt the following measures to treat sore nipples :

- Build up mother's confidence.
- Improve baby's attachment.
- Continuous breastfeeding.
- Reduce engorgement by expressing breast milk frequently.
- Treat for Candida if the skin becomes red, shiny, flaky, itchy, painful and soreness persists.
- Wash the breasts only once a day.
- Avoid using soap.
- Avoid rubbing breasts hard with a towel, which irritates the skin.
- Avoid applying medicated lotions and ointments on areola and nipples.
- Rubbing expressed breast milk on areola and nipples.

What to do if baby refuses breasfeed?

- Check if a baby is getting enough breast milk.
- Check baby's weight gain. This is the most reliable sign. For the first six months the baby should gain weight at least 500 gm. every month (125 gm. every week). If a baby gains less than that, look for the cause, it means he is not getting enough milk. Consult your doctor.

- Check baby's urine. Baby getting adequate milk supply usually passes dilute urine at least six to eight times in 24 hours. If a child urinates less than four times, consult your doctor.
- Babies urinating less than six times in 24 hours, usually may have concentrated, strong smelling and dark yellowish to orange urine

Age of the mother, sexual intercourse, menstruation, age of the baby, number of children, diet and effect of caesarian section do not affect the supply of breast milk. On the other hand there are many causes as below when a baby may not get enough milk :

- Psychological factors.
- Physical conditions.
- Use of contraceptive pills.
- Infrequent short feeds.
- Pregnancy stress.
- Use of alcohol and smoking.
- Tiredness.
- Poor attachment of baby and mother.
- Poor breast development.
- Retained pieces of placenta in the uterus.
- Lack of night feeds.
- The baby is or abnormal
- Mother is taking estrogen pills or diuretic.

Sick mother and breastfeeding

- A sick mother may continue breastfeeding. If she has been admitted to a hospital, admit baby with her.
- If the mother has fever, give her plenty to drink.
- If she is unwilling to breastfeed the baby, help her to express her breast milk four hourly and feed the baby by cup.
- In most of the cases where the mother is taking drugs, they leave very little effect on the milk. To stop breastfeeding is more likely to be dangerous than the effect of medicine. However, there are very few medicines, which may cause side- effects, usually to babies less than one month old. The effect is much

less in older babies. In case, the mother is taking anti-cancer drugs, it may be necessary to stop breastfeeding. In case the mother is taking psychiatric drugs or anti-convulsants, the breastfed baby will face weakness and drowsy.

- If the mother is being treated with radioactive substances, she should stop breastfeeding temporarily.
- Avoid using contraceptives which contain estrogens, and usually cause side effects such as abnormal sleepiness, unwillingness to feed and sometimes suffer from jaundice.

When baby refuses breastfeed

The prominent causes include illness, pain, wrong handling, sedation of drugs, blocked nose, sore mouth due to thrush or teething. Adopt techniques to breastfeed and reduce over-supply of milk as a result of poor attachment. Stimulate the breast so that it produces more milk than the needs. This will help the baby to feed from both breasts. When a newly born baby roots for the breast, he moves head from side to side as if refusing feed.

8
Vitamins, Minerals and Nutrient Diets

Vitamins are organic substances essential in small quantities for normal metabolism and health. Vitamins are classified under two groups as below :

1. Fat soluble : These are Vitamin A (retinol), Vitamin D and E (tocoferol) and Vitamin K.
2. Water soluble : These are Vitamin B (thiamine), Vitamin B_2 (riboflavin), niacin (nicotinic acid), biotin, Vitamin B_{12} (cyanocobalamin), folic acid and Vitamin C (ascorbic acid).

The following table will give an idea of vitamins and minerals :

Vitamins	*Best sources*	*Role*
Vitamin A	Milk products, green vegetables.	Needed for body membranes such as retina of the eye, lining of lungs and digestive system.
Vitamin B	Whole grains, enriched flour and cereals, nuts, peas and beans.	Ensures proper burning of carbohydrates.
Vitamin B_2	Milk and cheese.	Needed by all cells for energy.
Vitamin B_6	Whole grains and	Needed by red blood

(contd.)

Vitamin B_{12}	milk.	cells and nerves for proper functioning.
Pantothenic Acid	Dairy products.	Needed for red blood cells for the production of bones and marrow, and nervous system.
Biotin	Nuts and whole grains.	Needed for all cells and energy production in the body.
Vitamin C	Fresh vegetables and nuts.	Needed for skin and circulatory system of the body.
Vitamin D	All citrus fruits, tomatoes, raw cabbage, potatoes and strawberries.	Needed for bones, teeth and tissues in the body and their proper maintenance.
Vitamin E	Dairy products and sunlight (some vitamins are pruduced in the skin due to sun-exposure.	Required for the maintenance of blood calcium levels and growth of bones.
Calcium	Vegetable oils and several other food products.	Needed for tissues handling fatty substances and formation of cell membranes.
Phosphorus	Dairy products and green vegetables.	Essential for blood clotting and the Structure of the bones and teeth. Needed for the maintenance of body nerves and tissues.

(contd.)

Potassium	Dairy products, beans and peas and cereals.	Basic cells energy store, which is needed during growth of body.
Magnesium	Fruits and vegetables (avocados, potatoes, carrots, oranges, banana apricots, pineapple, grapefruit)	Major minerals in the body. Essential for fluid balance and cell reactions.
Iodine	Beans, peas, nuts, cereals and all green leafy vegetables.	Needed by cells, nerves and muscles in the body.
Iron	Iodized salt, kelp, seaweed, lettuce, pineapple juice and garlics.	Needed for thyroid gland.
Fluoride	Enriched cereals, millets, pulses and green leafy vegetables.	Needed for the oxygen carrying compound in the blood.
	Water, whole wheat, beans, peas and nuts.	Helps to protect teeth from decay. Needed for the structure of cell enzymes and cells to utilize oxygen.
Copper/Zinc	Whole wheat, beans, peas, nuts.	Needed for the structure of cell enzymes.
Chromium/ Selenium	Trace elements in foods.	Have role in the blood chemistry (required in minute quantity).

(contd.)

Molybdenum, Manganese and Sodium	Most of the foods, except fruit.	Essential for fluid balance, muscles contraction and nerve creation.

Required dietary daily allowance (RDA) for vitamins and minerals

Vitamin A	1 mg.
Vitamin B	1.0-1.4 mg.
Vitamin B_2	1.2-1.7 mg.
Vitamin B_6	Above 2 mg.
Vitamin B_{12}	3 mg.
Pantothenic acid	4-7 mg.
Biotin	100-200 mg.
Folic Acid	400 mg.
Vitamin C	60 mg.
Vitamin D	5-10 mg.
Vitamin E	8-10 mg.
Calcium	Required during growth.
Phosphorus	About 800 mg for adults.
Potassium	Whatever quantity obtained.
Magnesium	300-350 mg.
Iodine	10-18 mg.
Fluoride, copper, zinc	About 1.5 –15 mg.
Chromium, selenium	Minute quantity.
Manganese and sodium	1000-3000 mg.

Protein contents (in gm.) of food products (per 100 gm.)

Rice (Raw milled)	6.8
Wheat	11.8
Wheat flour (whole)	12.1
Wheat bread (white)	7.8
Wheat bread (brown)	8.8
Bengal gram (pulse)	20.8
Bengal gram (roasted)	22.5
Green gram	24.5

Red gram	22.30
Cowpea	24.0
Soya bean	42.20
Almond	20.80
Cashew nut	21.20
Ground nut	25.30
Cow's milk	3.2
Buffalo's milk	4.3
Milk (Khoya)	22.3
Skimmed milk powder	25.8
Agathi	8.4
Beans	7.4
Banana	1.2
Pomegranate	1.6
Wood apple	7.1
Raisins	1.8
Grapefruit/ musk melon	17
Guava	51
Mango ripe	34
Orange	48
Papaya	32
Pineapple	46
Pear/plum	52
Lemon juice with honey (250 ml.)	22
Carrot juice	120
Grape juice	115
Tomato juice	60
Soups (250 ml.)	16-35
Baked/boiled vegetables (100 gm.)	50-80
Raita (100 gm.)	50-80
Mint chutney (one teaspoon)	15-20
Ground nut	178
Fruit cocktail canned (120 gm.)	100

9
Tomours and Cancer in Women

What is Cancer?

It is a disorderly wild growth of tissue cells. If the process continues unchecked, the normal structure and function of an organ are destroyed. Cancer is a complex and life-threatening disease that required professional medical care. Some alternative remedies may actually worsen cancer if they are not used appropriately. Any organ of the body may be affected by cancer or a cancer-like growth. It is estimated that one in four people will at some time in their lives develop a cancer and that one in eight people lose his or her life as a result of cancer. Cancer is not contagious but some investigators think that certain cancers are associated with virus invasion and therefore might conceivably be transmissible.

Cancer in Men and Women

The incidence is approximately the same. However, certain types of cancer show up more often in one sex. For instance, lung cancer is more prevalent among men, breast cancer among women. An early treatment for all tumors is essential, as a non-cancerous tumor turn into a cancer and lives can be saved by the removal of benign tumors, which if left alone, might turn into cancer at a later stage. Cancer is on rapid increase due to increased pollution of air and water and greater contacts with dangerous carcinogens. Cancer occurs at any age, but more frequently in the latter half of the life span. It is seen, children, adolescents and young adults develop cancer less often than older people. But some investigators feel that stout people are somewhat more susceptible than thin people.

However, the person who submits to thorough health examination at regular intervals is better protected, since the presence of cancer may be detected at an earlier and more curable stage of its development. Cancer is not inherited, but many doctors feel that a tendency towards cancer may be inherited. There are practically no families in which some history of cancer can be found. Cancer exists throughout the world. However, cancer is influenced by environmental factors. People who live in areas of least pollution may have a lower overall incidence of certain types of cancer. There may be a greater incidence of lung cancer that exists among peoples who use to smoke too much.

Types of Cancer : Cancer is not one but many diseases. There are more than a hundred different types of cancer. According to a survey conducted by an NGO, the following estimated (approximate) cancer incidence and cancer deaths in both sexes have been observed :

Cancer site	Incidence in Women	Incidence in Men
Skin	3%	3%
Oral	2%	4%
Lung	11%	20%
Breast	28%	-
Pancreas	3%	3%
Colon & Rectum	16%	14%
Ovary	4%	-
Prostate	-	20%
Urinary	4%	10%
Uterus	10%	-
Leukemia & Lymphomas	7%	8%
All others	12%	18%

Cancer Site	Deaths in Women	Deaths in Men
Skin	1%	2%
Oral	1%	2%
Lung	20%	35%
Breast	18%	-

(contd.)

Pancreas	5%	5%
Colon & Rectum	14%	11%
Ovary	5%	-
Prostate	-	11%
Urinary	3%	5%
Uterus	4%	-
Leukemia & Lymphomas	9%	9%
All other	20%	20%

How does Cancer grow and spread?

The cancer cells outgrow the normal cells within the organ. They often use up most of the available nourishment and oxygen meant for the normal tissues, thus causing the normal tissues to starve and die. The cancer spreads through three main routes :

1. By direct growth and extension to surrounding structures.
2. Through the lymph channels to distant organs.
3. Through the blood stream to distant organs.

Cancer cells break loose from their site of origin and get into the lymph channels or blood vessels. The spread may be prevented from one part to the other by removal of the primary tumor when it is in an early stage of development. To find out if a cancer is spreading from its organ of origin, the microscopic examination of an wide surgical removal of primary tumor with surrounding normal tissues will reveal whether the cancer has been spreading. X-rays such as Bone Scans and CAT (Computerized Axial Tomography) Scan may exhibit the spread of cancer. On a slight finding of a lump anywhere in the body or the occurrence of unexpected bleeding from any orifice in the body is not a sure indication of a cancer. One should have thorough examination on finding a symptom. Remember, cancer doesn't often cause symptoms until it has existed for quite some time. That is why, an semiannual or an yearly examination is essential.

What is Biopsy?

The microscopic examination of a tumor or a piece of tumor tissue is known as biopsy. The suspended tissue is taken and is subjected to frozen section microscopic examination, when a preliminary report is obtained within 15 to 20 minutes. It takes about a week to get a detailed report. CAT scan is another new X-ray method for scanning the body and can pick up cancers deep within the body when they are in very initial stage. Cancer grows very slowly that the patient lives out his normal life span and dies of a related condition. Certain type of cancers, such as skin cancer is fully curable. Other forms of cancer vary according to location, duration of disease and its diagnosis. If timely diagnosed, cancer is curable. Cancers may be treated by surgery, various medications, chemotherapy and X-ray therapy. A combination of the three often gives better chance for recovery.

Sometimes, few cancers recur after a lapse of even ten years or so. If the cancer spreads beyond the point of origin, the chances for the recovery are markedly lessened. Surgeons always strive for complete removal of cancer, but sometimes the tumor spreads into vital organs that cannot be removed by surgery. X-ray or cobalt treatments, radioactive isotopes, chemicals or hormones may destroy those cells that have gotten beyond the original site of cancer. People suffering from cancer want to know the following points :

- The signs of Anemia : No, unless marked bleeding occurs from the tumor.
- Loss of appetite : No, unless tumor exists in stomach or esophagus.
- Weight loss : Usually not.

A surgeon always strive for complete removal of a cancer, but sometimes the tumor extends into the vital organs that cannot be removed. Other times, the cancer spreads so extensively that it goes beyond the help of a surgery. A surgeon cannot operate microscopically, and a few cells may have spread beyond the reach of his/her scalpel. A surgeon cannot tell that he has removed cancer completely.

How to minimize the chances of recurrence of cancer?

1. Wide, primary removal of the tumor.
2. Post-operative treatment with appropriate methods such as X-ray, radioactive substances, chemotherapy, or hormones.

Remember, diet has no role to avoid or with the recurrence of cancer. A patient having recovery from a cancer may return to normal life depending upon the location of the cancer and the form of treatment that was administered. But generally the majority of those who have recovered from cancer do return to normal or near normal activity. A cancer, sometimes have harmful effect upon a woman undergoing pregnancy, as it may reactivate the growth of the tumors in certain organs that are influenced by the hormones of the body. A semi-annual visit to a doctor for examination is most essential for a woman who has recovered from a cancer in past.

What is oncology?

Oncology is a branch of medical science dealing in tumors and malignant growths in the body. An oncologist is a physician who specializes in the treatment of cancer and allied growths. To treat cancer without surgery following measures are adopted :

1. Radiation Therapy and administration of radioactive substances such as iodine, phosphorus, gold etc.
2. The use of hormone injections and tablets. It has been observed that the breast cancer is most of the times is inhibited by male or female hormones. The growth of a prostate cancer is often inhibited by the administration of male hormones.
3. Chemotherapy is a treatment by administration of drugs and to kill cancer cells.
4. The modern techniques of X-ray and radioactive substances have improved the results remarkably.

What is chemotherapy?

Chemotherapy is a method of treating cancer and allied growths with chemicals. A physician who specializes in treating cancer and allied growths trained in internal medicine, in hematology (disorders of the blood and blood forming organs) and has knowledge of administration of hormones.

What is immunotherapy?

It is the prevention or treatment of disease through the production of immunity. A tremendous amount of research is presently taking place in the world. Since cancer is thought to be associated with virus invasion, this treatment eliminates cancer-producing agents (viruses).

Statistics using drugs and hormones in cancer treatment?

- More than 90% of children with acute leukemia can be benefited through chemotherapy.

- Nearly 70% of children with kidney tumors can be benefited from chemotherapy.
- About 70% of men with prostate cancer are benefited through the administration of hormones.
- Nearly 60% of women with breast cancer are treated through the administration of drugs and hormones.
- About 80% patients with chronic leukemia are benefited through chemotherapy.
- Nearly 80% of men with cancer of testicles benefit from chemotherapy.
- More than 40% of women with ovary cancer can be treated.
- It has been found that in case of bulk cancer cells in the body can be reduced through surgery, than the non-surgical methods of treating cancer, including radiotherapy, chemotherapy and hormone therapy are more effective. However, there are certain conditions, such as leukemia and lymphoma, those do not eradicate bulk tumor tissue in the body.

Food that contribute breast cancer

Eliminate the foods that contribute 40 to 60 percent of all breast cancer. More than hundred scientific studies show that saturated fat - the kind in red meat and dairy products can increase the risk of cancer. The saturated fat found in red meat and dairy products feed a tumor. If such fat are removed from your diet, you will slow the rate at which a tumor grows and perhaps even stop its growth. All dairy products, even those such as fat-free milk contain potential tumor-promoting growth hormones that are fed to cow to improve their milk production. The dairy industry uses many such hormones that leave adverse effect on the human breast tissue and promote the growth of breast cancer cells and cervical cancer. A recent survey reveals that the cause of the rapidly rising rate of breast cancer in India is due to increasing consumption of dairy products. It is advised that women suspected to have breast cancer should eliminate dairy products from their diets and instead to take daily 1500 mg. calcium supplement that contains vitamin D.

Few tips to beat cancer

- **Taking much sugar** : Do you know the sugar you eat: sucrose (refined white sugar) or fructose, maltose, or dextrose (natural sugars also used as commercial sweeteners) – it all turns into blood sugar or glucose. Some alternative practitioners believe that cancer cells rely on a metabolic process that is driven by glucose. It is advised that women suffering from a breast cancer should ban taking sugar and drinking much fruit juices.

- **Distilled water** : Drink water distilled by home water distiller as the distillation process applied by the distilled water manufacturers usually remove all possible carcinogens from your drinking water.
- **Drinking** : Alcohol is a carcinogen. Having drinks increases risk of developing breast cancer. The alcohol increases a tumor's growth rate. If you have been diagnosed with breast cancer, avoid drinking.
- **Smoking** : More than 30% of cancers are caused by inhaling tobacco, which is loaded with carcinogens. Tobacco creates free radical, unstable molecules that can damage DNA and trigger cancer. It burns up antioxidant vitamins such as vitamin C, which is cancer protective and erodes immune system. If you are a smoker, and have been diagnosed with breast cancer, quit smoking immediately, otherwise your cancer is more likely to spread.
- **Exercise** : Cancer thrives in an oxygen-poor environment. Mild exercise fights cancer. The breast cancer patients over 40 should not undertake exercise regularly and should be checked for cardiovascular risk factors. If the circulatory system of the patient is normal, she should start a walking program. Start with light walking, then gradually increase the pace and distance.
- **Stress reduction** : Mental stress with worried, overloaded mind weakens the immune system. A mental ease, calm and quiet mind, strengthens immune system and helps to resist cancer. The following ways help to reduce mental stress :
  1. Take a hot shower.
  2. Listen to calming music.
  3. Mediate, repeating a single thought.
  4. Be sexually intimate, either by having intercourse or just hugging and cuddling.
- **Genistein** : Studies show that eating more soy products may lower your risk of cancer. The most powerful anti-cancer substance in soy products is genistein, which helps kill cancer

cells, stop a tumor to spread through the body and keep a tumor away from growing blood vessels.

Soy contains natural estrogen, which balances out the excess estrogen in the body, helping to decrease breast pain and lumpiness.

- **Food** : High-fat diets raise estrogen levels in the body, whereas excess estrogen causes the build up of fluid and cellular tissue in the breast that leads to lumps and pain in the breast. On the other hand fiber escorts excess estrogen out of the body. Most vegetables (such as cabbage, kail, broccoli, sprouts and turnips) and fruits are rich in fiber as are whole grains and beans. High fiber contain indole-3-carbinol – a chemical that helps block estrogen from binding to breast tissue. The hormone progesterone may help balance the receptors in the breasts so that the large quantities can't be absorbed. Massage creams that contain real progesterone are available in the market. Massage the cream into your breasts, abdomen and thighs following the dosage recommend on the label or by your doctor (these creams sometime have side effect). It takes time for progesterone to decrease breast lumps and pain.
- **Caffeine** : Methylxanthine - a chemical in coffee and other sources of caffeine stretch blood vessels, irritate nerves and increase breast tenderness. Women suffering from breast cancer should decrease their caffeine intake from sources such as coffee, tea, cola, chocolate etc. in the week before their periods.
- **Massage** : A gentle massage can help improve circulation to the breasts and decrease pain. Make small, gentle, circular motions over the entire surface of the breasts, which decreases pain in the breasts. When you feel a cyst or a lump, massage gently around it, but never so hard that you irritate the tissue or cause any pain.

Is it breast cancer? : Although a malignancy may develop in any part of the breast, the majority of cancers occur in either the upper portion of the breast, toward the shoulder, or else close to the nipple. Breast cancer may occur at any time of life, but it is much more common between the age 35 and 65. After 65 the breast cancer is rare. When the cancer is present in the breast, there is usually one hard single lump, which may be fixed to the surrounding tissues. Usually there is no pain. In few cases there may be slight bloody discharge from the nipple, but this is not common. A slight discharge may also occur in some benign tumors. In any case, it is always wise to have the tumor removed by surgery.

Mammography : The technique of breast radiography is known as Mammography. The technique has three radiographic methods: film mammography, film screen mammography and Xero-mammography. Film and film screen mammography is based on the principles of soft-tissue radiography. Xero-mammography is an electrostatic process rather than a chemical process. The principles of Xerography and its applications in breast examination have been well described basically as a charged selenium plate is discharged by X-radiation in proportion to the amount of radiation reaching the plate. The Xero-radiographic image has several characteristics, such as has a wide recording latitude enabling the skin, nipple, base of breast and even chest wall be seen equally clearly on a single image.

Appearance of breast lesions

1. **Cysts** : Give rise to smooth, well-defined, anechoic, transonic lesions with distal enhancement and refractive edge shadowing
2. **Fibro-adenoma** : Presents a smooth rounded or lobulated lesion with homogeneous or varying echo levels sometimes associated with posterior enhancement. There are varying degrees of attenuation if coarse calcifications are present.
3. **Carcinomas** : Usually possess well-defined, irregular anterior and lateral margins but a poorly defined posterior margin, which becomes more obvious with increasing intensity of the ultrasound. A distal shadow is seen as a result of attenuation of the beam. The malignant mass shows low-level echoes as compared with normal breast tissues. Circumscribed cancers (usually of the colloid or medullary variety), however, may display a homogeneous echo pattern and posterior enhancement, thus stimulating lesions. These lesions are difficult to diagnose radio-graphically.

Miscellaneous Breast lesions : These include :

- **Carcinoma of male breasts** : Cancers of the male breast shows identical features to those of the female breast. Micro-calcification is not as common, however, an smooth circumscribed carcinoma are relatively more common in the male.

- **Paget's disease of the nipple** : The condition is usually associated with breast cancer. Radio-logically, there may be an irregular mass with or without micro-calcification or micro-calcification may be the only sign of malignancy.
- **Cysto-sarcoma Phylloides** : This is a cystic, fleshy tumor. It is usually a large, smooth, dense, lobulated lesion, which may contain coarse, irregular, flake-like calcification.
- **Fibro-adenosis (fibrocystic disease; mammary dysplasia)** : This benign condition is extremely common and is related to the menstrual cycle, usually combined with a palpable nodularity or thickening and tenderness of breast tissues. The symptoms may be associated with any radiology appearance of the breast including completely fatty glandular breasts with or without cysts or associated prominent ducts.
- **Sclerosing adenosis (lobular sclerosis, lobular fibrosis)** : It may present as a hard mass with or without associated breast discomforts.
- **Duct ectasia (secretory disease, periductal mastitis, plasma cell mastitis)** : This is an idiopathic inflammatory condition of the breast ducts. The condition followed by inflammation may present with nipple discharge at varying appearances, including serous milky and blood stained discharge. A painful lump is common. Radio-logically, the ducts are enlarged and sometimes trans-radiant due to increased fat content. The condition may give rise to fat necrosis.
- **Gynaecomastia** : In the normal male breast the mammogram shows a small faint linear density beneath the nipple. A low density opacity of varying size is seen. In this condition its differentiation from cancer of the male breast and its associations with systemic disease.
- **Galactograph** : A serious blood stained nipple discharge. It occurs frequently with duct ectasia and during the later stages of pregnancy and lactation. Greenish and the brownish nipple discharge are usually associated with duct ectasia and cystic disease. The condition should be thoroughly investigated even in the absence of palpable abnormality. This may lead to breast cancer.
- **Pneumocystography** : A breast cyst with the main indication of blood stained fluid on aspiration of a cyst. This indicates the presence of an intra-cystic papilloma or carcinoma.

Pneumocystography demonstrates the presence, position and extent of an intracystic tumor and usually a diagnosis of benign or malignant tumor can be made.

- **Indications of Mammography** : The use of mammography is in the investigation of symptomatic patients as a complementary method to clinical examination. Its clinical diagnosis to confirm patients with a palpable lesion either in the same breast or in the opposite breast. It is a useful complementary method of examination in patients with vague breasts symptoms, eczema of the nipple or nodular breasts. Accurate assessment of the response of the primary breast cancer is possible in cases treated with radiography or chemotherapy. Finally unsuspected cancers of the breast may be found on screening.

A Mammography and other Tests ?

Women feel hesitant about going for a mammogram. Remember, a check up is the only thing that stands between timely intervention and fatal disease to save your life.

What is mammography? : It is a technique of taking soft tissue X-rays. Two films of each breast are taken after adequate compression under an acrylic sheet by a radiographic. A mammography test must be conducted if you:

- Have pain, discharge or a lump in the breast.
- Would like to have a routine screening of your breasts.
- Have a family history of breast cancer.
- Are undergoing hormone replacement therapy (HRT).
- Feel a lump during self-examination or felt by a doctor during a routine examination.

A mammogram should be done under the advice of a doctor. It must be done after the month's menstrual cycle. An examination of breasts and the armpits is conducted during mammogram test. A mammography test is done in standing position with your breast resting on a flat platform. The breast is placed on the platform and flattened slightly for a short period of time by an adjustable acrylic sheet. The presence of a tumor or a cyst (if any) will be indicated. It will also indicate abnormal distortion of the internal structure of the breast.

How to prepare for mammogram? : You must have mammogram test when your breasts are least tender to lessen the discomfort from the X-ray: avoiding the week before your menstrual period. Go dressed for the examination wearing a two-piece outfit, preferably a skirt and blouse or a two-piece suit so that you may remove only your top when having examination. Do not apply a deodorant, a lotion or powder under your arms or near the breasts, which may hamper the performance of test. You must also carry the copies of your earlier mammography tests (if conducted in past) and show to the radiologist so that he may study the change (if any).

In case you are feeling uncomfortable due to pain while going for a test, take normal pain killer tablets with you or have in the beginning of the day before your mammogram. Cut down on caffeine and salt one to two weeks before a mammogram. Practice deep-breathe or meditation during the procedure. Deviate your intention away from the pain during the test. Relax muscles completely during the test and don't feel tensed. Try to speak up if you are feeling severe pain.

In case of a incorrect mammography technique or mammography limitations, the following errors may arise:

- Solid and cystic masses cannot be differentiated.
- Intra-cystic lesions cannot be diagnosed.
- Dense fibro-glandular parenchyma (loosely packed tissues) in young breasts may obscures masses.
- Benign lumps may appear malignant as a result of fibro-cystic mastitis, which may mask the margins of a lump.
- Overlapping structures may limit complete visualization of a mass.
- Evaluation of a tender breast is difficult and usually inadequate.

Dimensional Echocardiography

This test is conducted when a woman is prone to cardiac problems or suffering from valve lesions. It checks the structure of the heart (the walls, chambers, valves, aorta, pulmonary artery and the blood flow gradients). This test is conducted lying on the back, then turned to your left side. The contact jelly is applied to facilitate the procedure, followed by application of probes to the chest. There should be no pain or discomfort during the test. The result will show any abnormality in the structure of the heart and its parts. It will also diagnose the congenital heart disease, abnormalities of the pumping action of the heart, movements of heart muscles and the movement of the heart valves.

Electrocardiogram

This is a test to assess the electrical conductivity of the heart and its variations by a radiologist at the chest area on the advise of a doctor when the patients feel pain, discomfort or palpitations. This test is recommended before a major operation. The patient is asked to lie flat on the back, then applied contact gel and probes to the both hands, legs and the chest area for five to ten minutes. The result shows heart blocks and electrolyte abnormalities to help in the diagnosis of coronary artery disease, angina, thickening of heart muscle, abnormal heart rhythms and conduction defects of the heart.

PAP smear

PAP smear is a clinical examination of the cervix, followed by scraping of the cervical cells. In this examination no solution has to be applied, which may alter the state of the cervical cells. Don't panic if your doctor advises for a PAP Test, you could be just in time to prevent cancer. The test will be carried out by a gynecologist as a part of the routine check up in case of :

- Menstrual complaints.
- If there is constant discharge from the vagina.
- If you bleed after intercourse.
- If your doctor thinks your cervix is unhealthy.
- There are lesions and growths on the cervix.
- You are sexually very active.

Remember, not to indulge in sexual intercourse for 24 hours prior to the smear. Do not douche or use a vaginal pessary for 48 hours prior to the procedure. The cervix, and sometimes the vagina or uterine cavity will be checked during the test. The gynecologist checks the cervix, the vagina and the uterus cavity. Lie down on your back with your knees flexed and spread apart during examination. The gynecologist inserts the speculum or brush inside and a smear is taken out with the help of spatula, which is then spread on a slide. The examination is done with the fingers. There is usually no pain or discomfort while conducting this test. The result shows early detection of cancerous changes in the cells of cervix, vagina and endometrial cavity.

Don't douche if you are going to have a examination, even if you are embarrassed by vaginal odour. Douching often eliminates the evidence that is necessary to make a diagnosis, such as vaginal discharge that could indicate infection.

Dilation and Curettage Test

This a minor surgical test carried out by a gynecologist under anesthesia. The cervix is dilated by inserting progressively thicker dilators to make room for the insertion of the curette. This test is done to diagnose the cause of irregular uterine bleeding, post-menopausal bleeding, and to confirm cancer of the uterus, endometritis, infertility. Ashermann's syndrome and removal of retained products from the uterine cavity. Do not eat anything for minimum six hours before the test. In this test, the uterine cavity and the endocervical canal are examined.

The patient lies on back with knees flexed and legs spread apart. To carry out this examination, after the dilation (enlargement of cervical canal to allow the curette inside) the inner lining of the uterus cavity is scrapped with the curette and the material removed is sent for microscopic examination. The scrapping should be done under general anesthesia as there would be dragging ache in the lower abdomen. After the process there may be bleeding for a couple of days and a mild pain in the lower abdomen.

Pelvis Sonography

Sonography – a painless procedure to examine the uterus, ovaries, cervix and bladder relies on the sound waves to draw a visual picture with the help of an in-built computer. The process is safe during pregnancy, as it doesn't include radiation. A sonography must be done in case of the following conditions :

- Lower abdominal pain.
- Menstrual disorder.
- Infertility.
- Excessive vaginal discharge.
- Routine screening.
- To diagnose multiple pregnancy.
- To observe the growth of fetus.
- To ascertain the position of the placenta.

- To detect that no remains of the placenta after childbirth has been left in the uterus.
- To detect external abnormalities of the fetus.

Make sure that your bladder is full at the time of sonography test, as the bladder pushes the intestines up to facilitate viewing of the relevant parts. Do not pass urine for at least two hours before the test and drink as much water as you can. A thorough check up of the uterus, ovaries, cervix and bladder can be conducted by sonography. To sonography, apply contact jelly and move a sensor probe over the lower abdomen Sonography of the upper abdomen is done using sound waves to form a visual picture of the organs of the upper abdomen. It should be done when you suffer from :

- Abdominal pain.
- Prolonged fever.
- Inexplicable weight loss.
- To diagnose conditions related to the liver, gall bladder, pancreas, spleen, kidneys and lymph glands.

Do not eat food for at least three hours prior to the sonography. Sonography is a painless procedure, in which contact jelly is applied over the area and a transducer is moved over the abdomen and the organs to be viewed with the help of sound waves.

Endoscopy

It is a procedure to visualize internal parts of the body through endoscopes. Endoscopy is used to examine a variety of procedures as described below :

1. Gastroscopy : for the stomach.
2. Duedonoscopy : for the duodenum.
3. Calposcopy : for the colon or large bowel.
4. Laproscopy : for the abdomen.

It is possible to have a look at almost every organ of the body with the help of fiber-optics by endoscopy.

Laproscopy

In this procedure, with the help of introduction of a telescope into the abdomen, the intra-abdomen and pelvic structures can be viewed by the gynecologist to check disorders of abdomen, uterus, tubes, ovaries and surrounding pelvic peritoneum intestines and diagnose the following :

- Infertility in women.
- Endometriosis.
- Chronic pelvic pain.
- Ectopic pregnancy.
- Genital tuberculosis.
- Pelvic inflammatory disease.
- The beginning of ovarian cancer.
- To evaluate the response to the treatment.
- Tubal ligation (family planning operation).
- Tubal reconstructive surgery.
- Cauterization of endometriotic patches.
- The removal of the fallopian tubes, ovaries, ovarian cysts, intra uterine contraceptive devices (IUCD) lost in the abdominal cavity and fibroids.

For the examination the patient should lie on back with knees flexed and legs apart. Under general anesthesia, a small (about one centimeter) cut is made below the umbilicus, the abdominal cavity is filled with carbon dioxide gas and a telescope is introduced. A light source is connected to the telescope in order to make it possible to see the intra-abdominal organs. In case of emergency, surgery is carried out at the same time.

Hysteroscopy

In this procedure, a telescope is introduced into the uterine cavity after dilation of the cervix to make room for this introduction. The following examinations are carried out by the gynecologist :

- When the threads of Intra uterine contraceptive devices are not visible but are known to be within the uterine cavity.
- For removal of fibroids.
- For tubal ligation by blocking the tubal openings for family planning.
- To check uterine cavity.

The patient should lie on the back with knees flexed and legs apart. Under local or general anesthesia, a direct visualization of the uterine cavity lining and a scraping is removed for biopsy.

Calposcopy

This is a direct visualization of the outside of the cervix (exocervix) under microscopic examination. Get it done, if the PAP smear is abnormal or the cervix seems unhealthy or where lesions on the cervix cannot be pinpointed. In this procedure, lie on the back with knees flexed and legs apart. The calposcope is focused on the cervix to enable visualization. The abnormal area is marked out and acetic acid solution (1%) is put on the cervix and the junction of the aceto-white and non-white area is marked out. The treatment should be done by an experienced gynecologist.

10

Allergies, Liver & Kidney Disorders

Allergy - Common female disease among women

Allergy is a state of abnormal sensitivity to a substance or substances that ordinarily cause little or no irritation. Almost anything that we touch, swallow or inhale may cause an allergy response. Substances that produce allergies are caused allergens. Among the most common allergens include pollen of trees, grasses, dust, animal hairs, certain foods, drugs, dyes, cosmetics (especially perfumes), chemicals, antitoxins etc.

Symptoms : The most common symptoms of an allergy are sneezing, paroxysms, nasal stuffiness, wheezing, shortness of breath, itching of the skin, swelling, vomiting, diarrhea, abdominal cramps, headaches, severe rashes and redness and other symptoms.

The effects : Serious complications may be avoided by treating allergies in their early stages. The most serious allergic diseases are the following :

- **Hay fever** : It is a respiratory allergy caused by sensitivity to pollens or molds or both. The main symptoms of hay fever include: inflamed itchy skin, weepy eyes, clogged or runny nose. Infections of the sinuses are commonly associated with hay fever. Asthma may also develop in winters. Hay fever get into the body when inhaled pollens or molds. Hay fever is not contagious, but the tendency is definitely inherited. Sometimes, year-round condition exists, which is also known as allergic rhinites with symptoms, such as the itchy, watery eyes, sneezing, and running nose conditions throughout the year.

- **Perennial allergic rhinitis (Vasomotor rhinitis)** : There are three methods of treatment :
  1. Coseasonal method.
  2. Preseasonal method.
  3. Perennial method.

Consult a doctor in case of allergic reaction. There are medicines to bring about prompt relief from the reaction.

- **Bronchial asthma** : It is a common allergen, such as pollen, mold spores, house dust, animal hair, foods or drugs. Asthmatic attacks usually occur in the early morning hours with common symptoms, such as wheezing, suffocation, hard dry cough and difficulty to expel air from the lungs. There is often swelling in the mucous membranes of the bronchial tubes and in smaller bronchioles within the lungs. The following treatments for asthma are suggested :
  1. Finding an allergen that has caused asthma.
  2. Giving steroid medications.
  3. To relieve acute attacks, injections of adrenalin or epinephrine are given.
  4. The inhalation of special medications to relieve bronchial spasm.
- **Eczema (dermatitis)** : It is a skin allergy often occurring in infants and generally caused by food sensitivity. Consult doctor in case of such allergic reaction.

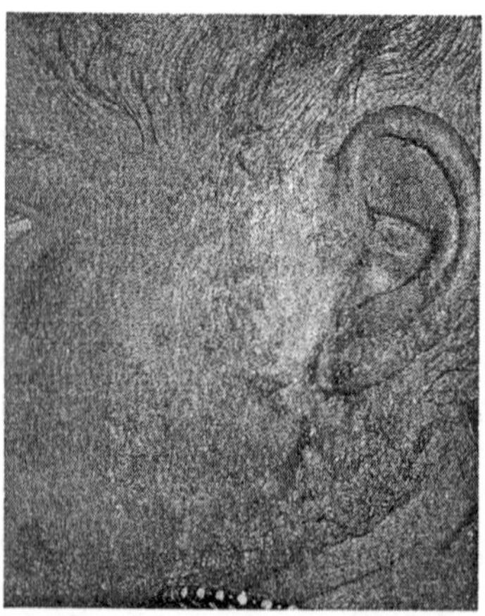

It is caused by exposing the skin to a substance, to which the patient is hyper-sensitive. The symptoms of dermatitis are itching and redness of the skin with swelling, blisters, oozing, crusting and scaling. The allergy may occur at one place or the entire body. The common substances that may cause dermatitis are chemicals, plant oils, cosmetics, mouthwashes, medicines, clothing, plastics, dyes etc.

- **Hives (urticaria)** : This skin allergy is characterized by wheals of various sizes and number on the skin surface. These wheals are swellings, which may cause intense itching, usually occurring at the lips, face, tongue, throat, eyelids, ears or any other part of the body. Hives are generally caused by an allergy to a food or a drug. Fish, seafood, highly seasoned foods and aspirin are the most frequent causes. Itching is the most distressing symptom.
- **Contact dermatitis** : Chemicals, plant oils, cosmetics, deodorants, mouthwashes, medicines, clothing, plastics, dyes etc. are the substances to cause contact dermatitis. The appropriate treatment is to give antihistaminic drugs and application of medication to relieve skin irritation. Frequently, it is necessary to resort to the use of steroid, such as cortisone.
- **Migraine and food allergy** : Disorder of the stomach and intestines due to foods to which the individual is sensitive is caused the digestive allergy. Belching, nausea, vomiting, abdominal pain, constipation, diarrhea and sores in the mouth are the prominent symptoms of this allergy. The allergic reaction may be immediately, even within few minutes or delayed for hours after food has been eaten. The treatment includes the following :
    1. The elimination of offending substances.
    2. Giving antihistaminic or other drugs to relieve the attack.
- **Insect allergy** : A person can be allergic to the bites of bees, hornets, wasps and yellow jackets. The persons can be treated prophylactically; and can be tested with the extracts of the insects and then hyposensitized with appropriate extract. Various patent extracts are now available to treat the allergy instead of extracts of a particular insect.
- **Physical Allergy** : An abnormal reaction caused by some physical agent, such as heat, cold, light or mechanical irritation.

The reaction is usually of two types: the contact reactions and the reflex reactions.

1. The contact reactions : occur at the sight of contact with physical agent.
2. The reflex-like reactions may be generalized or developed in remote tissues of the body.

To treat a physical allergy, the following measures are suggested :

1. Expose the patient to a small degree of heat or cold or other irritant for some time daily.
2. Daily bath (cold or hot, according to season).
3. Application of antihistaminic drugs to bring about desensitization.

Anemia

Iron-deficiency anemia very common in women is easy to treat, which causes decline in energy level in the body. Four out of ten women are generally seen suffering from iron deficiency with the following symptoms :

1. They are pale complexioned and feeling cold much of the time.
2. Their menstrual flow soak a tampon or sanitary pad every hour and their menstrual period lasts for more than a week, suffering from menorrhagia-an excessively heavy or long menstrual flow. Heavy bleeding during periods must be reported to the doctor immediately.
3. In case there is rectal bleeding; must see a doctor.

The following precautions should be taken to correct iron deficiency :

- Improve your diet and lifestyle. Have iron-rich foods.
- Vitamin C enhances absorption and helps the body to absorb the non-heme iron in plant foods. Alternately take a supplement of 1,000 to 2,000 milligrams of vitamin C with each meal.
- Cut back to alcohol and sugar. Beer, wine and other alcoholic beverages, which deplete the body of B-complex vitamins and some minerals that can worsen anemia. Reduce your sugar intake as well.

Drug Allergy

The patient suffering from drug allergy must find out the cause of allergy. By avoiding the substances that cause an allergic reaction can be prevented. Most allergists believe that the tendency to develop the disease, rather than the disease itself is inherited. A child whose parents are allergic is much more likely to develop an allergy than one whose parents are not allergic. Most of the allergies are rarely fatal. However, allergy due to a drug may prove fatal. Allergies are not over contagious, and are not transmitted from person to person by contact. To conduct an allergic test, the serum obtained from the blood of patient is injected into several sites in the skin of a non-allergic individual and tests are done.

Bladder Infections

You should see a doctor immediately :

- If you have blood in your urine.
- A fever that doesn't go away.
- A fever and pain near one or both kidneys.

You may be suffering from kidney infection and you may need a antibiotic treatment (in consultation with doctor). Any one with recurrent bladder infections should see a doctor for a thorough check up to detect possible structural problems, such as narrowing of the urethra, the tube that carries urine out of the bladder that can be causing the infections. Women who have recurrent bladder infections should be evaluated for hormone imbalance, which can also cause the problem.

Treatment for bladder infection :

- Vitamin C, Vitamin A and bioflavonoids strengthen the inner surface of the bladder, making it harder for the bacteria to stick.
- The mineral Zinc strengthens the immune system, helping it fight off the infection. A daily dose 30 mg. is recommended during infection.
- The herb dandelion is a powerful diuretic that increases the flow of urine to help flush out bacteria and strengthen the immune system.
- Honeymoon cystitis is a serious bladder infection that occurs after frequent intercourse. An homeopathy remedy

'Staphysagria' can help clear it up. You may consult a homeopathy doctor for the treatment.

- Lie on a slant board and start rubbing your tummy just above the pubic bone. The massage takes weight off the bladder and improves bladder circulation. It also stimulates urine flow. Do the massage for 10-15 minutes once a day.

Chronic Pain

They are common among women. There are dozens of different conditions that cause chronic pain, including arthritis, chronic headaches, back pain, fibromyalgia and repetitive strain injury. A doctor's check up is necessary for the treatment. The usual treatments are the following :

- The natural substance 5-hydroxytryptophan (5-HTP) increases serotonin levels (neurotransmitter-brain chemical) to eliminate the pain of fibromyalgia, migraine, headaches and arthritis. A daily dose up to 200 mg. is recommended.
- Vitamin B6 helps clear up chronic pain and chronic pain syndromes.
- Spice turmeric helps to reduce joint pain and swelling, stiffness and chronic pain of arthritis without the side-effect.
- Bromelain is a proteolytic enzyme - a substance that digest proteins and eliminates small blood clots.
- Inadequate levels of zinc in the body can cause chronic pain and inflammation. For chronic pain a daily dose of 500 mg. is recommended.

Diabetes

Diabetes occurs because the immune system attacks and kills the cells of the pancreas, the organs that produces the hormone insulin, which ushers blood sugar (glucose) out of the blood stream and into the cells of the body. To make up for the shortage of insulin, the diabetics of minute (Type I) disease must take insulin injections (with the recommendation of doctor). About 5-10% diabetics have type I disease (also called juvenile diabetes). It can occur at any age (even in teenage). The main symptoms of Type I diabetes are the following :

- Frequent urination.
- Increased appetite and thirst.

- Fatigue.
- Heavy weight loss.
- Decreased consciousness (possible leading to coma).
- In case of severe symptoms, consult a doctor promptly.

The following treatments should be taken :

- Avoid cow's milk.
- Gluten is a protein found in wheat, rye, oats, barley and other grains. Remove the gluten from the diet (especially, in case of child patient).
- Avoid all foods containing the grains mentioned above.
- Exercise for 30-40 minutes at least three to four times a week to cut insulin needs by 20-25%. Aerobic exercise, brisk walking or jogging help a lot.

Type II diabetes is a serious illness that should always be monitored by a doctor. Its symptoms include :

- Increased thirst.
- Increased urination.
- Increased appetite.
- Dry mouth.
- Vomiting.
- Diarrhea.
- Blurred vision.
- Rapid or irregular heartbeat.
- Dizziness.
- Unintentional weight loss.
- Recurrent urinary tract infections.

The following precautions/treatments should be undertaken :

- Reduce sugar intake.
- Get a variety of whole foods and try to eat every color each day.
- Supplements containing essential fatty acids, such as flaxseed oil can help repair the cellular damage caused by consuming too much sugar.
- Exercise twice a day, every day.

Kidney Stones

Kidney stones can be caused by a number of serious diseases. Nearly 70 to 80% of kidney stones are composed of calcium oxalate crystals, while another about 10% are made of uric acid crystals. You need to know the type of stone you have, because each type requires different preventive approach. To analyze the sediment in your urine, you must know whether it contains traces of either calcium oxalate or uric acid crystals, and choose the treatment that is right for you. You must see your doctor immediately if you have an attack of kidney stone :

- Accompanied by severe pain.
- The pain does not relieve by drinking large amounts of fluids.
- There is blood in your urine.
- You have fever accompanied by pain.
- You have pain near the kidneys, located in your lower back near the end of the rib cage.
- You are unable to pass urine.

11
Genital Diseases

There are many diseases related to female genital organs, but some of the serious ones concerning vulva, vagina and the cervix are described in this chapter.

Vulvar diseases

1. Bartholin's glands

A vulvar disease, causing abscesses or cysts due to infection in one or both Bartholin glands, resulting in swelling and or abscess formation. Usually, the pain occurs during reproductive years.

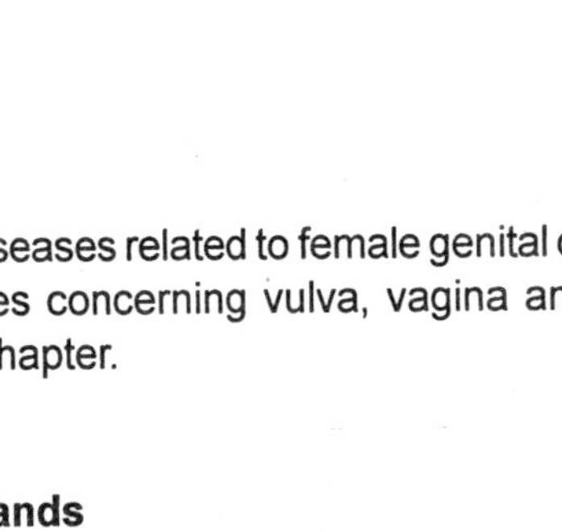

Abscess of Bartholin's gland

The signs and symptoms include cystic painful swelling of labia on vulva diagnosed by cellulites, nacrotizing fascitis, masonephric cysts of the vagina, lipomas, fibromas, hernias, hydrocele, neurofibroma and sebaceous cyst.

To prevent the disease, avoid or reduce exposure to sexually transmitted disease (STD) and vulvar trauma. Generally, clear or yellow or blue color smooth smaller cysts are seen at the base of the labia majora.

2. Contact vulvitis

A vulvar irritation caused by contact with an irritation or allergan (usually during reproductive or menopausal years) caused by feminine unhygiene, effect of deodorants and use of soaps, tight-fitting and synthetic under-garments, tampons or pads, perfumes, scented toilet paper, laundry soap, latex condoms, lubricants, topical contraceptives, sexual aids, semen remaining in vagina and soiling of vulva by urine or faces.

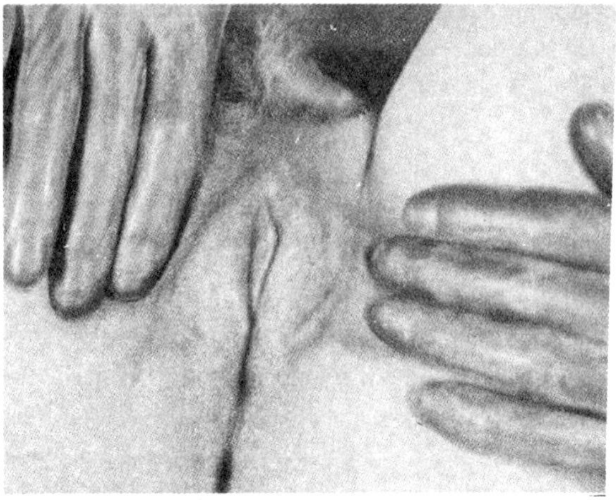

The signs and symptoms include severe dermatitis of vulva and reddening of vulvar skin accompanied by itching or burning.

Diagnostic approach: include vulvar dermatitis, atrophic vulvitis, vulvar dystrophy, pinworms, psoriasis, seborrheic dermatitis, neuro-dermatitis, impetigo, hidradenitis suppurative and vaginal secretions. Apply Eucerine crine to reduce itching, which rehydrate the skin.

3. Dysareunia insertional

Pain occurs with the sexual penetration, which may lead to severe vaginal spasm that inter-fere with penetration. An average 15% women during the reproductive age suffer from it. It is caused due to congenital factors, systitis, hermorrhoid's, insufficient foreplay, inadequate lubrication, phobias, pelvis muscle spasm, scarring due to episiotomy, surgical repairs, vulvitis, proctitis trauma, urethral diverticula, urethral syndrome, urethritis, vaginismus, herpes vulvitis and vestibolitis.

Signs and symptoms include burning or pinching discomfort generally localized to the vulva, perineum or outer portion of vagina.

Treatment includes vaginal lubrication, pelvic relaxation exercises, modified sexual techniques to reduce pain during intercourse and improved position during intercourse.

4. Female circumcision

Removal of part or external genital organs including labia majora, labia minora and/or clitoris.

The signs and symptoms are the following :

1. Scarring and deformity of the external genitalia structures.
2. Obstruction to result in amenorrhea or dysmenorrhea.
3. Dyspareunia/orgasmic dysfunction/libidinal dysfunction.

The disorder can be diagnosed by burn injuries, inter-sex conditions and imperforate hymen.

Treatment include surgical opening of fused/scarred genital tissues, menstruation hygiene and episiotomy required at the time of childbirth.

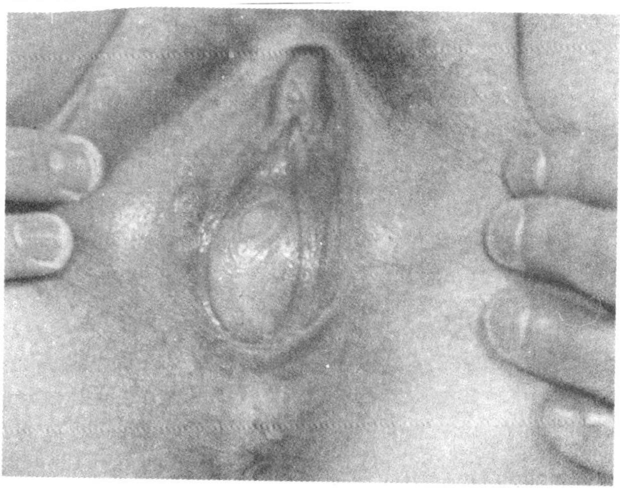

Possible complications are bleeding, infection, urinary retention, pain, sexual dysfunction, urinary-tract infections, retrograde menses and pelvic inflammatory diseases.

5. Hidradenitis suppurative

A chronic, unrelenting, refractory infection of the skin and subcutaneous tissues, which causes inflammation of aprocrine glands with sinus and abscess formation involving axilla, vulva and perineum usually during reproductive (not before puberty).

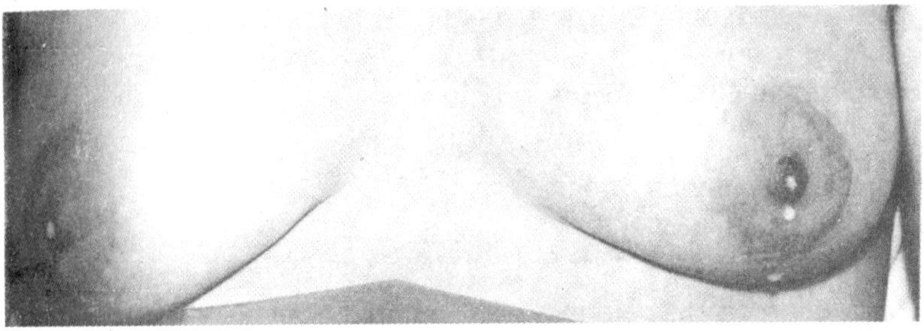

Signs and symptoms include recurrent and chronic inflammation on labia with pain and foul smelling discharge or sometimes formation of abscess. It may be diagnosed by sexual transmitted disease.

The disorder may cause conditions such as dysparenia and Volvodynia to be diagnosed by a biopsy. It may cause inflammation of aprocrine glands, cystic dilation, inspissation of keralin material and causes formation of abscesses.

General measures for the treatment of this disease include perinal hygiene, sitz's bath administering antibiotics, topical steroids, oral contraceptives and use of anti-androgens and isotretinoin. Avoid formation of scarring, abscesses, infection and sexual dysfunction.

6. Hymenal stenosis

Thickening or narrowing of hymenal opening resulting difficulty in intercourse caused by congenital narrowing of the hymen or scarring after surgery or trauma. It can be diagnosed by vulvar vestibulatis, vaginismus and vulvitis.

Evaluation, gentle digital dilation and surgical excision are general measures to treat this disease. If not timely treated, it may cause complication of sexual dysfunction.

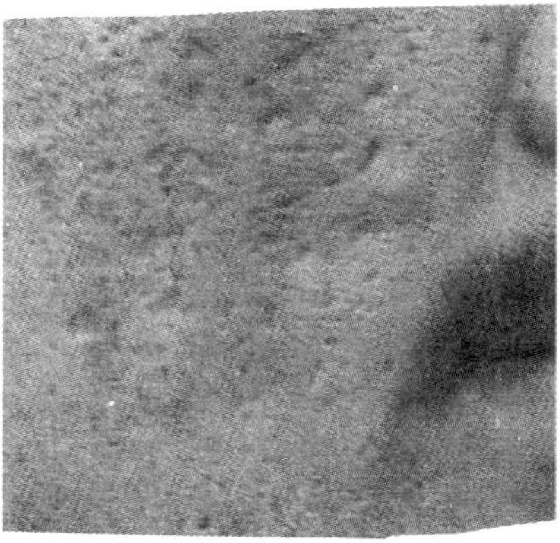

7. Hyper-plastic vulvar dystrophy

Thickening of vulvar skin over the labia majora, outer aspects of labia minora and clitorial areas with inflammation.

The signs and symptoms of disease include vulvar itching, white appearance of vulva, fissuring and excoriations. The disease can be diagnosed by vulvar cancer, chronic mycotic vulvitis, psoriasis, vulvar pruritis and dyspareunia.

To treat the disease, perineal hygiene, stress reduction, sitz bath, reducing candidiasis or contact allergy are the general measures. The following precautions should be taken :

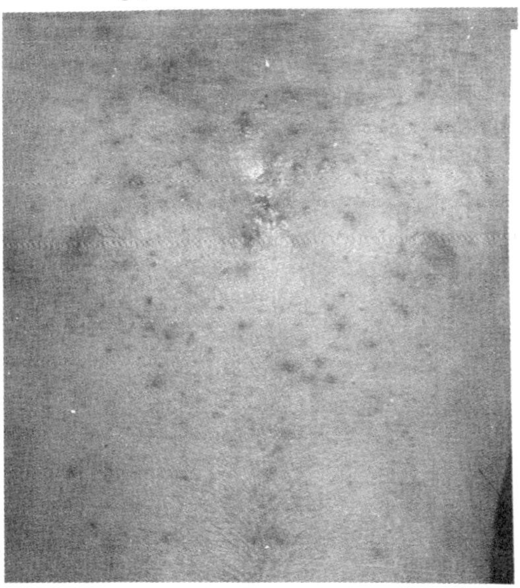

1. Wear white gloves during night to avoid tissue danger due to scratching.

2. Avoid itch/ rash scratch.
3. Use perineal soothing agent to reduce itching.
4. Vulvar cancer can be a possible complication, if not treated properly.

8. Imperforate hymen

It results from abdomenalities in the development of canalization of mullerian ducts.

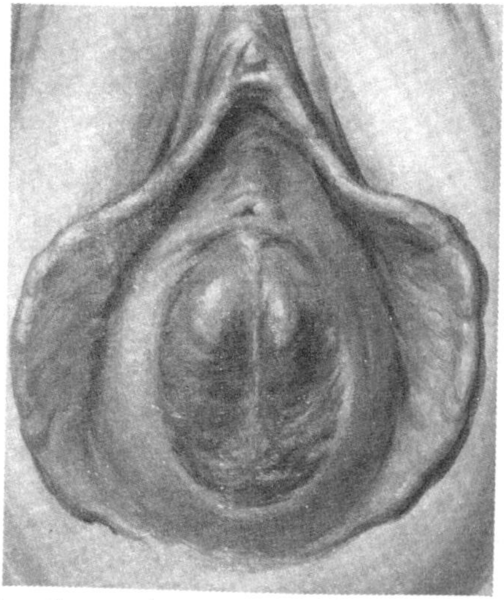

Vaginal obstructions, primary amenorrhoea, abdominal pain and hematocolpos are few signs and symptoms of the diseases, which can be diagnosed by vaginal agenesis and hermaphroditism (to be detected by ultra-sonography of the upper genital tract).

To treat this disorder, incision of hymenal membrane and drainage of vaginal canal are important measures. If not treated timely, it may lead to serious complications such as hymenal scarring and narrowing after surgical excision.

9. Labial adhesions

It causes by local inflammation resulting in labial infections or irritation.

Fusion of labia majora just below the clitoris, retention of urine resulting in irritation, discharge and odour are signs and symptoms which can be diagnosed by inter-sex, female circumcision, sexual abuse, urinary tract infection and vaginal bleeding.

General measures to treat labia adhesions include perineal hygiene, sitz bath and use of topical estrogen cream. If not treated timely, complications such as vaginitis and formation of vaginal cyst may arise.

10. Lichen planus

The causes of this disease are unknown.

Red erosion and ulceration of vulva, oral lesion in labia minora and post-coital bleeding are common signs and symptoms, which can be diagnosed by amebiasis, behcet's syndrome, candidiasis, dermatophyte infection, lichen sclerosus, neurodermatitis, vulvitis and psoriasis.

To treat the diseases, measures such as evaluation, local cleansing, antipruritis, retinoids griseofulvin and surgery are adopted. If not treated properly there is possibility of formation of vulvar lesion.

11. Lichen sclerosus

A chronic condition of vulvar skin with inflammation, generally during late reproductive to early menopausal.

Signs and symptoms of disease include intense itching, scratch marks or fissures extending around the anus.

The diagnostic approaches are hyper-plastic vulvar dystrophy, scleroderma, vitiligo, preget's disease, vulvar candidiasis and carcinoma.

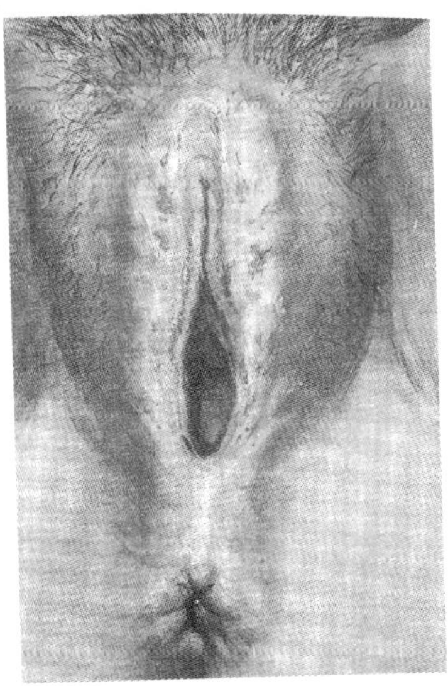

General measures to treat this disease are perinal hygiene, cool Sitz Bath, moist soaks, wearing loose fitting clothes and application of petroleum jelly. If not treated timely, complications such as vulvar cancer, scarring and narrowing of the introitus may arise.

12. Vulvar cancer

Presence of ulcer and lesions mostly in the age group of 60 to 70.

Itching, irritation, cracking and bleeding of vulva are the common signs and symptoms of disease. To detect, biopsy of suspicious lesion or vulvar biopsy is required. The illustrations show carcinoma of the clitoris, carcinoma of leukoplakia, sarcoma of the labium and metastatic hypermephroma.

13. Vulvar hematoma

Swelling of one or both labia because of interstitial bleeding occurring at any age and caused by straddle injury, sexual abuse, subject to rape, water skiing, vaginal surgery, delivery of child, varicose veins of vulva and sports activities.

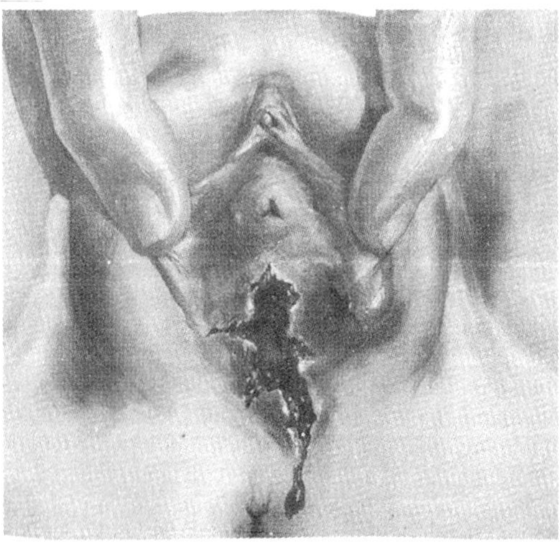

Signs and symptoms include painful swelling of one or both labia, dark blue or black discoloration of vulva and bleeding from vulva generally diagnosed by appearance of cysts or abscess, varicose veins on vulva and hydradenitis suppurative.

Measures to treat this disease are analgesis, application of ice packs and surgical drainage in case of rapidly expanding hematomas.

14. Vulvar lesions and cysts

The skin of vulva varies similar to skin elsewhere in the body. The tissues of vulva have close interactions with the fluids, hormones and microbes in the body. The skin of the vulva contains hair follicles,

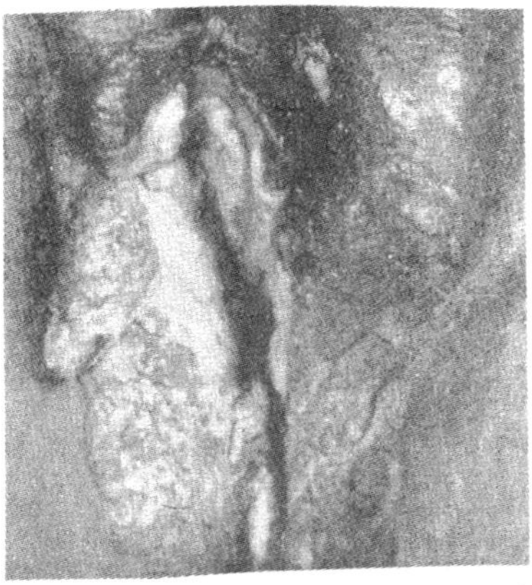

sebaceous, sweat and apocrine glands. The vulva is affected by inflammatory and dermatologic skin diseases such as atopic dermatitis, intertrigo, hidradenitis, psoriasis, seborrheic dermatitis, Fox-fordyce disease, Fifth disease, Crohn's disease, viral infections and parasites.

The signs and symptoms of disease include irritation, vaginal secretions, fleshy tumor of vulva and recurrent urinary loss. The type of lesions and cysts which appear on vulva due to folliculitis and furunculosis include herpes genitalia, tinea eruris, psoriasis, senile atrophy, kraurosis valvae, leukoplakia, lichenification, varicose veins, angioneurotic, edema, elephantiasis, diabetic, vulvitis, trichomaniasis, moniliasis, Bartholin's disease, sebaceous cysts, inclusion and canal disorders.

Vaginal Diseases

1. Cystocele/ Urethrocele

Loss of support for the anterior vagina rupture, prolapse of the urethra (urethrocele) or bladder (cystocele) is caused due to loss of normal tissue integrity as a result of trauma such as childbirth, obstetric injury, surgery etc.

The signs and symptoms include asymptomatic, pelvic pressure or heaviness, stress, urinary infections, bulging of tissue at vagina opening, urethral diverticulum, cysts, tumour or abscess, uterine prolapse and hernias.

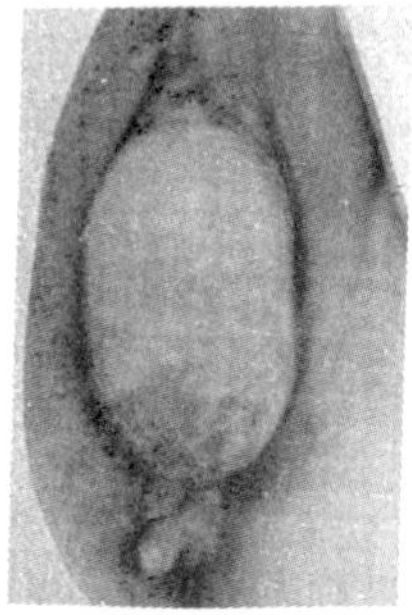

Measures, such as weight-reduction, treatment of cough (if present), topical estrogen replacement or therapy, pessary therapy, pelvic muscle exercises and surgical repair are recommended for treatment. The following precautions are necessary :

1. Avoid heavy lifting and straining.
2. Have a check on vaginal bleeding and breast cancer.

2. Enterocele

Occurs due to rupture or pro-lapse of the vaginal walls after abdominal or vaginal hysterectomy. Weight reduction and surgical repair are the main remedial measures.

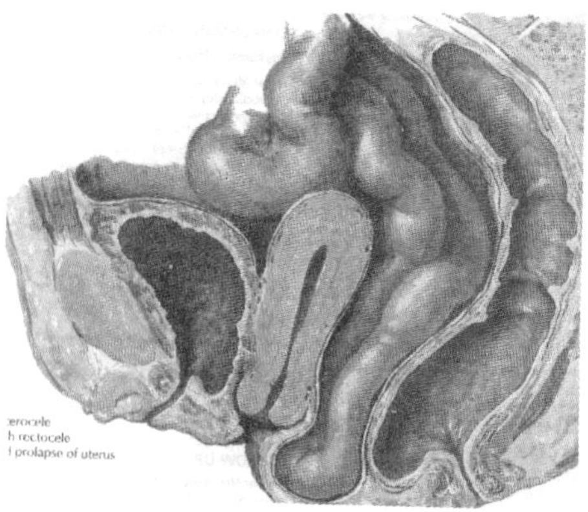

3. Rectocele

Failure of the normal support mechanism between the rectum and the vagina, which result in herniation of the posterior vaginal wall and underlying rectum into the vaginal canal as a result of childbirth, obstetric injury and surgery due to obesity, heavy lifting and intrinsic tissue weakness.

The main signs and symptoms of this disease are bulging of posterior vaginal wall and difficulty in passing stool. The disease can be diagnosed due to rectal cancer, vaginal cyst after episiotomy and uterine pro-lapse.

The measures to treat disorder are weight - loss, treatment of chronic cough (if present), systemic estrogen replacement, pessary therapy, pelvic muscle exercises and surgical repair.

4. Sarcoma botryoides

Tumor arising from cervix are usually seen on the vagina of young girls that cause vaginal bleeding and mass which resembles a cluster of grapes, urethral pro-lapse, vaginal polyp and indo-dermal sinus tumor. The treatment may be done by surgical excision.

5. Vaginal cysts

A common disorder in females from adolescence to middle reproductive years generally caused by factors e.g. episiotomy or obstetric laceration and gynecologic surgery.

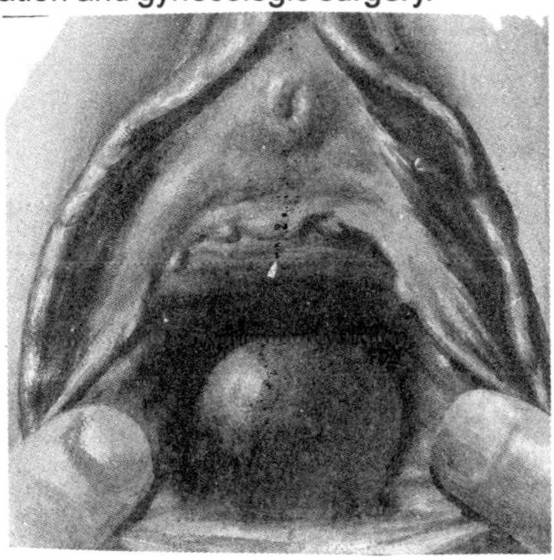

The signs and symptoms of this disorder include asymptomatic, dyspareumia and cystic mass lesions (ranging from one to five cm.) found in the lateral vaginal wall. The disease can be diagnosed by urethral diverticulum, vaginal adenosis, perirectal abscess and vaginal fibromyoma.

Surgical excision is the only reliable treatment.

6. Vaginal dryness

Loss of normal vaginal moisture results in irritation, itching or pain during intercourse. This may occur due to inadequate or inappropriate sexual stimulation, sexual phobia or pain more commonly in menopausal women.

Vaginal dryness, itching or irritation and inflamed vaginal tissues are some of the signs and symptoms, which can be diagnosed by vaginitis, vulva vestibulitis and lichen sclerosis.

Topical moisturizing, lubrication of vagina, estrogen replacement therapy, counselling regarding sexuality, foreplay and use of water soluble lubricants before intercourse are few prominent measures. If not treated properly, it may lead to vaginal lacerations, infections, vulvar excoriations and sexual dysfunction.

7. Vaginal laceriation

It is caused due to sexual trauma generally in reproductive age as a result of intercourse, injury, sexual assault, penetration by foreign objects that cause virginity, vaginismus, post-partum, post-menopausal vaginal atrophy, hysterectomy and use of alcohol and drugs.

Signs and symptoms of this disorder include vaginal bleeding, acute pain during intercourse and persistent pain after intercourse. The disease can be diagnosed by cervical polyp, menstrual bleeding, threatened abortion, episiotomy and vaginal surgery.

To treat this disorder, have pelvic rest and avoid sex until healing occurs.

8. Vaginal Prolapse

Loss of normal support mechanism resulting in vaginal wall-down in vaginal canal. In extreme cases vagina become everted beyond the vulva outside the body. It is usually caused because of childbirth, surgery, intra-abdominal pressure, chronic cough, heavy lifting, intrinsic tissue weakness and atrophic changes resulting from estrogen loss.

Signs and symptoms of this disorder include conditions such as urinary incontinence, pelvic pain, uterus dyspareunia, inter-menstrual or post menopausal bleeding, cystocele, urethrocele, rectocele, bartholin cyst, vaginal cyst or tumor.

The beneficial measures to treat this disorder are pessary therapy, surgical and estrogen replacement therapy. Avoid estrogen therapy if undiagnosed vaginal bleeding exists.

9. Vaginitis atrophic

Atrophy of vaginal tissues caused by the loss of ovarian steroids, which generally grips post-menopausal women above age 50, and is usually caused as a result of surgery, chemotherapy, radiation or natural cessation of ovarian function.

Signs and symptoms of the disease include vaginal dryness, burning and itching, pain or bleeding during intercourse and appearance of thin, shiny, red epithelium with a smooth surface. The disease can be diagnosed by vaginal infections, vulvitis, hot flashes and flushes, sleep disturbance.

Use of vaginal moisturizer and lubricants when involved in intercourse and oral or injectable estrogen treatment is usually recommended.

10. Bacterial vaginitis

A vaginal infection caused by an over-growth of normal or pathogenic bacteria which causes irritation and inflammation among females between 15 to 50 years age, generally due to suffering from diabetes, pregnancy and debilitating disease, smoking, excess number of sexual partners, use of vaginal contraceptives, oral sex, unhygienic menstruation practice and douching.

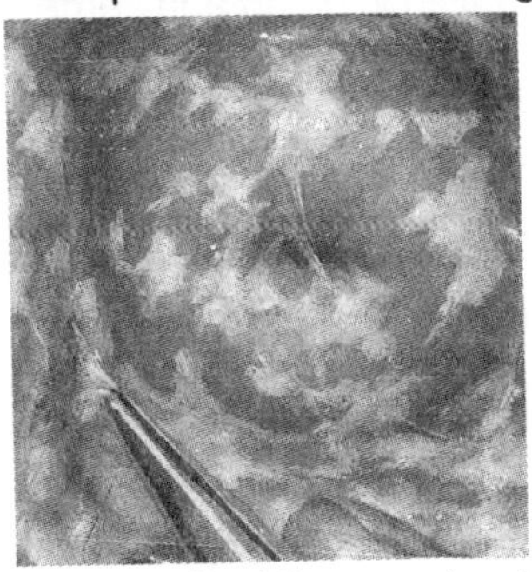

Perinal hygiene and medical therapy (oral and topical with the consultation of a doctor) are important measures to treat this disorder. If neglected, the possible complications include cystitis, cervicitis, infections of the skene's or bartholin's glands, pelvic inflammatory disease, pelvic pain, infertility, increased risk of upper genital- tract infection, premature delivery and premature rupture of the membranes.

11. Vaginitis-monilial

A vaginal infection caused by ubiquitous fungi found in the atmosphere are common inhabitants of the vagina, rectum and vaginal mouth. It usually occurs in females between age 15 to 50 years. Nearly 80 to 90 % cases are caused by candida albicaus and the remaining due to candida glabrata or candida tropicals generally due to stress, diabetes, depression, topical contraceptives and warm and moist environments.

Signs and symptoms of disease include vulvar itching or burning, scratching, external dysuria, dyspareunia, tissue erythema, edema, vulvar excoriations and white to yellow thick discharge which can be diagnosed by bacterial vaginitis, trichomonas vaginal infection, allergic vulvitis, atrophic vulvitis, vulvar dermatoses and pinworms.

Following are the important measures to treat the disease:

1. Perineal hygiene to keep the affected area clean and dry.
2. Avoid wearing tight synthetic undergarments.
3. Avoid topical steroid preparations.

12. Vaginitis trichomonas

A vaginal infection common in females of age between 15 to 50, generally caused by the following reasons :

1. Multiple sexual partners.
2. Vaginal pH (less acid in blood and semen).

Signs and symptoms of this disease are the following :

1. Vulvar itching or burning.
2. Thin runny yellow-green to grey odour discharge.
3. Dysuria, dyspareunia and edema of vulva.
4. Sexually transmissible infections, which can easily be diagnosed by physical examination or by microscopic examination of vaginal secretion in normal saline.
5. If not treated properly, complications such as cystitis, pelvic inflammation diseases, infertility and pelvic pain arise.

The disorder can be cured by medical treatment. Consult a doctor immediately.

Diseases of Cervix

1. Abnormal Pap smear intra-epithelia lesion

It consists of carcinoma in cervical generally in reproductive age, which is caused due to exposure to HPV and STD asymptomatic.

Signs and symptoms of this disease are associated with conditions such as vaginitis, cervicitis, cervical dysplasia, CIS, invasive carcinoma of cervix and endocervical adeno-carcinoma.

Important measures to treat the disease are :

1. Pap smears examination at four to six month interval for two years.
2. Cryotherapy.
3. Electro-cautery and electro-surgical loop excision.
4. Laser ablation or conization.
5. Avoid HPV infection.

2. Carcinoma in cervix

The thickness of epithelium is replaced with dysplastic cells with invasive carcinoma usually occurring in the age early 30s caused by herpes virus, early sexual activities, multiple sexual partners, smoking, oral contraceptives and early childbearing.

The signs and symptoms include asymptomatic, abnormal cervical cytology and abnormal colposcopy.

The measures to treat the disease are: standard hysterectomy, ablative therapy and cryosurgery, CO2 laser therapy and radical electrocautery.

3. Cervical cancer and carcinoma

Almost all cancers of cervix are carcinoma. The disease is common in women between the age 40 to 60 caused by early sexual activities, multiple partners and presence of sexually transmitted viral infections. Signs and symptoms of disease include abnormal Pap Smear, vaginal bleeding, dark vaginal discharge, post-coital bleeding, back pain, loss of appetite, weight loss, bleeding lesion, inguinal lymph nodes, swelling of legs. The disease can be diagnosed by cervical erosion, cervical polyp, condyloma acuminata and Nabothian cyst. Chemotherapy is curative measure of the disease.

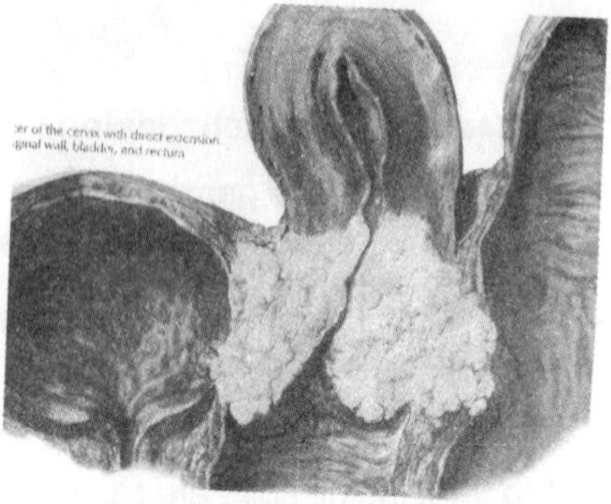

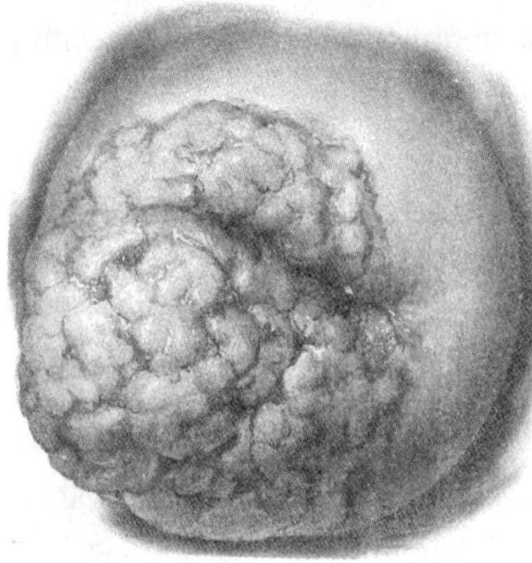

4. Cervical erosion

Loss of epithelial surface on vaginal portion of cervix usually caused by traumatic reasons such as fingernails, sexual appliances, diaphragm, pessary or other instrumentation.

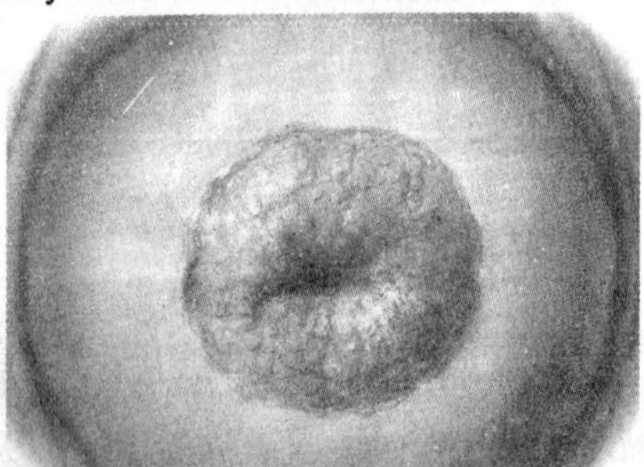

The signs and symptoms of disease are irregularly shaped lesions, bleeding tissues resulting in post-coital spotting and increased discharge. The disease can be diagnosed by ectopy (cervical eversion), herpes simplex, cervicitis, carcinoma under the epithelium surface, syphilis, cervical polyp and chronic cervicitis.

5. Cervical polyps

Fleshy tumors arising from the cells of the cervix generally in the age group of 40 to 50 in women having the history of the cervical infection and used to oral contraceptive resulting inflammation.

Signs and symptoms include asymptomatic, inter-menstrual spotting, post-coital spotting and a smooth, soft, reddish purple to cherry red friable mass (upto 4 cm size) at the cervix, which bleed on slight touch.

The disease can be diagnosed by cervical cancer, cervical eversion and cervical erosion, which may also result in conditions such as intra-menstrual bleeding, post-coital bleeding and leucorrhoea (white vaginal discharge). A Pap smear test is essential.

6. Cervical stenosis

Narowing of the cervical canal which may result in complete or partial obstruction. The damage is caused by cone-biopsy, electro-cautery, cryocautery, radiation, infection, neoplasia atrophy and sometime due to congenital reasons.

The signs and symptoms of this disease include pre-menopausal dysmenorrhea, abdominal bleeding, amenorrhea, infertility, uterine enlargement, post-menopausal asymptomatic, hematometra or pyometra which may result in endocervical cancer or endometrial cancer and uterine leiomyometa.

Treatment measures such as symptomic therapy, nonsteroidal anti-inflammatory drugs, dilation of the cervix under ultrasound guidance cures the disease.

7. Cervicitis

Acute or chronic inflammation of the endocervical glands or ectocervix usually during reproductive age and in adolescents till

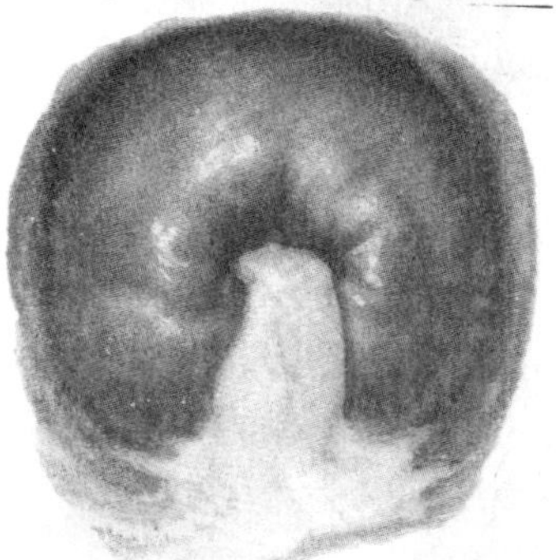

early 20s, is caused by exposure to sexually transmissible infections, multiple sexual partners, post-partum period, herpes simplex and trichomones vaginalis.

Signs and symptoms of this disease include asymptomatic, a yellow discharge with white blood cells, cervical neoplasia, cervical erosion, cervical eversion, post-coital bleeding, premature rupture of membrane in pregnancy, pelvic inflammation, dyspareunia, premature labour and pre-maturity.

Seek the help of your doctor for treatment when the disease is diagnosed.

8. Nabothian cysts

Retention cysts occur closure of a gland opening generally during reproductive age. These are raised white to blue to yellow bumps 3 mm. to 3 cm. in diameter, causing chronic inflammation of the cervix, followed by mucus-filled cysts and cervical cancer.

9. Uterine atony (Postpartum)

Loss of uterine tone after delivery that often presents as postpartum hemorrhage. The hemorrhage is seen in about 5% deliveries. It is caused due to the loss of the normal uterine contractile forces. The risk factors include multiparity, uterine overdistention, prolonged labor, prolonged oxytocin stimulation, retained placental tissue and chorioamnionitis.

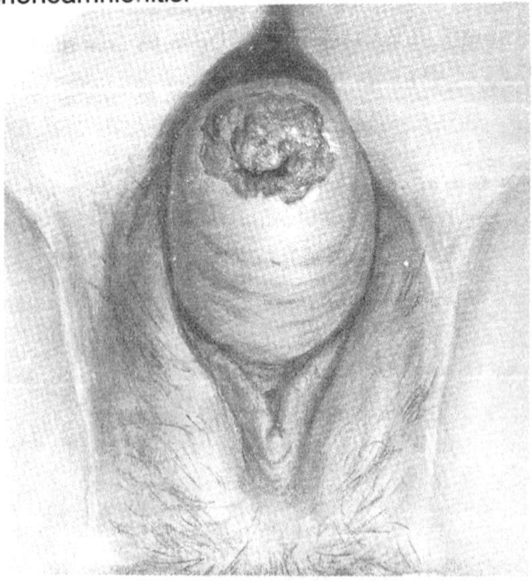

Signs and symptoms of this disorder include bright red vaginal bleeding, loss of uterine tone palpable on abdominal examination, tachycardia, hypotension and vascular collapse.

Diagnostic approach : can be diagnosed by retained placental fragments, genital tract lacerations (Cervical and vaginal), uterine rupture, uterine inversion and coagulopathy.

General measures : Uterine atony should be suspected in a patient with excessive bleeding after delivery of placenta. To treat this disorder, massage the uterus fundus. The bladder should be drained to allow the uterus to contract and to assess urinary output.

10. Uterine rupture

Breech of the uterine wall, that may result in significant maternal or fetal morbidity or mortality. Rupture of an intact uterus doesn't occur on rare occasions. In many cases it prevails in patients with a previous cesarean delivery or of patients for whom vaginal birth after cesarean delivery fails. The main causes include abnormal healing of previous uterine scar, mechanical disruption of the uterine wall weakened by previous surgery, congenital anomalies or abnormalities of placentation, traumatic rupture of the uterus and effect of an accident, which results in injury to both mother and fetus.

Signs and symptoms include abrupt fetal distress, vaginal bleeding, abdominal pain and maternal circulatory collapse. It can be diagnosed by uterine dehiscence, placental abruption, umbilical cord prolapse, adnexal torsion and pulmonary or amniotic fluid embolism. An immediate operative delivery is required as a measure.

Venereal and Reproductive Organ Diseases

There are many types of venereal diseases in women. But there are few major diseases related to sex and are frequently picked up through sexual intercourse with someone who already has the disease. Prostitutes and call girls are the usual source of infection in any community. Men and women who want to be healthy and strong will naturally avoid all contacts with such opposite sex. Certainly no sensible young man or woman would want to have sex relations with such sick people – many of them usually are infected with syphilis or gonorrhea, often having both diseases at the same time – both are foul body and soul-destroying disease. But because of careless living on the part of many young people the diseases are spreading rapidly today in spite of advances in modern medical science.

Syphilis

Syphilis is one of the greatest scourges ever to hit the human race. It is a dangerous venereal disease caused by a tiny corkscrew-shaped germ called a spirochaete, which is transmitted from one person to another mainly through sexual contact. In some cases syphilis is acquired through contaminated material and even through injections or blood transfusion, if the germs are present in the blood. If a mother is infected with syphilis, the germs may find their way into the child's body before birth.

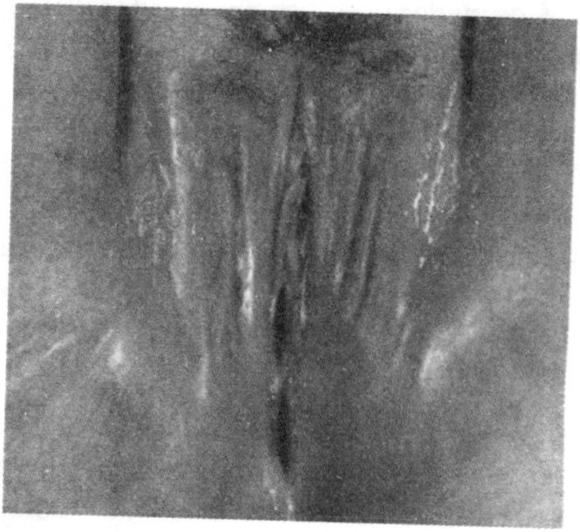

In the male there may be painless sore on the penis lasting several weeks. In female there may be a sore deep in the vagina, but because there is no pain the woman may not be aware of it. This early primary lesion is known as a chancre. At first the germs are confined to this one area, later they invade the blood stream and are carried to all parts of the body causing a mild rash on the skin. This is the secondary stage of disease, which remains for a long period of time in the latent form. The disease can be discovered with blood test. In the later stage, tumors or swellings (especially on genital organs in both sexes) may appear in various parts of the body and there may be severe inflammation and degeneration. The nervous system is often affected with disastrous results. Syphilis involves brain and the spinal cord severely affecting frequent headaches, loss of memory, tremors of the lips, tongue, fingers and hands, and the changes in the pupils of the eyes.

Another form of degenerative disease due to syphilis is known as 'tabes dorsalis'. In this disease syphilis germs attack the nerve roots coming from the spinal cord. Severe gastric upsets are common. There may be vomiting and acute abdominal pain lasting for hours or even days. Large ulcers may develop on the toes, heels, soles, and there may be a thickening and splintering of the bone in the knee joints. There is often a loss of normal bladder control in the later stage of this disease. In some cases a large swelling may develop under the skin in several places. These may also occur in the inner organs of the body such as stomach and liver.

Syphilis in newly born babies

Pregnant woman suffering from syphilis may pass on the disease to her unborn baby growing in fetus. If proper treatment is not taken, the disease may strike the unborn child resulting in serious conditions. Soon after birth, the bones of the baby may appear somewhat deformed. It affects the liver, spleen, brain, central nervous system causing the child to be retarded both mentally and physically. The syphilitic mother runs the great risk of recurrent abortions and still birth due to the infection, damaging the placenta and the growing embryo. Large doses of penicillin usually destroy the germs of syphilis, particularly during the early stage of the disease.

Gonorrhea

Gonorrhea is another venereal disease transmitted by sexual contact with opposite sex. It is caused by a tiny bean-shaped germ called gonococcus. Many adult women carry the germs for a long

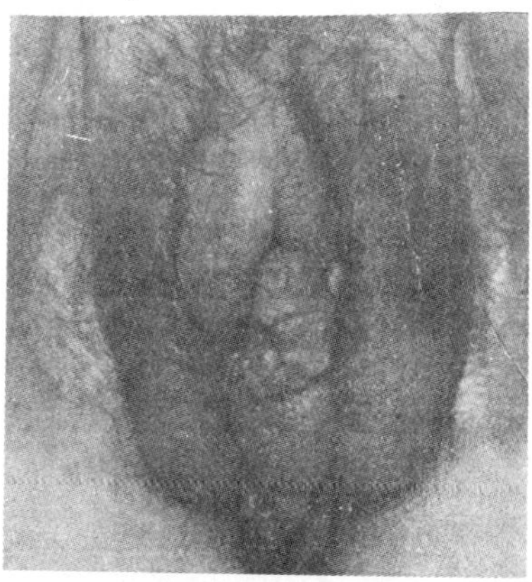

period of time without realizing that they have disease and may readily transmit the germs during sexual intercourse. If a mother happens to be infected with gonorrhea, there is great danger of the new-born infant contracting the disease during the process of birth. Unless the infant is properly treated, he / she become mentally retarded or blind in later life. In young children, particularly in little girls suffering from this venereal disease, there may be marked redness and swelling of the genital organs with burning on urination. Signs and symptoms of this venereal disease include :

1. Persistent pus discharge from vagina.
2. Inflammation of entire genital passage, both in male and female.
3. Burning and discomfort.
4. Burning on urination.
5. Sense of urgency and frequency of urination
6. A profuse greenish yellow discharge.
7. In the female the glands around the opening to the vagina may be hot and swollen.
8. Presence of thick yellow discharge all the time present around the opening of vagina.
9. In males the end of the penis may be red and swollen

Causes of the disease are as following :

1. Transmitted by sexual contact with opposite sex.
2. Contracted from contaminated hands, instruments, clothing, contaminated toilet seats and bath water.

Complications : Complications arising from the disease include the following :

1. Sterility results from this serious infection.
2. In the female, fallopian tubes may become closed by an abscess and the inflammation may spread to the whole female pelvis.
3. In males, the prostate gland becomes infected and there may be narrowing of the urinary canal resulting in slow urination.
4. There may be fever, nausea, vomiting and severe pain in the lower abdomen.
5. Many cases of suspected appendicitis are later found to be due to gonorrhea.

6. If the germ invades the blood stream there may be inflammation in the larger joints, such as knees, ankles, elbows as well as inflammation in the eyes.

Treatment : Penicillin or Terrimacin are the best drugs for treating this disease strictly under the advice of a doctor.

White discharge

The secretions from the uterus and upper portion of the vagina flows down and are reabsorbed in the lower part of the vagina. Usually the female organs of a growing girl operate without any thing unusual occurring. But there are times when the girl may be troubled by an excessive white discharge known as leukorrhoea (or whites), which is not a normal occurrence. She should seek the counsel of her doctor. However, a slight discharge is not unusual at ovulation or during times of strong sexual excitement. But if there is intense itching, the trouble may arise from certain organisms, such as trichmonas or some other type of infection. Pinworms are another source of irritation in the vagina, particular in young girls, which should be referred to a doctor for treatment. But before treatment is begun, all the organs should be thoroughly examined to rule out the presence of gonorrhea or even cancer.

Genital herpes

Herpes simplex virus produces the infection and it is passed on through sexual contact. The following sign and symptoms are observed :

1. Symptoms of fever, body-aches and weakness.
2. Vaginal discharge and irritation.
3. Urinary burning and enlarged lymph nodes.
4. Different sized vesicles and reddish ulcers are noticed in the vulva region.
5. Few blebs and ulcers in the vaginal mucous membrane.

Causes and the treatment: Women who practice anorectal sex develop lesions in the area around the anus and higher up in the rectum.

AIDS

AIDS virus increase the risk of common and rare infections and may be transmitted hetero-sexually or by infected blood transfusion.

Being sexually transmitted the virus can be transmitted from man to man, man to woman, woman to man and infected mother to the child. Hetero-sexual transmission in promiscuous individuals has been observed with frequent exchange of partners.

Signs and symptoms: These include fever, loss of weight, diarrhea, extreme fatigue, glandular enlargement, tumors, severe toxicity and lack of resistance to fight infection.

Treatment: There is no effective treatment for AIDS. However, use of condoms reduces risk.

Ovarian Diseases
Clear cell carcinoma

Description: An ovarian tumor made up of cells containing large amounts of glycogen (which give a clear or hobnailed appearance). These tumors may also arise in the endocervix, endometrium and vagina. This disease is often seen in women between 40 to 75 year age.

Causes : Unknown. It may arise from mesonephric or mullerian elements.

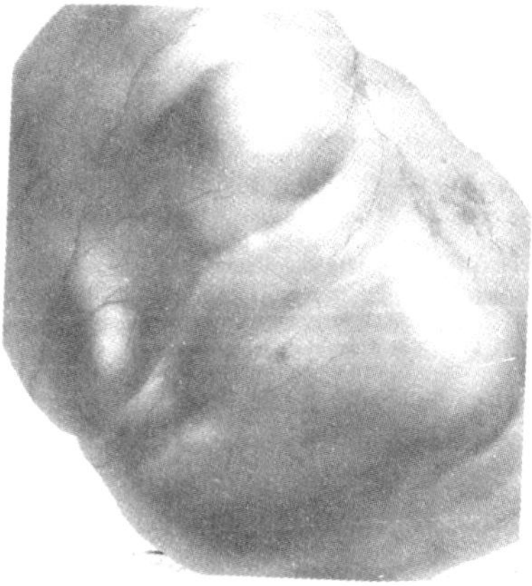

Signs and symptoms : Include the following :

- Asymptomatic.
- Pelvic mass up to 30 cm., partially cystic with yellow, gray and haemorrhagic appearance.
- Papillary projections generally giving a velvety appearance (40% of tumors are bilateral).

Diagnostic approach : Can be diagnosed by physical examination and imaging with differential diagnosis as following :

- Benign adnexal masses (corpus lutenum and follicular cyst).
- Nongynecologic pelvic masses.
- Hepatic, renal or cardiac disease resulting weight loss and ascites.
- Endometriosis.
- Hydrosalpinx.
- Ectopic pregnancy in case the woman is pregnant.
- Gastrointestinal malignancy.
- Pedunculated leiomyomata.
- Pelvic or horseshoe kidney.

Remedial measures : These include :

- Surgical exploration and extirpation (including the uterus and contralated ovary).
- Adjunctive chemotherapy.
- Radiation therapy.

Dysgerminoma

Description : An ovarian tumor made up of germ cells and stroma. The tumor is also found in the male testes. Nearly 90% sufferers are usually older than 30 years age and the remaining are generally prepuberal girls. The causes are unknown. Signs and symptoms include asymptomatic and adnexal mass with a gray white or cream colored cut surface.

Diagnostic approach : The following diagnosis are observed :

- Benign adnexal masses (corpus luteum, follicular cyst),
- Endometriosis.
- Hydrosalpinx.
- Paratubal cyst.
- Appendiceal abscess.
- Ectopic pregnancy.
- Pedunculated leiomyomata.

- Pelvic or horseshoe kidney.
- Nongynecologic pelvic masses.

Remedial measures : Include the following :

- Evaluation, supportive therapy based on symptoms.
- Surgical exploration and resection in case of a tumor is confined to one ovary.
- Preservation of the uterus and other ovary is possible to preserve fertility.
- Multiagent chemotherapy.

Ectopic pregnancy

Description : Pregnancy implants outside of the endometrial cavity, which takes place in the ovary, fallopian tube, abdominal cavity or cervix. Nearly 40% cases are seen in women between the age 25 to 35 years. The main cause is tubal damage that results in the fertilized eggs being improperly transported, causing implantation outside the uterine cavity.

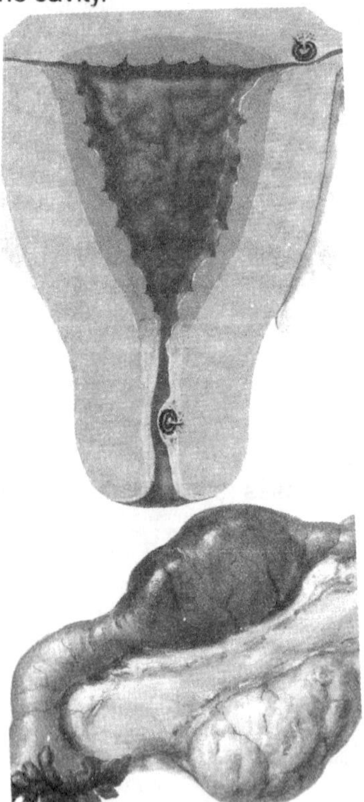

Signs and symptoms : They include the following :

- Amenorrhea and uterine softening.
- Acute abdominal pain.
- Evidence of intra-abdominal bleeding including hypotension and collapse.
- Adnexal mass (with or without tenderness).
- Vaginal bleeding.
- Signs of peritoneal irritation.
- Absence of a gestational sac.
- Abdominal pregnancy may be asymptomatic.
- Pelvic inflammatory disease.
- Infertility.
- Recurrent abortion.

Diagnostic approach : They are the following :

- Appendicitis.
- Degenerating fibroid.
- Dysfunctional uterine bleeding.
- Endometriosis.
- Gastroenteritis.
- Mosenteric thrombosis.
- Ruptured corpus luteum cyst.
- Salpingitis.
- Septic abortion.
- Threatened or incomplete abortion.
- Torsion of an adnexal mass.

Epithelial stromal ovarian tumors

Description : The most common type of ovarian tumor, derived from the surface epithelium and ovarian stroma are usually occurring between the age 20 to 50 years. The causes are usually unknow, with risk factors as the family history, high-fat diet, advanced age, nulliparity, early menarche, late menopause, oral contraception, high parity and breast feeding reduce risk.

Signs and symptoms : They are the following :

- Asymptomatic.

- Weight loss.
- Increasing abdominal girth despite constant or reduced caloric intake.
- Ascites
- Adnexal mass (partly solid massed in patients over 40).
- Vague lower abdominal discomfort.

Diagnostic approach :

- Functional cyst (corpus luteum, follicular).
- Endometriosis.
- Hydrosalpinx.
- Paratubal cyst.
- Appendiceal abscess.
- Ectopic pregnancy.
- Pedunculated leiomyomata

Germ cell tumor

It is most common type of ovarian tumor, which contain cells that echo the three layers of embryonic tissue or extraembryonic elements, usually occurring in females of age less than 30 (many times seen in teens and twenties). The causes of tumor are unknown.

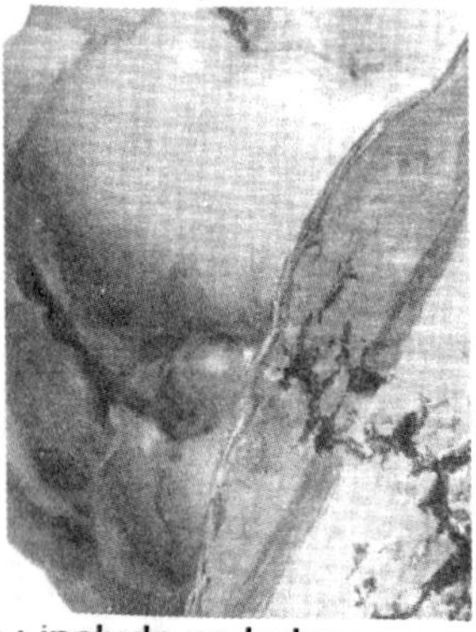

Signs and symptoms : include as below :

1. Asymptomatic.
2. Ovarian enlargement.

Diagnostic approach: It can be diagnosed by endometriosis, benign adnexal masses, hydrosalpinx, paratubal cyst, appendiceal abscess, ectopic pregnancy, pedunculated leiomyomata, pelvic or horseshoe kidney and nongynecologic pelvic masses.

Remedial measures : are surgical exploration and resection, followed by chemotherapy.

Granulosa cell tumors

It is a sex cord stromal tumor of the ovary, which often secretes estrogen. The main cause of this tumor is unknown. The signs and symptoms include enlarging or ruptured adnexal mass, abnormal menstrual patterns (menorrhagia and amenorrhea) and postmenopausal bleeding.

The disorder can be diagnosed by benign adnexal masses, paratubal cyst, appendiceal abscess, weight loss (due to hepatic, renal or cardiac disease), ectopic pregnancy (among reproductive age women), gastrointestinal malignancy, increased estrogen causing breast tenderness, menstrual disturbances and isosexual pseudoprecocity.

Remedial measures: include surgical exploration and resection followed by chemotherapy.

Mucinous ovarian cysts

A group of benign and malignant epithelial tumors of the ovary up to 30 cm. or greater in size, usually occur during the reproductive age (between 30-60 years). Nearly 15-20% tumors turn to ovarian cysts and 6-10% to ovarian cancers. Usually, the causes are unknown. The common risk factors include family history, high-fat diet, advanced age, early menarche, late menopause, higher economic status and oral contraception.

Signs, symptoms, diagnosis and remedial factors: Asymptomatic, vague lower abdominal symptoms and adnexal mass (size up to 50 cm) are the common symptoms of this disorder, which can be diagnosed by benign adnexal masses, endometriosis, hydrosalpinx, paratubal cyst, appendiceal abscess, ectopic pregnancy, pedunculated leiomyomata and nongynecologic pelvic masses. Surgical exploration and extirpation followed by chemotherapy is prominent remedial measure.

Ovarian cancer and cysts

The detail of ovarian cancer has been described in detail in a separate chapter. This is usually caused by high fat diet in advanced age usually in high economic status families. Breastfeeding, however,

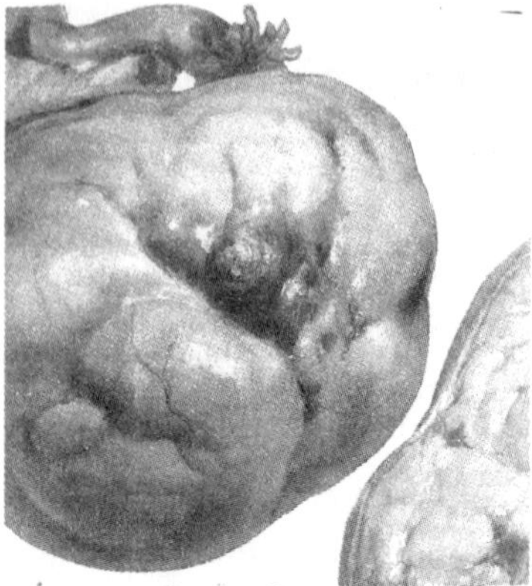

Ovary Cancer

reduces the risk. Usually, weight loss, ascites, increasing abdominal girth, adnexal masses and vague lower abdominal are prominent signs and symptoms. The disease requires surgical exploration and extirpation followed by chemotherapy. A cystic growth within the ovary, generally arises from epithelial components and most often benign. The most important objective of the management of an ovarian cyst is the timely diagnosis of its type and origin. A rapid evaluation and intervention may be necessary.

Pelvic infection

It is a serious, diffuse, frequently multi-organism infection of the pelvic organs that results in significant morbidity. Nearly 85% cases are found in sexually active women of menstrual age. The main causes of the disease include due to venereal diseases, the effect of bacteria, multiple sexual partners, effect of douching, infection of genital tract and bacterial vaginosis. Usual signs and symptoms of disease are pelvic pain and tenderness, elevated white blood cell count, irregular vaginal bleeding or discharge, nausea and vomiting and cervical discharge. It may be diagnosed by ectopic pregnancy, torsion, bleeding, appendicitis, endometriosis, enteritis, diverticular abscess and cholecystitis.

Sertoli-lydig cell tumor

It is a rare sex cord tumor of the ovary usually in women older than 30 years. The tumors vary in size but generally are 5-15 cm. in diameter. The causes are unknown. The sign and symptoms include asymptomatic, adnexal enlargement, abdominal swelling, abdominal pain, ascites, amenorrhea, loss of female secondary sex characteristics, suffering from acne, hirsutism (unwanted hair on body), temporal balding, deepening of voice and clitoral enlargement. The disease can be diagnosed by adrenal virilizing tumor, paratubal cyst, endometriosis, appendiceal abscess, follicular cyst, pelvic or horseshoe kidney, nongynecologic pelvic masses and ectopic pregnancy.

12 Health Problems during Pregnancy

Disorders during pregnancy

During pregnancy a woman may develop many disorders, which are generally common among all women. Precautionary measures can put check to further development if timely taken care. Aches and pains are seen most common problems a pregnant have to face. In the past, when women became pregnant, they were often treated like invalids. They were forbidden to carry out their normal activities and after an delivery, were kept in bed for two weeks. Their list of aches and pains was longer and more serious. Now this has changed and the pregnancy is no longer regarded as an illness. If you take sensible care of yourself, you may actually feel better than usual while pregnant. But for some women it is still a time which makes them worried.

Pregnancy is a good time to increase your body awareness. It should not become a period of constant worrying. A good way to avoid this is to build up a regular exercise program that is well integrated into your everyday life. Develop a self-confidence-emotional as well as physical, which will enable you to cope with pains and aches. Remember, the first priority to feel best and to make sure that :

- You are healthy.
- You are taking a well-balanced and healthy diet.
- You are doing enough exercise, that shouldn't make you tired.
- You are getting good sleep and relaxation. A deep warm bath

can often soothe away tiredness and tension and giving you a chance to appreciate your changing figure of your body.

- You are not taking any medication, even the mild one, without consulting your doctor.
- You are taking responsibility for your body now, will help you to feel ready for the labor and to participate actively in the birth of expected baby.

1. Morning sickness

Generally in the early stages of pregnancy a woman gets vomiting sensation, normally in the morning and as such, it is usually termed as morning sickness. Generally a woman with tender and weak constitution has this trouble more frequent. Healthy women have little such feeling, which usually start in the beginning of sixth week after conception or after two weeks beyond the schedule date of regular menses. This sensation may start a little early or late. Usually, it starts in the morning and subsides by afternoon and a few women continue to have this sensation even till evening. There is nothing to worry about this casual disorder. Six to eight weeks after conception, this sensation ceases without any treatment. The following treatments help to relieve to great extent :

- Keep yourself safe from any sort of constipation. When the rectum is clear 'lawan bhaskar churan' (a harmless patent ayurvedic product) should be continued during this period. You may consult your doctor, if the condition is severe.
- If milk is given mixed with a little lime water, it gives good results.
- One part each white sandal powder and amla powder when mixed to two parts sugar candy and one teaspoon honey is a good home remedy.

Generally, this vomiting sensation continues till the fetus starts movement in the stomach. It is not necessary that there must be vomiting after sensation. Only the nausea remains for a long time. This usually happens due to extra pressure on the limbs and organs of a pregnant woman. Moreover, the pressure of embryo falls upon the organs, muscles and the nerves of a expectant mother.

If the vomiting sensation is abnormal, it develops the following diseases :

- Spasms in stomach.

- Inflammation in hands and feet.
- Pain in the backbone and thighs.
- Headache, insomnia, constipation and thirst.
- Blood in vomiting, fever, grains over the tongue and inside the throat.
- Pain in the stomach.
- Swelling on the feet.
- Bile trouble increases; it sometimes results in an abortion.
- Frequent urination occurs due to nausea and this state continues for 10-12 weeks after conception.

2. Constipation

It is most common disease among all pregnant women and is very harmful during pregnancy. the repeated trouble of constipation records that the bowels are not working properly. The accumulation of faeces may diffuse poison in the blood. Constipation develops during pregnancy due to pressure of the embryo and weakening of intestine.

The following treatments are recommended :

1. In case of constipation, start taking light and easily digestive food.
2. Take lemon juice in hot water in the morning before going to toilet.
3. Try to drink as much water as you can during the day and one glass of water before retiring
4. Takc castor oil along with hot milk, if constipation continues.

3. Piles

Like constipation piles develop due to faulty eating and poor bowel habits. Taking highly spiced food, increased intra abdominal pressure, irritation to the stomach and intestines are some of the basic causes for the disorder. The following treatments are recommended :

1. Application of anti-hemorrhoid ointment.
2. Avoid taking highly spicy food.
3. Consult your doctor for the treatment.

4. Blood Pressure

The pressure exerted by the blood on the walls of arteries depends on the forcible action of heart, resilience of blood vessels and viscosity of blood etc. Tension, worry, lack of relaxation, environmental noise, obesity, over-eating, faulty functioning of kidneys, anger, excessive salt in diets, smoking, intake of alcohol and excitement are some of the causes of high blood pressure (hypertension). A normal blood pressure fluctuates between 110/70 and 130/86.

5. Breast inflammation

During pregnancy some inflammation of the breast is a common disorder. The inflammation further passes towards throat and sometimes a woman starts belching. Due to soreness in the throat a woman loses the taste of her mouth.

6. Stomach pain

Most of women during pregnancy feel stomach pain due to increased weight of the embryo as a result nerves are stained causing pain. It may result in a miscarriage. Normally, this pain starts in the evening and remains up to the night. In some cases the pain is so much that a woman feels her whole body burning. These pains sometimes continue in all successive months.

To treat this disorder, massage stomach slowly with ghee. It will relieve pain and swelling as well.

7. Liver pain

Liver pain generally starts in the night only; suddenly starts from the back and then passes to the right shoulder. During this pain a woman finds relief if her stomach is pressed. The cause of pain is usually accumulation of acidity in gall-bladder. In most of the cases it is difficult to intermediate between liver pain and kidney pain. But normally the kidney pain starts from the kidney and passes upwards and one feels middle pains in the breast. Aniseed juice gives much relief.

8. Pregnancy toxaemia

It results in sudden increase in weight, swelling of the body, a rise in blood pressure, an appearance of albumin in urine, breathlessness, constant thumping of heart and an abrupt occurrence of bleeding. A high protein low fat diet, control of blood pressure followed by diuretics to flush out urine, relaxed state of mind, light morning and evening walks, a good sleep at night and light yogic exercises would help.

9. Gastritis

A common condition among pregnant, who start feeling inflammation in breast and throat. To cure this disorder, have old rice, gourd vegetables, papaya, coconut water, barley water, mineral water, amla sauce, kidney bean, ghee. Sugar, wheat and milk.

10. Dyspepsia

Generally the digestive system of a woman during pregnancy doesn't function properly, and the result is dyspepsia. The woman doesn't digest the food properly and starts belching.

11. Headache and tension

Tension in the neck is often caused by holding your neck incorrectly and by tense, raised shoulders. You may be unaware of these postural faults until you begin to feel uncomfortable. Pull your shoulders down and the back of your neck will lengthen upward. Try to maintain this good posture throughout the day. Practice the neck and shoulder exercises turning your neck up-down, left and right daily. Ask your partner to massage your neck, shoulder and the face to relieve headache and tension. If these headaches are severe or persist during pregnancy, see your doctor for advice.

Sometimes, due to severe headache the eyes get reddish. In some cases even the tongue becomes stiff and if due care is not taken in an early stage, this develops into hysteria, epilepsy or eclampsia. In the beginning some laxative should be given to stop chronic constipation trouble. Generally when the bowels and rectum is clear, this pain will subside in a short time.

12. Pain between the shoulders

This is usually due to tension and the typical bad posture of pregnancy (usually arched back and tens shoulders). Correct your balance. Do a few backward shoulder circles to help release knots of tension.

13. Swollen hands

Many pregnant women wake up with slightly puffy hands, but this generally disappears when they begin to move about. If you are troubled by this, take off any tight rings before you go to sleep. Circle your hands from the wrist, flap them up and down and stretch your fingers out regularly to stimulate your circulation. If the swelling persists, report to your doctor.

14. Tension or pain in the chest

Pain under the rib cage can be caused by the growing baby pressing the ribs out. Lift your rib cage up and outward to give your self the maximum space for breathing comfortably.

15. Backache

This is one of the most common problems of pregnancy-your back vulnerable because of the extra progesterone, which softens the ligaments supporting the spine. Always bend your knees when lifting anything heavy. Bad posture is the most likely cause of general discomfort in the back. Do pelvic tilts regularly. Frequent backaches may be caused by weak abdominal muscle.

If you are in pain, stop whatever you are doing. Pain is always a warning signal and should not be disregarded. It is best to lie on a firm surface-preferably on the floor. Put one small cushion under your head and another under your hips; relax your shoulders, arms and hands. Bend your legs, do a pelvic tilt and press your back into the floor. Two minutes routine for backache is as following :

- Forward pelvic tilt.
- Side to side tilting.
- Circling your hips all round.
- Twisting your shoulders.

16. Shooting pain in the legs

Sudden shooting pain in your groin or down one leg when you walk is probably due to pressure from the baby. Stop and rest, breath slowly until the pain goes away. Take more rest : have a nap every day, or at least lie down or sit with your feet up an hour every day.

17. Heartburn

This is a common complaint that seems to be most noticeable towards the end of pregnancy. Increased production of the hormone progesterone slackens the muscle tone of the gastro-intestinal tract and allows the reflux of gastric juices into the esophagus, causing the burning sensation. The following care is necessary :

- It is better not to get too tired and hungry before eating.
- Do eat slowly.
- Try eating small snacks every two hours.
- Don't have your main meal too late at night.
- More rest and good posture help.
- Lift your spine, making as much space between your pelvis and ribs as possible. Do exercises to strengthen your abdomen.
- Try sleeping with an extra pillow or prop the head of your bed up slightly.

18. Sciatica

Extra progesterone may be the culprit in pregnancy for this pain, felt in the sciatica nerve, running from the lower back through the buttocks and down the back of the legs. Find time for extra rest, lying on your side with a pillow between your thighs. The sufferer should undertake light exercises for the buttocks.

19. Too much of spittle

Soon after conception, extra formation of spittle starts and sometimes a woman gets tired of spitting. Drink milk with sugar-candy and parched rice mixed in it. Always take light food.

20. Insomnia

Generally, women who exhaust their strength and energy in feeding the embryo, develop troubles like insomnia due to over weakness. Due to delicate state of mind, she can neither sleep in the night, nor in daytime. Ultimately, it is followed by fever and a woman loses her appetite also. If proper treatment is not given there remains a possibility of miscarriage. The following remedial treatments are suggested :

- The best treatment is to avoid reasons, which lead a woman towards insomnia.

- Mix equal quantity of pumpkin oil, poppy seed oil to half the quantity of camphor and massage the head with this mixture.
- Massage head with any of these oil: Brahmi oil, Narayan oil or Mahanarayan oil.

21. Premature separation of placenta

Placenta previa or the premature separation of placenta, are the two worst diseases against which special care should be taken during pregnancy. The placenta in spite of coagulating in the upper part of the uterus, it coagulates near vaginal orifice. During the advanced stage of pregnancy when the vaginal orifice starts widening, and the time of actual delivery approaches, the portion of the placenta, which has already coagulated near the vaginal orifice, gets burst and it is immediately followed by hemorrhage. This disorder generally develops during first pregnancy, but disappears slowly during successive pregnancies. The second stage is known as premature separation of the placenta. Take the patient to the hospital immediately.

22. Pain in the lower belly

A weak pregnant woman may have this problem due to infection in pelvic organs or a urinary problem.

23. White vaginal discharge

It is noticed generally due to a local infection of the vagina or cervix. Symptoms of severe itching, burning and heavy yellowish flow are visible. Anti-fungal creams are usually recommended.

24. Blood-stain discharge

It may be due to infection or erosion of the cervix. A severe vaginitis producing blood-stain discharge is an alarming sign of problem pregnancy.

25. Dark spots and pigmented lines on the skin

The texture of the skin is affected during pregnancy, which becomes fairer or darker due to action of sex hormones. They are generally seen with patches of dark spots on the face and neck or pigmented lines on various parts of the body including neck, back, abdomen and the upper thighs due to stretching of the skin or hormonal load on the blood. The areola (skin around the nipple on the breast) usually becomes darker with the symptoms of striae and pigmented lines. Do not feel anxiety over this, you will go back to your original skin condition without permanent scars few months after the delivery of baby.

26. Anemic condition

Most of the women suffer from shortage of blood, which is termed as anemic condition. In the 12th and 32nd week this condition reaches its climax. If an expectant mother fails to take sufficient iron, she may fall a victim to anemia. Include maximum fruit, green vegetables etc. in your diet to supplement iron.

27. Varicose veins

The extra progesterone in your body relaxes the muscle in the walls of your body, increase the risk of varicose veins developing. These can appear on the legs or in the vulva (the opening of vagina) or in the anal passage, where they are called hemorrhoids. If you have hemorrhoids, take care to avoid constipation and straining. Consult a doctor for medication. If neglected, hemorrhoids can be extremely painful.

Varicose veins usually subside after the baby is born, but they do tend to return with each pregnancy. Some women are more prone to them than others. Avoid sitting with your legs crossed and whenever you can, sit or lie with your feet up. Don't stand if you can sit, or sit if you can lie down. Circle your ankles as often as possible to aid your circulation and keep fit. Do not wear any tight elastic round your legs.

28. Cramps

These can be painful and annoying if they wake you up in the middle of night. There is no proven remedy, but you might try a calcium and vitamin D supplement along with extra intake of milk. The trouble usually starts in the 4th month from conception when the pain shoots up often during night when asleep. The trouble develops due to deficiency of minerals and vitamins in the body. The pain develops in waist, stomach, buttocks, legs and muscles. You may try the following remedies :

- Massage whole body with 'Narayan' oil. Massage can be comforting too.
- If the cramps are in your foot, bend it upward. When the cramp subsides, do some ankle circles or stimulate the circulation.

- If your ankles remain puffy, check with your doctor; there is nothing to worry about.

29. Swollen legs and ankles

Some women suffer from swollen ankles during pregnancy, especially in hot weather. Flat, comfortable shoes help – try not to wear high heels too often. Rest with your feet up as often as possible. Try simple exercise for the legs and feet. If your ankles are still puffy, check with your doctor; there is nothing to worry about.

30. Obstruction of urine

It causes when uterus shifts its place and is pushed back developing pressure on the kidney, affecting normal flow of the urine. As a result of obstruction in urine there is feeling of pain, inflammation in the urethra and the uterus due to accumulation of blood or pus or swelling.

31. Incontinence

The bulk of the uterus presses down on the pelvic floor and leaves little space for the bladder, so it's normal to empty your bladder often. If you leak a little urine when you sneeze or cough, it's a warning signal that your pelvic floor needs strengthening. This condition can be prevented or cured by regular practice of pelvic exercises, which strengthen the muscles of pelvic floor.

32. Itching pain in vagina

The trouble is common among those who have trouble of regular secretion. The itching causes sometimes due to semen remaining in the vagina after sexual intercourse. Too frequent sex should be avoided during pregnancy. Avoid too much scratching of the genital organs and if the secretion touches the anus, itching pain and swelling spreads.

33. Hydramnios

It usually develops in the 5th or 6th month after conception and sometimes results into miscarriage. In the uterus there is a small membrane, which is full of animistic fluid, in which a fetus develops. The disease develops due to swelling in the membranes. Usually, the placenta orifice gets closed due to inflammation and pain or the orifice of the placenta is closed from the beginning.

34. Jaundice

Very common in pregnant women. It is an ailment due to obstructed functioning of the liver. Better consult a doctor.

35. Diarrhea

All women in pregnancy do not have this disease, but those who are careless towards their digestive system and who allow to accumulate foeces, fall a victim to this disease.

Sometimes, this disease attains such a stage that there arises a possibility of miscarriage. There are several Ayurvedic medicines to deal with the disorder.

36. Dysentry

Diarrhoea or phyratic diarrhoea in later stages develops into dysentery. In dysentery sometimes blood passes with stools. In the early stages, try medicines already prescribed for diarrhoea with an addition of butter milk or skimmed milk along with it. There are several naturopathic medicines for the treatment of dysentery. The stomach can be easily cleaned by taking castor oil. Sometimes, due to the pressure of the embryo, the veins below the bowel gets puffed due to additional pressure on the intestine veins, and a woman falls a victim to piles.

37. Cough

Dry food, fast eating, dust entering in the mouth and nose, pressure on the lungs due to development of embryo are prominent causes, which develop cough to a woman during pregnancy. The ordinary cough may turn into a whoping cough and there is always danger of a miscarriage due to this.

Black pepper powder mixed in honey, candy and ghee should be given to treat cough. Better consult a doctor.

38. Heart trouble

Pregnancy often proves harmful to women suffering from some heart disease. It doesn't mean that a woman having some heart disease is incapable of pregnancy. But if the heart is too weak, after consulting a doctor, it is better to have a forced abortion. This condition sometimes at the time of delivery may prove fatal to a woman.

13
Overweight and Healthy Diets for Women

Useful Tips to Fight Overweight

Why overweigh?

Overeating is the sole cause for overweight. In other words, total caloric intake exceeds total caloric needs.

What's the effect of glandular disorders on overweight?

Glandular disorders have rare effect for overweight. Most of obese women seen overweight are usually over-eaters.

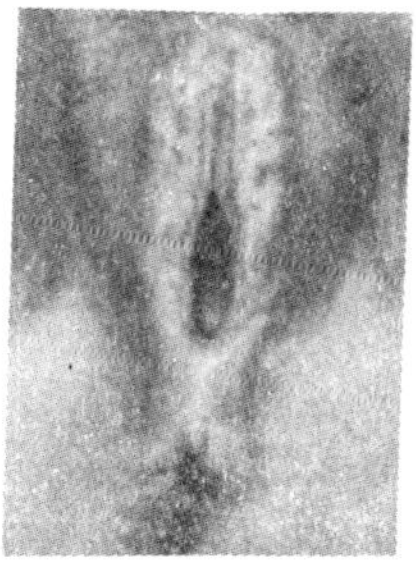

What is the effect of administering thyroid extract to reduce weight?

Thyroid glands control the metabolic rate and excessive dose may have a harmful effect and damaging the heart.

Should injections be given to reduce weight?

Doctors administer injections for reducing weight, which consist of diuretic drugs that leave temporary results, because they cause water loss in the body rather than decrease in fat tissue. There is no permanent weight loss due to such injections.

To what extent the weight can be reduced by medication?

There are few medicines that cut the appetite temporarily to enable the patient to take less food but their result is not long lasting.

What are these weight-reducing drugs?

These drugs usually belong to the amphetamine group, such as Benzedrine, Dexedrine, etc. There are also certain cellulose products, which give the patient the sensation that stomach is full. In fact, such cellulose products are harmful.

What is the effect of physical exercises for weight loss?

Physical exercises play an important role for weight loss. However, short, irregular spurts of activity are ineffective.

What is the best way to lose weight?

To eat well-balanced, medically approved low-caloric diet.

All obese person must lose weight?

Those suffering from ulcers or other intestinal upsets should lose weight gradually under close medical supervision.

What is the hereditary effect on obesity?

A child born and brought up in a family of heavy eaters, usually become a big eater influenced by environments and tend to become obese.

Inspite of dieting, when there is no weight loss?

Such people do not diet carefully or at sufficiently low level of caloric intake. For desired result to reduce weight, adhere to a prescribed diet.

Will all overweight people who diet properly lose weight?

They wMill lose weight, if their caloric intake is less than their caloric need.

What is the relationship between life span of a person and obesity?

Longevity is decreased in direct proportion to the degree of obesity.

What is relationship between overweight and coronary heart disease?

The evidenced reveal that coronary heart disease is much higher among people who are obese and who eat high-fat diets.

What is cholesterol?

A fatty substance found in certain foods and chemical analyses of blood. Cholesterol level varies in different people.

What is relationship between incidence of coronary heart disease and blood cholesterol?

Study reveals that those having higher ratio of blood cholesterol have tendency towards a greater incidence of coronary heart diseases.

What type of fatty food a woman should avoid?

Vegetable foods are not much harmful to increase blood cholesterol as compared to animal fats, which should be avoided as far as possible.

Are massages, baths and standardized weight reducing gadgets help to lose weight?

They have no much affect upon weight loss of a person except psychological influence, unless they eat low-calorie diet.

Should people dieting strenuously take vitamin supplements?

If they are on an unbalanced weight-reducing diet, vitamin supplements are required. However, a weight-reducing well-balanced diet doesn't need additional vitamin supplements.

Effect of smoking on weight gain?

Smoking has a tendency to cut one's appetite. But usually those people who stop smoking are seen divert towards sweets, fried foods and calorie increasing diets instead of cigarette smoking and start gaining weight.

Effect of taking alcoholic beverages on obesity?

An average glass of alcoholic drink contain about 100 calories and stimulate appetite.

Does strenuous dieting tend to make one nervous?

Only to those persons, who feel frustrated by eating less than their desire.

Weight-reducing diets cause constipation?

Sometimes, occur because the total mass of food intake reduces. Seek medical advice in order to aid bowel evacuation.

Should children as well as adults go on low-calorie diets to lose weight?

It is very important for children to maintain normal required weight as poor eating habits among children make them obese not only in childhood, even when they are adult. Children can be made to gain weight by establishment of habits, which lessen food intake, such as :

- Avoiding excess physical activity.
- Avoiding emotional strain on them.
- Not to punish or threatening them.

Excess weight-loss is harmful?

It is.

Those having excess weight are more prone to develop diabetes and heart diseases?

It is. Even tumors and cancer are more common among the obese than among the thin.

What is the effect of salt on weight loss?

Salt-restriction permits a greater loss of fluid and therefore has a greater weight loss. However, this is a temporary loss.

Is it possible to reduce extra weight only from hips?

There is no efficient means for losing weight from a particular area of the anatomy. All such claims are baseless. However, exercises to stimulate muscles of the hips will help to reduce extra flesh on the hips.

What are common causes for underweight?

- Chronic infections or diseases such as tuberculosis, kidney ailments, chronic liver disorders etc.
- Glandular imbalance such as excessive activity of thyroid glands or malfunctioning of the pituitary glands.
- Poor eating habits usually associated with an irregular life, excess physical activity and less sleep.

Does emotional strain affects weight and what's the best way to gain weight?

Usually people under emotional strain eat less, resulting in lose weight. Underweight people must eat more calories than they use. A thorough search must be carried out to make sure there is no infection or a physical cause for the underweight.

When the weight doesn't increase apart from eating large quantity of food, what would be the cause. What is the best way to gain weight?

Eating too much low-caloric value food doesn't increase weight. Such people should be placed upon foods containing higher caloric value such as cream, eggs, carbohydrates, butter etc. They may also burn up more energy with more-than-normal amount of sleep.

Following tips help to gain weight :

- Eat several full meals a day consisting of foods containing high-caloric value.
- Develop eating habits with four or five meals a day instead of three meals a day.
- Do not feel emotionally upset. Find out the psychological cause and attempt to eliminate it.

What are the medications that can aid one to eat more?

There are stimulants to increase the appetite, but generally their affect is unsatisfactory.

1,000 calories Reducing Diet

Food	*Include*	*Avoid*
Breads :	2 thin slices of whole wheat or enriched white bread.	Hot bread, coffee, cake, waffles, sweet rolls.
Cereals	None	All
Soups	Clear broth, vegetables soups Made of skim milk/ vegetables.	Creamed or thickened soups.

(contd.)

Meat, fish, eggs or cheese	Small quantity of chicken, ham, kidneys, liver. 1 egg Dry cottage cheese	Fatty meats, Fried meats, fish canned in oil. Cheese, pot cheese.
Vegetable	From 5% vegetable group up to 12 gm. carbohydrates.	Dried beans, dried peas.
Potato/substitute	None	All
Fats	2 tsp butter and 2 tsp cream	Any other
Fruits	Fresh, unsweetened equivalent to 30 gm. carbohydrates.	Sweetened, frozen or canned fruit, avocado, dried fruit.
Desserts	Unsweetened custard of skim milk and eggs, unsweetened gelatin.	Cakes, cookies, ice cream pastries, puddings and other rich desserts.
Sweets	None, except saccharin.	All
Beverages	Coffee, tea, 1 cup skim milk.	Carbonated beverages, other sweetened drinks, whole milk.
Miscellaneous	Condiments, salts and spices.	Alcohol, catsup, chili, cream, sauce, gravy, nuts, pickles.

Low-salt Diet (High Blood Pressure)

Foods	*Include*	*Avoid*
Breads	Salt-free bread and crackers	Any made with baking soda, salt and baking powder.

(contd.)

Cereals	Salt-free cereals, puffed rice, puffed wheat, shredded wheat.	Any other cereal.
Soups	Salt-free broth or cream soup.	Soup made with salt.
Meat, fish, eggs or cheese	Any meat, fresh water fish without salt, 1 egg.	Salted meats, canned meats or fish, all cheeses.
Vegetable	Any canned, cooked or raw vegetables without salt.	Vegetables prepared with salt. Vegetables such as sprouts, cucumber, cabbage, onions, dried peas, green peppers, radishes, turnips, cauliflower and broccoli.
Potato/substi-tute	Potato, macaroni, noodles, rice-all prepared without salt.	Fried potatoes, potato chips.
Fats	Salt-free butter, 1/3 cup cream, lard oil, salad dressing and vegetable fat.	Salted butter, salted salad.
Fruits	Any juice, canned, cooked or raw fruit.	Dried fruit with sodium benzoate.
Desserts	Salt-free desserts, custards, custards, gelatin, ice cream, unsalted fruit pie, puddings, rennet desserts.	Desserts prepared with salt, baking powder or egg white.
Sweets	Candy, jam, jelly without sodium benzoate, sugar, syrup.	Jam or jelly containing sodium benzoate.

(contd.)

Beverages	Carbonated beverages, coffee and milk.	Soft water.
Miscellaneous	Cocoa unsalted, cream sauce, herbs, spices and vinegar, and unsalted nuts.	Catsup, chili sauce, gravy, mustard, olives, peanut butter, pickles, popcorn and salt.

Low-fat (Low-cholesterol) Diet

Foods	*Include*	*Avoid*
Breads	Any (without eggs, butter or milk).	All made with butter, eggs or milk.
Cereals	Any	None
Soups	Vegetable soup without milk.	Cream soups, meat soups.
Meat, fish, eggs or cheese	Chicken, lean ham, fish (not oily), egg white, dry cottage cheese, pot cheese and farmer cheese.	Fatty meats, glandular meat, fish canned in oil, egg yolk and all other cheese.
Vegetable	Any cooked without butter or fat.	None.
Potato/substitute	Potato hominy, macaroni, rice all cooked without fat or cream.	Noodles made with egg.
Fats	Vegetable cooking fats and oils.	Animal fats, butter, cream lard, suet.
Fruits	Any.	None.
Desserts	Angel food cake, gelatin, ices.	Ice cream, pastry, coca cola and pie.

(contd.)

Sweets	Jam, jelly, sugar and hard candy.	Candy made with butter cream, chocolate, cocoa.
Beverages	Buttermilk, skim milk, coffee, tea and carbonated beverages	Whole milk, cocoa and chocolate.
Miscellaneous	Popcorn, salt, spices and vinegar.	Cream sauce, gravy, butter popcorn.

High-Residue (High-Roughage) Diet

Foods	*Include*	*Avoid*
Breads	Whole wheat, graham, dark rye.	White enriched and toast.
Cereals	Whole-grain cereals.	Refined cereals, corn, rice wheat, dry cereals prepared from cooked oatmeal.
Soups	Cream soups, vegetable soups.	Bouillon, broth.
Meat, fish, eggs or cheese	Tough meat containing fibers.	Bacon, tender meat, fish, fowl, canned fish, eggs, and cheese.
Vegetable	All especially lettuce, celery, cabbage, endive etc.	None.
Potato	Hominy, unrefined rice.	Potatoes, macaroni, noodles and refined rice.
Fats	Any other.	Butter, cream and margarine.
Fruits	All including fruit skins.	None.

(contd.)

Desserts	Desserts containing fruits and nuts.	All plain cakes, cookies, custards, gelatin, ice cream, pies and puddings.
Sweets	Candy containing fruit or nuts, and jam.	Hard candy, honey, jelly, sugar and syrup.
Beverages	Coffee and milk.	Carbonated beverages and decaffeinated coffee.
Miscellaneous	Nuts, olives, pickles, popcorn.	Cream sauce, gravy, peanut butter, spices and vinegar.

High-Residue (Low-Roughage) Diet

Foods	*Include*	*Avoid*
Breads	White, enriched or fine rye bread, white crackers and toast.	Whole wheat, graham, dark rye bread.
Cereals	Refined cereals, corn, rice, wheat, dry cereals prepared from cooked oatmeal.	Whole-grain cereals.
Soups	Bouillon and broth.	Cream soup, vegetable soup.
Meat, fish, eggs or cheese	Tender meat, fish, fowl, eggs, and cheese.	Tough meats containing fiber.
Vegetable	None	All especially lettuce, celery, cabbage, endive, etc.
Potato/substitute	Potatoes, macaroni, noodles, refined rice.	Hominy and unrefined rice.

(contd.)

Fats	Butter, cream and margarine.	Any other.
Fruits	None	All including fruit skins.
Desserts	All plain cakes, cookies, custards, gelatin, ice cream, pies, pudding.	Desserts containing fruit or nuts.
Sweets	Hard candy, honey, jelly, sugar syrup.	Candy containing fruit or nut and jams.
Beverages	Carbonated beverages, decaffeinated coffee.	Coffee and milk.
Miscellaneous	Cream sauce, gravy, peanut butter and vinegar.	Nuts, olives, pickles, popcorn and relish.

Low-Purine (Gout) Diet

Foods	*Include*	*Avoid*
Breads	All	None
Cereals	All	None
Soups	Milk soups from vegetables.	Bouillon, broth, consomme.
Meat, fish, eggs or cheese	Fish, fowl, shellfish, meats eggs and cheese.	Kidney, liver, meat extracts, sweet bread, sardines, gravy and broth.
Potato/substitute	Potatoes, hominy, macaroni and rice.	Fried potatoes, potato chips.
Fats	Butter or substitute in moderation.	None

(contd.)

Vegetables	All	None, except in case of obesity.
Desserts	Simple cakes, cookies, custards, gelatin desserts and puddings.	Mince pie.
Sweets	All	None, except in cases of obesity.
Beverages	Carbonated beverages, coffee, milk, milk drinks and tea.	None
Miscellaneous	Condiments, cream sauce, nuts salt and spices.	Alcohol, gravy and yeast.

Full Liquid Diet

Foods	*Include*	*Avoid*
Breads	None	All
Cereals	Strained farina, cornmeal or oatmeal gruel.	Any other.
Soups	Broth, strained cream soups.	Any other.
Meat, fish, eggs or cheese	Raw eggs in beverages.	Any other meat, fish, fowl or cooked eggs.
Vegetable	Tomato juice, soups and carrot juice.	All others
Potato/substitute	None except puree in soup.	All
Fats	Butter, cream and margarine.	Any other.

(contd.)

Fruits	Strained fruit juice.	Any other.
Desserts	Thin custards, plain gelatin desserts and ice cream.	Any other.
Sweets	Sugar and plain sugar candy.	Any other.
Beverages	Carbonated beverages, coffee, tea, milk and milk drinks.	None.
Miscellaneous	Spices salt.	Any other.

Diet for Allergic Patients (Elimination Diet)

Foods	*Include*	*Avoid*
Breads	Quice bread, yeast bread, crackers (all without eggs)	Bread, rolls containing eggs.
Cereals	Any except chocolate flavored.	Chocolate-flavored cereals.
Soups	Any made from allowed foods. Unusual soups.	
Meat, fish, eggs or cheese	Any meat or fowl except fresh pork and cottage cheese.	Fresh pork, fish.
Vegetable	Seasonal vegetables, all canned or cooked vegetables.	Seasonal vegetables such as corn and tomatoes.
Fats	Butter, cream, french dressing without pepper, lard and oil.	Salad dressings with pepper or eggs.

(contd.)

Fruits	Seasonal fruits, all canned or cooked fruits.	Fresh seasonal fruits such as fresh berries or melon.
Desserts	All cakes, cookies, gelatin, ice cream and puddings.	All baked custards containing chocolate, cocoa and eggs.
Sweets	Hard candy, honey, jam, jelly, sugar and syrup.	Candy with chocolate, egg or nuts.
Beverages	Carbonated beverages, coffee and milk.	Cocoa, coffee and tea.
Miscellaneous	Cream sauce, gravy, salt, spices and vinegar.	Cocoa, chocolate, nuts, pepper and favoring.

Low-Carbohydrate Diet

Foods	*Include*	*Avoid*
Breads	Two slices of plain bread.	Any other type of bread.
Cereals	$^1/_2$ cup of cooked cereal daily.	Cereals with sugar added.
Soups	Cream of vegetables.	Thickened soups.
Meat, fish, eggs or cheese	Any plainly cooked food.	Those cooked with excess gravy.
Vegetable	Vegetables in 5% or 10% grouping.	Vegetables in 15% or 20% grouping.
Potato	None —	Potatoes come in 15% grouping should be avoided.

(contd.)

Fats	Any	None.
Fruits	Any canned or cooked fruits without sugar or fresh fruit.	Ordinary canned fruit, dried or frozen food.
Desserts	Gelatin sweetened with saccharin.	Cakes, pastries, pies and ice cream.
Sweets	Saccharin.	All others.
Beverages	Coffee, tea and milk.	Carbonated and other sweet beverages.
Miscellaneous	Condiments, pickles, spices and vinegar.	Beer, catsup, cream sauce, gravy and sweet pickles.

High Calorie Diet

Bread :	Any bread, especially whole-grain or enriched bread.
Cereals :	Any, especially whole-grain or enriched cereal.
Soups :	Any.
Meat, fish, egg or Cheese :	Minimum one egg and two servings daily of meat, eggs or cheese.
Vegetables :	Any canned vegetable (cooked or raw).
Potato :	Any potato or substitute.
Fats :	Butter, cream, lard, margarine, oil and salad dressing.
Fruits :	Canned, cooked, dried or fresh fruits.
Desserts :	Cakes, cookies, ice cream, pies, puddings and others.
Sweets :	Candy, jelly, sugar and others.
Beverages :	Any beverage those high in calories.
Miscellaneous :	Condiments, gravy, nuts, salt, spices and vinegar.

Caloric value of important food products in day to day life

Product	*Fibre*	*Carbohydrates*		*Fat content*
		Sugar	*Starch*	
Milk (whole)		4.8	3.8	
Milk (skimmed)		4.8	0.1	
Butter			82.0	
Cheese		0.1	33.5	
Yoghurt		6.2	1.0	
Egg (boiled)			10.9	
Egg (fried)			19.5	
Fruit cake	2.8	43.1	14.8	12.9
Rice (white cooked)	0.8		29.6	0.3
Pasta (white cooked)			25.2	0.3
Bread (white)	2.7	1.8	47.9	1.7
Bread (brown)	5.1	1.9	42.9	2.2
Roast chicken				14.0

14
Definations of Medical Terms

Abortion	Interruption of pregnancy.
Abscess	Collection of pus in the body tissues.
Acne	Skin disorder involving the sebaceous glands.
Acne Rosacea	A chronic inflammatory congestion of the cheeks and nose, characterized by redness, dilation of blood vessels and formation of papules and pustules.
AIDS	Full form : Acquired immunity deficiency syndrome. Acquired immunity is something the body develops after it has overcome a disease or through inoculation.
Acute disease	One, with symptom of more or less violent character, such as fever and usually of shorter duration.
Acromegaly	Abnormal enlargement of bones of head, hands, feet and face due to change in the endocrine glands.
Adipose	Tissue, is a fatty layer found below the dermis.
Adolescence	The period of growth from 12 to 21 years of age.

Adrenalin	A powerful hormone produced by the adrenal glands.
Albumin	A protein substance found in most animal and plant tissues.
Allergy	Sensitivity of an individual to a specific substance, such as horse dust.
Alopecia	Patchy baldness.
Amino acids	Chemical compounds out of which proteins are formed.
Amoeba	A microscopic animal consisting of one single cell.
Amniotic sac	Fetal membrane surrounding the unborn infant.
Anemia	Deficiency of red blood cells.
Aneurysm	Bulging or rupture of blood vessel wall.
Ankylosis	Stiffness of joint.
Anorexia	Loss of appetite.
Antibiotic	A chemical substance having the power to retard the growth of certain germs.
Antidote	Medicine for counteracting the effects of poison or disease.
Antitoxin	Substance formed in the blood stream, capable of combating certain poisons within the body.
Anaethetic	Causes absence of sensation.
Antispasmodic	Relieves or checks spasms.
Antiemetic	Relieves vomiting.
Aperient	Causes bowel movement.
Aphrodisiac	Arouses sexual desire.
Analgesic	Relieves or stops pain.

Anodyne	Relieves pain.
Anticoagulant	Prevents clotting.
Aerobic	Use of oxygen to create energy in muscles.
Aorta	The large artery that carries blood from the heart to the rest of the body.
Apoplexy	Brain hemorrhage or stroke.
Arteriosclerosis	Hardening of the arteries.
Asepsis	Freedom from germs and infection.
Atrium	Auricle or upper chamber of the heart.
Alveolar glands	Milk producing glands in the breast.
Alkaline	A water-based solution having a pH greater than 7.0 on the pH scale.
Anatomy	The study of the structure of the body and what it is made of (such as bones, muscles and the skin).
Antiseptics	Kill bacteria or slow their growth, but they are not disinfectants.
Anus	Final part of large intestine.
Arrector pili	A small involuntary muscle attached to the under of the hair follicle. The muscle can cause goose flesh when you are frightened or subject to cold.
Astringent lotion	Are designed to remove oil accumulation on the skin.
Athlete's foot	A contagious disease caused by a fungus.
Asteatosis	A condition of dry, scaly skin characterized by absolute or partial deficiency of sebum due to old age or some bodily disorders.
Auricularis	Anterior, muscle in front of ear; whereas posterior is a muscle behind the ear.
Autoclave	The most popular method of physical sterilization by steam.

Barium	An opaque chemical compound used in taking X-ray pictures. It helps to visualize internal organs.
Balsam	Healing or soothing agent.
Barbiturate	A sedative drug.
Benign	Tumor or a condition, which is not malignant or cancerous.
Botulism	A severe form of food poisoning.
Bronchoscope	An instrument used to examine the bronchial tubes and to remove foreign objects lodged therein.
Bunion	Swelling of the main joint of the great toe.
Bursa	A saclike cavity filled with fluid.
Bacteria	They are minute, one celled vegetable micro-organism found nearly everywhere. (microbes that can cause illness and disease.
Bactericides	Kill harmful bacteria.
Birthmark	A small or large malformation of the skin due to abnormal pigmentation or dilated capillaries.
Blackheads	They are caused by a hardened mass of sebum formed in the ducts on to the sebaceous glands.
Boil	An acute infection of a hair follicle producing pain.
Blood	A nutritive fluid circulating through the circulatory system in the body.
Basal layer	Deepest layer of epidermis.
Bladder	Organ that stores urine.
Bicep	Muscle of the front of the arm.

Brain	Organ of central nervous system.
Bone	Dense connective tissue forming the skeletal system.
Blue nails	Nail disorder caused by poor blood circulation.
Blue light	Used on oily skin that is bare. It contains few heat rays, soothing to the nerves and produces good skin tone. It has some germicidal and chemical benefits. Useful for mild cases of skin eruptions.
Boric powder	It is used for its bactericidal and fungicidal properties in powder, mouth washes, soaps and skin fresheners.
Bromidrosis	Foul smelling perspiration usually noticeable in the armpits or feet.
Bruised nails	Dark purplish spots due to injury or bleeding under the nail.
Bulla	A blister containing watery fluid similar to vesicle, but larger in size.
Barium	An opaque chemical compound used in taking X-ray pictures. It helps to visualize internal organs of body.
Bronchoscope	An instrument used to examine the bronchial tubes and to remove foreign objects lodged therein.
Catalyst	A substance used to alter the speed of a chemical reaction.
Cell	A growth; basic units of all living things including bacteria, plants and animals.
Calorie	Unit of heat used to measure the energy value of food.
Capillary	A tiny blood vessel, finer than a human hair and connecting a vein and artery.

Carbohydrates	Energy foods, such as starches and sugars.
Carcinoma	Malignant or cancerous tumor of the skin or internal organs.
Cardiac	Pertaining to the heart.
Caries	Dental decay.
Calmative	Agent that has calming or tranquilizing effect.
Carminative	Relieves gas from intestines.
Catheter	A thin rubber or plastic tube.
Cholecystectomy	Removal of gall-bladder.
Cholesterol	A chemical substance found in fats and oils; also in bile and gall-stones. It is essential to every cell in human body.
Coagulant	Causes clotting.
Chemistry	The science that deals with the composition, structure and properties of matter, and changes under different chemical conditions.
Chronic disease	Long duration disease usually mild but recurring.
Chloasma	Characterized by increase deposits of pigment in the skin.
Contagious disease	The disease that can be spread from one person to the another.
Corium	The underlying or the inner layer of the skin.
Corrugator	Muscle beneath the frontalis and draws the eyebrow down and in. It produces vertical lines, and is the muscle used for frowning.
Cortex	The middle or the inner layer which gives strength and elasticity to the hair. It is made up of fibrous substance formed by elongated

	cells. This layer contains the pigment that gives the hair its color.
Crust	The accumulation of the sebum and pus, mixed perhaps with epidermal material.
Cutis	The underlying or inner layer of the skin.
Cyst	A semisolid or fluid lump above and below the skin.
Carotene	Yellow pigment affecting the color of the skin.
Cerebellum	The small brain.
Cilia	Tiny hair attached to a cell.
Cirrhosis	Inflammation of the liver, usually due to alcoholism.
Concussion	Narrowing or constriction of the aorta.
Coma	An unconscious state from which the patient cannot be aroused.
Congenital	A condition existing from one's birth.
Conjunctivities	Inflammation of the membrane covering the eye.
Curettage	Scraping process to remove the contents of a body cavity.
Cyanosis	Bluish discoloration of the skin caused by a diminished supply of oxygen.
Dehydration	Abnormal loss of body fluids.
Delirium	State of mental confusion and excitement.
Dermatitis	Inflammation of the skin.
Diarrhea	Loose, watery stools.
Diastolic	Lower level of the blood pressure within the arteries at the moment when the heart is at rest.

Diuretic	A medicine that releases large quantity of urine.
Derma	The underlying or inner layer of the skin.
Ducts	Tubes.
Dermatitis	An inflammatory condition of the skin. It is an skin infection that develop from allergies to ingredients in cosmetics, antiseptics, cold waving lotions and aniline derivative tints.
Depressant	Agent which reduces nervous activity.
Depurative	Agent that purifies, particularly the blood.
Digestive system	Body system associated with the intake and output of food and drinks.
Diaphoretic	An agent that producesperspiration.
Diuretic	An agent that increases the flow of urine.
Dermatology	It is study of the skin, its nature, structure, functions, diseases and treatments. Dermatologist is a medical skin specialist.
Diagnosis	It is the recognition of a disease by its symptoms.
Disease	It is any departure from a normal state of health.
Diaphragm	A muscular partition that controls breathing, separates chest from the abdominal region.
Digestion	The process of converting food into a form that can be assimilated by the body.
Dysentery	Inflammation and ulceration of the lower part of the intestines, resulting in bloody or mucus filled stools.
Dysmenorrhoea	Painful or difficult menstruation.
Dystrophy	Progressive weakness of a muscle.

Eczema	A skin disease with itching and redness.
Electrocardiograph	Diagnostic instrument used to record the electrical current generated in the heart.
Embolism	Obstruction of a blood-vessel by a blood clot or foreign substance from some other area.
Embryo	Earliest stage of human life before birth.
Emphysema	Abnormal presence of gas or air in body tissues.
Endemic	A disease which is present more or less continuously in a community.
Endocarditis	Inflammation of the inside lining and valves in the heart.
Enzyme	Complex organic substances secreted by living cells which important in digestion and other bodily functions.
Epithelioma	A malignant tumor originating in the skin or mucus membrane.
Estrogen	Female sex hormones produced in the ovaries.
Eczema	An inflammation of skin, of acute or chronic nature presenting many forms of dry or moist lesions.
Endocrine glands	Ductless glands that have secretions called hormones delivered directly into the blood stream, which in turn influences the welfare of the body.
Epidermis	Outer layer of the skin.
Excretory system	Including the kidneys, liver, skin, intestines and lungs that purifies the body by eliminating waste matter.
Exhalation	Carbon dioxide is expelled.

Embryo	Earliest stage of human life before birth.
Emetic	Causing vomiting.
Emollient	Agent used externally for a softening and soothing effect.
Emphysema	Abnormal presence of gas or air in body tissues. Widening of the air sacs in the lungs.
Fibrillation	Rapid twitching of the valves of the heart.
Flatulene	Air or gas in the stomach or intestines.
Fetus	Unborn child after third month of conception.
Fomentation	A hot, moist pack or application to the body.
Fracture	Broken bone.
Febrifuge	Reduces or stops fever.
Gamma globulin	A protein produced in the blood with special properties for combating disease.
Fissure	A crack in the skin penetrating into the dermis.
Felon	An infection and inflammatory condition of the tissues surrounding the nail.
Formulas	Mixture of two or three ingredients.
Freckles	Small yellow to brown colored spots on the skin exposed to sunlight and air.
Fungi	Vegetable parasites including all types of fungus and mold.
Fungicides	Destroy fungus.
Frontal	Bone of the forehead.
Gastric	Pertaining to the stomach.

Gangrene	Death of part of the body tissue due to loss of normal blood supply to the affected area.
Gene	The biological units of heredity contained in the chromosome.
Geriatrics	A branch of medicine dealing particularly with the health and welfare of the aged.
Granule	A minute particle in the hair melanin.
Gall-bladder	Accessory organ of the digestive system.
Genitalia	Reproductive organs.
Granular layer	The layer of the epidermis lying directly above the stratum germinativum.
Hemoglobin	Substance that allows the blood cells to carry oxygen and carbon dioxide.
Holistic	The complete person-the whole self-body, mind and soul.
Hormones	Chemical messengers produced by endocrine glands.
Horny layer	The top layer of the epidermis consisting of dead, flat, hard cells.
Hepatic	A drug which works on the liver.
Hemostatic	Halting bleeding.
Halitosis	Offensive breath.
Hallucination	A mental impression having no foundation in fact.
Heartburn	Burning sensation in upper abdomen and chest.
Hypochondriac	One who is constantly over anxious about his health.
Hypertension	Elevation of the blood pressure.
Herpes simplex	A recurring virus infection; commonly called fever bristle.

Histology	The study of the minute structural parts of the body.
Hyper hidrosis	Excessive perspiration caused by excessive heat or general body weakness.
Hypertrophy	An overgrowth of the nail, usually in thickness rather than in length caused by local infection.
Insulin	Hormones produced in the pancreas.
Iris	Colored part of eyes.
Inorganic	The branch of chemistry deals with all substances that do not contain carbon.
Inhalation	Oxygen is absorbed into the blood.
Immunity	The ability of the body to destroy bacteria.
Infestation	Worms, insects and mites that attack the body.
Integumentry system	The skin, hair and nails.
Infarction	Death of a localized area of the heart due to sudden stoppage of blood supply to the involved area.
Infestation	Worms, insects and mites that attack the body.
Inoculation	Introduction of a virus into the system to produce a form of the disease and thus secure immunity.
Isometric	Static muscle contraction, without movement at a joint.
Isotonic	Active muscle contraction with movement at a joint.
Jaundice	Yellow skin due to presence of bile.
Kidneys	Two bean shaped organ that produce urine.
Laceration	A wound or tear of the skin or deeper tissues.

Laxative	Causes bowel movement.
Lactation	The period during which milk is produced.
Leucorrhoea	A whitish discharge from the female genital organ.
Leukaemia	A blood disease in which the white blood cells increase enormously in number. The condition is known as cancer of the blood.
Leukocytes	White blood cells.
Ligament	A tough band connecting bones or other tissues of the body.
Lymph nodes	Small gland where certain white blood cells are produced.
Lactic acid	The waste product of energy production in a muscle.
Liver	Largest internal organ.
Malignant	A condition leading to death, as from cancer.
Mastitis	Inflammation of the breasts.
Menopause	Change in life.
Menstruation	Periodic discharge of blood from vagina in females.
Metabolism	The process of chemical and physical change taking place within the cells of the body during the building up and breaking down of the tissues.
Metastasis	Spread of cancer cells from one part of the body to another.
Microbe	A germ.
Macule	Discolored spot or patch on the surface of the skin, such as freckles. These are neither raised nor sunken.

Mold	A type of fungus infection caused when moisture is trapped.
Miliaria rubra	Also known as prickly heat. It is an acute inflammatory disorder of the sweat glands characterized by an eruption of small red vesicles and accompanied by a burning and itching of the skin.
Mantle	It is deep fold of the skin in which the nail root is embedded.
Mucus	Lubricating fluid secreted by the mucus membranes of the body.
Mammary glands	Female breasts.
Mentalis	Muscle at the top of chin.
Monocytes	White blood cells.
Melanocytes	Cells which produce melanin.
Minerals	Food that provides the body with the nutrient needed to maintain its functions.
Mole	A small brownish spot or blemish on the skin. They range in color from pale tan to brown or bluish black.
Nephritic	A medicine which acts on nervous system to calm the nerves.
Miscarriage	Interruption of pregnancy, spontaneous abortion.
Myocardium	Heart muscle.
Myxedema	Condition due to thyroid deficiency.
Nephritis	Inflammation of the kidney.
Neuralgia	Pain in nerve.
Neurasthenia	A neurosis characterized by abnormal fatigue.
Neuritis	Inflammation of the nerves.

Neurosis	Emotional disorder caused by some inner conflict.
Node	A knot or swelling.
Naevus	A small or large malformation of the skin due to abnormal pigmentation or dilated capillaries.
Nerves	Long, made up of fibers that carry messages to and from various parts of the body.
Neurology	It is the branch of anatomy that deals with nervous system and its disorders.
Obesity	Overweight caused by accumulation of excess fat in the body.
Origin	Fixed point of attachment of a muscle to a bone.
Oedema	An abnormal amount of fluid in the body tissues, such as in the legs and ankles.
Ova/ovum	Eggs.
Osteoporosis	Thinning of the bones.
Otosclerosis	Progressive type of deafness.
Ovulation	Release of the ripened egg from the ovary, occurring each month midway between the menstrual period.
Oxytocin	Hormones produced in the posterior lobe of the pituitary gland.
Oxygen	Vital gas breathed into the body from the atmosphere. (A chemical element that is necessary to life).
Pacemaker	A section of the heart wall that controls the rate and rhythm of the heart-beat.
Palpate	To examine by touch.
Palpitation	Rapid throbbing pulsation of the heart.

Pancreas	Main digestive organ of the body.
Pathological	Concerned with disease.
Pellagra	A deficiency disease characterized by sores around the mouth.
Pericardium	Fibrous bag surrounding the heart.
Peristalsis	Wave-like muscular contractions of stomach and intestine walls.
Phlebitis	Inflammation of the veins.
Placenta	An organ developed in the uterus through which the unborn child obtains its nourishment.
Plasma	Liquid part of the blood.
Plastic surgery	Restoring normal appearance of skin following an injury.
Platelets	Tiny fragments of cells essential to the clotting of blood.
Pleura	Tissue covering the lung.
Pneumonia	Acute inflammation of the lung.
Podiatrist	Specialist in care of feet.
Polycythaemia	An excess of red blood cells.
Polyp	A small, soft tumor attached by a slender stalk to the surface of the mucus membrane.
Prostate	A sex gland surrounding the neck of the bladder in the male.
Prothrombin	One of the blood clotting factors in the blood.
Pruritus	Intense itching.
Psychosis	A serious mental disorder.
Psychotherapy	Treatment of mental and emotional disorders.

Puberty	The time when a boy or girl begins to become sexually mature.
Papillary layer	Top layer of dermis that connects the lower layer of epidermis.
Parasites	Animal or vegetable organism which lives on or within another.
Purgative	Any agent that causes bowel relief.
Pectoral	Relief for chest and lungs ailments.
Penis	Male sex organ.
Parathormone	Hormones produced in parathyroid glands.
Respiration	The act of breathing.
Rhinitis	Inflammation of the mucous membranes of the nose, as seen in cold weather and hay fever.
Sclerosis	Hardening of the tissue.
Sebaceous	Pertaining to the oily or fatty matter secreted by the skin glands.
Seizure	A sudden attack of pain or disease condition.
Senility	The mental and physical weakness of old age.
Sloughing	The separation of dead from living tissues caused by decay or decomposition.
Systole	The contracting phase of the heart's action.
Systolic	Upper level of the blood pressure indicating the greatest force exerted by the heart.
Stomachic	An agent that stimulates, strengthens and tones the stomach.
Tachycardia	Rapid heart-beat.
Tetanus	An infectious disease characterized by tonic spasm of the voluntary muscles.

Thrombosis	Clogging of blood vessel caused by the formation of a clot.
Tourniquet	A tight band used to stop bleeding.
Toxin	A poisonous substance produced by the action of micro-organism.
Umbilicus	Navel or depression in center of the abdomen.
Varicosity	A swollen twisted vein.
Wassermann	Blood test to determine presence of syphilis.

15
Women Health Remedies

Asthma

Asthma is a chronic and complicated condition, which require immediate medical attention. The following symptoms are the possible signs of this dreaded disease:

- Shortness of breath.
- Severe coughing and wheezing.
- Tightness in the chest.
- Excessive yawning or extreme fatigue

In the under-40 age group, in 90% cases asthma is triggered by an allergy such as grass pollens, animal fur, dust, fumes, odour and an improper diet that lacks all the nutrients they need. After the age 40, in over 50% cases asthma is caused due to some form of lung infections or disorder such as emphysema. Asthma patients should use doctor-prescribed inhaler immediately when having an attack. If you still cannot breathe easily after using inhaler, get in touch with the doctor without delay. The following precautions or remedies help stop or reduce asthma attack:

- Control over cigarette smoking: Asthma patients should avoid smoking. Asthmatics should not smoke, this is particularly important in the winter season. Sometimes, in the house smoke, especially in winter months, it leads to a worsening of asthma. Asthma patients should not work on wood stove and chimneys while cooking.
- Asthma can be caused by stomach reflux: A condition in which acid backs up into your esophagus from your stomach, when

the contents in the stomach may leak out a little and drip down into your airway while sleeping. Prop your bed up and elevate the pillow while you are lying to prevent the dripping. Take an antacid at bedtime to cut down acidity.

- Stay indoors when it is cold outside: Make sure to keep your mouth and nose covered with a scarf or mask covering your mouth when going outside so that you may end up breathing in warm, humid environment.
- Breathe in a warm, dry climate.
- Magnesium is recommended as a useful mineral nutrient for asthma patients, relaxes and opens the bronchial tract-the airway to the lungs.
- Fatty acids reduce lungs inflammation. The lungs become inflamed during asthma attack, which makes it harder to breathe. Fish and flaxseed oil are rich source of fatty acids.
- Swimming is the ideal exercise for asthmatics. Keep your mouth closed and breathe through your nose.
- Use auto air conditioning wisely. Air conditioning may be good for asthmatics but not if it is bringing outside air in, as it brings with it pollen and cool, air is bad for asthma.
- Stay out of the kitchen, as smelling the foods you are sensitive can bring an asthma attack.
- Beware of food additives (especially metabisulfite found in beer, wine, dried fruits, apricots and possibly monosodium glutamate) can trigger asthma.
- Use nettle to relieve from nasal allergies.
- Concentration on breathing properly can help stop an asthma attack. By drawing more air into your lungs, relaxing your body, controlling anxiety and panic, you can significantly reduce the severity of asthma attacks. Let your body feel the rhythm of the breath and your heart. Continue for 10 to 15 minutes.
- Have anti-asthma diet. Fish contains oil that reduces the airway inflammation of asthma. Onions, ginger and garlic strengthen the immune system, which thins mucus. Fruits and vegetables, healing components in food help control harmful free radical molecules in the body. Sea vegetables deliver lot of protein and minerals. Fruits high in vitamin C and beta-carotene, such as dark green, leafy vegetables help fight inflammation. High-

fat, high-salt condiments are unhealthy for people with asthma. Eat more fish, drink milk and have soy meal. High salt condiments, high fat, spices and lemon juice are unhealthy for people with asthma.

Arthritis

Arthritis is the oldest known ailment among women. The primary symptoms of arthritis are the following:

- Pain.
- Stiffness.
- Swelling in and around the joints.
- Limited movement of affected body organs that last more than two weeks.

There are many medical treatments that can help control arthritis pain, such as medication and surgery, but both may be ineffective and even damaging. Here are few steps recommended for the professional care and relief of arthritis:

- Controlling stress through relaxation techniques.
- Lose weight, gain relief. A complete diet plan and nutritional supplements designed to alleviate arthritis pain and also to reduce weight. The more overweight you are, the more stress and pressure you place on your joints. This increases the stress on the cartilage, which interferes with the bone, thus increasing the incidence of inflammation, swelling and pain.
- Detecting and eliminating food allergies that may cause complicating disease.
- Treating fungal, bacterial and viral micro-organisms, such as the fungus candida that may complicate the disease further.
- Removing toxic overload from the body.
- Stretch gently for strength and mobility. Yoga teaches movement with proper joint alignment, which helps bringing deformed joints back to normal position as appropriate muscles are lengthened and strengthened. Yoga exercise is the key to restore health to arthritic joints.
- Learn to relax.
- Water exercises are excellent to relieve arthritis.

- Turmeric boosts the healing power of glucosamine, which reduce the pain and inflammation of arthritis.
- Ginger is another spice with scientifically proven anti-inflammatory powers. Eat plenty of fresh (preferably raw) ginger.
- Use ice to prevent pain on the joints.
- Use heat to reduce pain. When joints become hot, swollen and tender, heat is the best solution.
- Take fish oil capsules. Fish oil supplements reduce the pain.
- Rub 'Mahanarayan oil' on the skin of the area having pain and causes immediate relief. But it is not a permanent cure. The oil penetrates the skin and softens pain-causing deposits in the bones.
- The herb 'Guggul' relieves arthritis pain. The herb travels to the arthritis bone and removes the imbalances that are causing the stiffness, swelling and inflammation.
- Avoid vigorous exercise, which do not result in curing joint inflammation. But it do improve the walk time, physical activity and health status of the participant. Some women put the baby to their joints, which is harmful for arthritis patients. Experts advise to follow light aerobic program, cycling or swimming gently.
- Unfortunately, sleeping pills, tranquilizers and narcotic painkillers can become part of life for a woman suffering from arthritis, which end up creating many problems than they solve. Consult a physiotherapist to recommend treatment to relieve pain.
- Boost your vitamin C intake as in most of cases remedy for someone with rheumatoid arthritis patients will be intake of sufficient vitamin C contents. Lack of this vitamin can aggravate rheumatoid arthritis.
- Avoid hydrogenated oils, which interfere with the metabolism of fatty acids. These oils are found in margarine, peanut butter, most cooking oils and several other processed products such as snack chips, baked goods and salad dressings.
- Massage for arthritis pain, working the muscles that are attached to the tendons leading to your painful joints. In case of arthritis in hands for women engaged in household work, always massage the forearms from the wrists to elbows, using a compression technique.

- Vegetable juices such as carrot juice, tomato juice, celery juice and cabbage juice reduce pain for many patients suffering from arthritis. You may seek advise of a doctor to suggest one suitable for you.
- Acupressure therapy cures arthritis pain. This encourages the flow of blood, which, lubricate the joints, carries away toxins and reduce pain, swelling and inflammation. In acupressure, the spine is a major affected part of the body along which chi circulates in the body. The increase of flow of chi in the spine helps to increase the flow of chi in entire body and can ease the arthritis pain all over the body. Roll a hand towel lengthwise into a tub. Lie on a bed with the towel underneath your back on the right side of and parallel to the spine, directly under the ridge of muscles. Acupressure points on the hands are more sensitive than the areas around them. Hold the pressure on each point for minimum four to five breathes. Then move the towel on the left side of your spine and press the points on your left hand.

Age spots

Brown spots start to pepper the backs of your hands when a woman reaches in forties or fifties. These are also called as sun spots, as are generally caused by direct exposure to the sun's ultraviolet radiation, which damage the color producing cells of the skin. In fact age spots are a cosmetic problem, not a medical or health-threatening condition. They can be medically removed by the following methods:

- The process of bleaching.
- Applying liquid nitrogen.
- By laser surgery.
- Consult a doctor if the area around a spot has turned black and irregular in shape. This condition is known as signs of melanoma.
- Aromatherapy helps the spot to fade or lighten. The essential oils of lemon have bleaching properties that eliminate the age spot. Add three drops of oil to carrier oil, preferably almond oil and apply the mixture to the spot twice a day for a couple of months.

- A mixture of honey and yogurt create natural bleach that can help lighten age spots. To a teaspoon of plain yogurt, mix thoroughly a teaspoon of honey. Apply a mixture to the hands, let it dry and wash it off after half an hour. Hands are the organs in a human body from where ageing starts.

Alzheimer's Disease

Alzheimer's (a brain disease) devastates mental, emotional and physical functioning in human body. This disease is usually treated by a neurologist by increasing levels of acetylcholine–a brain chemical responsible for memory and administering vitamin E (recommended intake 2,000 international units a day of the d-alpha tocopherol form of the nutrient as per consultation of your doctor). Alzheimer's disease may be treated by the following methods:

- Nutritional counseling.
- Brain-supportive nutritional and herbal supplements.
- Physical exercise.
- Mind-body stress control technique, which include meditation, psychological counseling etc.
- Replacement of hormones such as testosterone and growth hormones.
- The nutrient phosphatidylserine (daily dose 300 milligrams) taken as per your doctor's advice improves mental capacity.
- The nutrient Coenzyme Q 10 (daily dose 200 milligrams) is vital for producing energy in neurons and throughout the body.
- Eat plenty of cold-water fish and help protect brain cells.

Athlete's Foot

A condition caused by an organism that lives on the skin and breeds under warm, moist conditions. Sweaty footwear is most often responsible for this disorder. This is an acute form of dermatitis. The common symptoms include the following:

- Cracked skin.
- Red, swollen, sore and oozing blisters.
- Intermittent burning sensation.

The inflammation is not dangerous, but it can lead to bacterial infection if not treated properly. The following treatment is recommended:

- Use soothing compresses to cool the inflammation, ease the pain, lessen the itching and dry the sores. Mix two tablespoons Burrow's solution in ½ liter cold water and apply solution with cotton cloth 3 to 4 times a day.
- Soak your foot in a solution of 2 teaspoons salt mixed to ½ liter water for 5 to 10 minutes until the problem clears up.
- Apply an anti-fungal cream on your feet as recommended by your doctor.
- To avoid fungus on your feet, especially between the toes, apply baking soda paste. To make paste mix 1 tablespoon of baking soda to lukewarm water and rub on the site of fungus, then rinse and dry.
- Toenails are breeding spots for the fungus. Scrape the undersides clean every second or third day with a orange stick.
- After the infection has cleared up, apply anti-fungal cream or lotion regularly.
- Avoid use of plastic shoes and footwear; they trap perspiration and create a warm, moist spot for the fungus to grow. Keep your feet dry and clean. Give your shoes a little time in the sun to air out.
- Powder your toes frequently.

Consult a doctor immediately in case of:

- Inflammation which proves incapacitating.
- Swelling occurs in the foot or the leg at any time during the attack, and you develop a fever.
- Pus appears in the blisters or the cracked skin.
- Dab regular, plain yogurt on the infected areas. The yogurt helps reduce the symptoms of athlete's foot and is soothing to the skin.
- Rub two to three drops of garlic oil on the affected areas of your feet to kill foot fungus.
- Vitamin C is the best nutrients for strengthening the immune system. Start treatment with 250-milligram capsules for the first week, increase to 500-milligram dosages the second week, then to 1,000 milligrams in the third week. If you develop diarrhea or loose bowel movements due to possible side effect

of large doses of vitamin C, go back to the quantity of dose at which you do not have the problem.

Chapped lips

Rough, dry, flaking, chapped lips are as natural as the weather. If your lips remain dry all the time, your body needs more water. To hydrate your lips, you need to sip hot water, which usually dilates body's circulatory system. Dryness, redness or scaling of lips are the signs of getting lips chapped. The following remedial measures are suggested if you have chapped lips:

- Calcium, magnesium and fatty acids make an ideal remedy for chronically dry, chapped lips.
- Apply cocoa butter, which is non-toxic, rich in emollients and moisturizing agent, which protect, soothe, re-hydrate dry, chapped lips.
- Essential oils of lavender and sandalwood help to reduce inflammation, redness, and moisturize dry, chapped lips.
- Avoid eating processed foods, which make lips dry and flaky. A high-potency multi-vitamin and mineral supplement may correct the problem.

Backache

Back pain (usually lower back pain) is very common among women generally due to a ruptured disc or other spinal problems. The back pain comes in two forms You should seek medical assistance, if you have:

- Intense pain that travels down your legs or radiate from your spine.
- There is sudden weakness in your leg or foot
- Have loss of control of your bowels or bladder.

Some backs need immediate doctor's attention in case of:

- Back pain that comes on suddenly without a reason.
- Back pain accompanied by other symptoms such as fever, stomach cramps, chest pain and difficulties in breathing.
- Chronic pain that lasts more than two weeks without any relief.
- An acute attack of pain that lasts for more than two to three days without any relief.

- A back pain that radiates down your leg to your knee or foot.

The following measures are taken to relieve back pain:

- Exercise is the best way to cure chronic back pain.
- Swimming is great exercise for the back.
- Try ice massage on the spot for 5 to 8 minutes depending upon the condition. It helps reduce swelling and the strain on your back muscles.
- Hot and cold treatment is the best to relieve back pain. Do 30 minutes of ice, followed by 30 minutes of heat treatment, and keep repeating the cycle.
- Stretching a sore back will enhance the healing process of backache.
- Sleep on a bed that doesn't sag in the middle when you sleep on it.
- Develop fetal attraction. Sleep like a baby if you sleep on your side and stick a pillow between your knees.
- Take an aspirin a day to relieve back pain, which is often accompanied by inflammation around the site of the pain.

Knee Pain

Knee pain-a common disorder in women makes life miserable. The knee is composed of two bones balancing on one another and lashed by muscles and connective tissue. Usually weight-bearing joint in the body makes the knee prone to arthritis, injuries and pain. You must see an orthopedist for diagnosis and treatment of knee pain, swelling or tenderness, which occurs within 24 hours of an injury or a pain. An cffcctivc medical treatment for knee pain is reconstructive or neural-fascial therapy-which include a series of injections into the knee joint that helps stabilize tissue and strengthens the joint, cartilage, ligaments and tendons. The following remedies are recommended to eliminate knee pain:

- Exercise on the floor eliminates misalignment that causes knee pain. Just walk bare-feet back and forth in a straight line for five minutes two to three times a day.
- Reflex therapy helps cure a knee pain. Mix one drop of lemongrass essential oil with four to five drops of vegetable oil and massage gently the affected area with fingertips to

regenerate nerve tissues. Massage once or twice a day until the pain is relieved.

- Pressing an acupressure point in the middle of the crease in the back of knee releases a lot of inflammation from knee injuries.

Neck and shoulder pain

If you have sudden acute neck pain, seek medical help immediately. There are various movements and therapies to change muscular patterns that can cause chronic neck and shoulder pain. Therapies that may help relieve chronic neck and shoulder pain include chiropractic treatments, acupuncture and massage to correct muscles and bones, and relieve neck and shoulder pain.

- Proper breathing by exhaling completely relieves the tension and pain. Residual carbon dioxide in your lungs as a result the tight, painful neck and shoulder muscles deprive of oxygen in the muscles and cause tension and pain.
- Relaxation relieves pain in the body. Lie flat on well-carpeted floor placing chin and forehead in line. Bend your knees by resting your calves on the seat of a chair. Place your hands on your ribs. This will relieve tension and pain from your neck and shoulders.

Bad Breath (Halitosis)

Remember, brushing and flossing your teeth regularly can clean up some of the oral bacteria that commonly cause bad breath. Chronic type of bad breath may be caused due to many different types of diseases, such as:

- Cancer
- Kidney failure
- Diabetes.
- Tuberculosis
- Syphilis (a venereal disease)
- Dehydration
- Zinc deficiency
- Some drugs, including penicillamine and lithium.

To test your breath, cup your hands on the mouth and breathe into them with a great, deep, haaaaaa. Sniff, if it smells bad, then you smell bad. To relieve bad breath the following measures are taken:

- Rinse your mouth out when you can't brush. After having meals, get a mouthful of water, which will wash the smell of the food from your mouth.
- Eat three meals a day. Often a bad breath can be caused by irregular food habits. Bad breath is caused by the side effects of fasting or by having a poor diet.
- Swallowing water when having meal outside is another method to save from bad breath. You can excuse yourself from the dining table. Take a sip of water and circulate it across and around your teeth. Then swallow bits of food.
- Use tongue scraper. A lot of odor-producing bacteria as well as some smelly, decaying food particle covers the surface of your tongue. Scrape them off with a tongue scraper- a U shaped device, which drag over the length of your tongue to collect bacteria and food particles accumulated over the tongue.
- Odorize your digestive tract with chlorophyll, which relieves from bad breath caused by digestive problems in the stomach and intestinal tract, can cause mouth odor.
- Activated charcoal is a natural breath sweetener, which can clean out your insides and sweeten your breath. Take one capsule a day until the problem is solved. If the results are not encouraging consult a dentist.
- Digestive enzymes break down bad breath. Lack of digestive enzymes cause poor digestion resulting in bad breath.
- Herbs such as ginger, coriander, cumin, anise seeds, cloves and fennel are common herbs that can deodorize intestinal tract.

Bladder Infection (urinary tract infection)

You should see a doctor immediately if you observe the following symptoms:

- Blood contents in your urine.
- Have a fever and pain near one or both kidneys.
- When postmenopausal women have recurrent bladder infections, generally due to hormone imbalances.

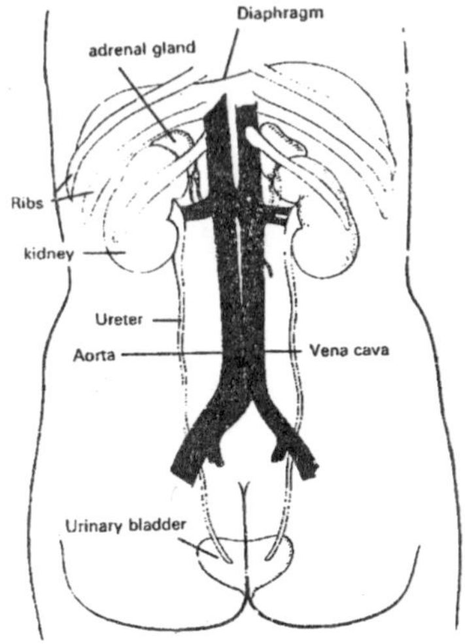

Urinary Tract Infection

- Have frequent urge to urinate (cystitis).
- Have burning, itching and painful urination.
- Feel nausea or vomiting.
- Have pain in the lower back or flank.

More than 40% women suffer from bladder infections caused by bacteria known as E.coli that exists in vagina and make their way to the urethra-the tube through which urine flows. Nearly 20% women are seen usually suffering from recurrent infections. The disorder is more common among over-sexy women and newly weds.

The following treatment is suggested:

- Wiping from front to back helps prevent infection from recurring, as you want to move bacteria away from-not towards the vagina and opening of the urethra.
- Go to the bathroom before having intercourse, which helps to flush out bacteria present in vagina. Remember, many times bacteria might be pushed into the bladder during intercourse.
- Always go to the bathroom after the intercourse as sometimes bacteria present on male organ can massage present at the opening of urethra push bacteria into the bladder. Urinary tract

infections are more common in sexually active women and the sex act with such women lead to accumulation of bacteria on male organ. It is seen a bladder infection occurs after frequent intercourse.

- Practice good hygiene and in case you don't remove bacteria in the perineal region between vagina and rectum, you may run the risk of repeated infections. Avoid douching as far as possible, which sometimes introduce bacteria into the vagina or replace them with infectious E. coli bacteria.
- Wear dry, cotton underwear. Avoid tight pants that reduce ventilation.
- Drink cranberry or blueberry juice and lot of water to flush out the bladder and rid of the infection.
- Vitamin C and vitamin A strengthen the inner surface of the bladder. (Daily dose of 1,000 to 4,000 milligrams of vitamin C and 50,000 international units of vitamin A).
- Antibiotic drugs (recommended by the doctor) relieve infection.
- Mineral zinc strengthens immune system and fights urinary tract infection.
- The herbs dandelion increases the flow of urine to help flush out bacteria besides strengthening immune system.
- If you develop honeymoon cystitis, usually an bladder infection occurs after frequent intercourse.
- Here is a natural way to get rid of bladder infection: Lie on a slant board and start rubbing your tummy just above the pubic bone for about 10 minutes. The massage improves bladder circulation and stimulates flow of bacteria-ridden urine.
- Take a hot bath in case of a inflammation due to bladder infection.
- Women prone to frequent bladder infection should use pads instead of tampons during menstruation period.

Blood Pressure

Nearly 70% women are seen suffering from a high or low blood pressure. If left untreated, blood pressure tends to rise slowly and steadily over a number of years.

Sometimes, a very high blood pressure strikes all of sudden, with diastolic pressure reaching over 130 mm Hg. and systolic pressures can reach 250 mm Hg. or more. This condition is known as malignant hypertension, which can damage blood vessels in the kidneys, eyes or brain if left untreated. There are dozens of powerful medications for lowering the blood pressure. If your blood pressure is 160/100 or higher, you may need pressure lowering drugs as well as natural remedies.

The cause of your high blood pressure may be hidden emotions if you:

- Develop high blood pressure suddenly-almost overnight.
- Have high blood pressure but no risk factors as: overweight or having a family history of hypertension.
- Develop high blood pressure at a very early age.
- Have uncontrollably high blood pressure.
- Often have recurrent high blood pressure

To treat hypertension, following measures are seen helpful:

- Aerobic exercise for 30 minutes four times a week relaxes artery walls and decreases stress. It also helps to lose weight.
- Scientific studies reveal that garlic eaten fresh or in supplement form help lower the high blood pressure.
- Avoid artery-hurting saturated foods, red meats and dairy foods However, eat fish daily if you are non-vegetarian. Take seven capsules daily of a high potency fish oil, with the recommendation of your doctor).
- Magnesium gluconate (recommended dose 500 to 1,000 milligrams a day) helps to lower blood pressure.
- High potassium fruits and vegetables are helpful to lower high blood pressure. Eat at least two bananas a day. Fruits and vegetables supply plenty of fiber, which lower blood pressure.

Low Blood pressure (hypo-tension)

For some women, the problem is not high blood pressure but rather low blood pressure, which cause suffering women dizzy spell or even faintness when they stand for too long or indulge in over work. A low blood pressure may cause:

- A weakness.
- Fatigue.
- Headaches.
- Fainting

In many cases, hypo-tension is caused by the medications a patient takes for hypertension, which include diuretics, alcohol, tranquillizers and antidepressants. The following measures are taken if you are suffering from a low blood pressure:

- Eat smaller, more frequent meals.
- Sleep on a slant. Sleep with the head end of your bed elevated 8 to 12 inches above the feet end.
- Talk less as far as possible.
- Don't worry when you are outside the home, you may get fainted due to anxiety.

High Cholesterol

Uncontrolled high cholesterol can be a serious health threat. Have your cholesterol level tested every six months. In case the total cholesterol reading is 200 or higher, the cholesterol level must be tested every three months. Cholesterol produced in a human body helps to build new cells, produce hormones and insulate nerves. You daily intake of cholesterol should be limited to 300 milligrams.

A high cholesterol level having a mushy, yellow fat-related substance circulating in the bloodstream is harmful. The excess builds up on artery walls, it can clog arteries and restrict blood flow, possibly leading to a heart attack, stroke or angina pain. The following supplement excess formation of cholesterol:

- Niacin: also known as nicotinic acid lower cholesterol in the body. Start off with low doses (up to 100 milligrams a day), then gradually increase the dose. But be aware that a sudden drastic increase in niacin can produce severe intestinal disorders and abnormal liver function. The treatment should be taken up strictly in consultation with a doctor.
- Vitamin C and Vitamin E: Vitamin raises the levels of protective HDL (high-density lipoprotein), especially in elderly people. The cholesterol level drops by consuming extra vitamin C through pectin-rich diet. Fruits and vegetables such as citrus

fruit, tomatoes, potatoes, strawberries and spinach-all these are very rich in vitamin C. Use of vitamin E increases HDL levels. It is very useful for people with high blood-fat levels.

- Calcium: supplements the health of your bones. 1 gm. of calcium taken daily for eight weeks lowers cholesterol level in the body. According to a study, 2 gm. calcium taken a day reduces cholesterol by 25% in a year.
- Watch your weight thoroughly. Your diet should consist of 2/3rd fruit and vegetables, cereals and whole grains, and only one-third of your calories should come from meat and dairy products.
- Cut the fat from your diet, which have an bad effect on cholesterol levels as below:
    1. Saturated fat elevates blood cholesterol.
    2. Polyunsaturated fat lowers blood cholesterol.
    3. Dietary cholesterol can contribute to elevate blood cholesterol to a lesser degree than saturated fat. Cut down foods having much saturated fat such as meat, butter, cheese and hydrogenated oil, and replace these items with fish, poultry, low-fat dairy products and polyunsaturated oils (corn, safflower and soybean).
- The substances such as tea, lemongrass oil, barley, rice bran also help combat high cholesterol.
- Regular exercise decreases the buildup of cholesterol blockage inside the arteries. It also helps body's ability to clear fat from the blood.
- Garlic and onions can reduce harmful blood fats.
- Cut back on coffee and smoking.

Corns and calluses

Corns, common among housewives and working women, are the ugly little bumps and lumps of dead skin cells on the feet as a result of friction and irritation between feet and shoes. Calluses are your body's way of protecting you from pressure. When the pressure increases, the callus gets thicker and thicker. People having calluses live easily than with painful corns between and on toes.

What to do in case of blisters?: The footwear that pinches gives you blisters. Shoes should not be loose, as constant rubbing can also give rise to blisters. The following precautions are essential in case suffering from blisters:

- Till the blisters has dried, do not wear the same shoes.
- Use a talcum powder and keep it dry.
- Cover blisters when you are going out, but otherwise air it properly.
- Use an antiseptic cream over blisters.
- Do not temper with the blister yourself but consult a doctor.
- Do not try to puncture blister yourself, it can infect your skin.

There is threatening by corn at the place where one gets blister. If the same defective shoe is being worn repeatedly and a blister is left untreated, you will develop corns. Make sure you change your footwear frequently. Scrub corns hard with a pumice stone and massage thereafter. Usually, the corns on the sole of the feet are painful and give trouble. Better consult a doctor. Never be tempted to remove the corn by attempting to cut it with a pair of scissors.

Cracked nails. sweaty toes, foot odor, enlarged veins, cracked heels, rough skin, tanned toes, swollen feet, bunions and fungal infection are some of common problems in women. Cracked nails often happen as a result of neglecting your toenails. Sweaty toes can pose a lot of problems and acquire a peculiar odor. The following care should be taken:

- Wash your feet often with cold water.
- Use a skin astringent on the soles of your feet.
- Sprinkle little talcum powder before wearing a closed shoe.
- Do not wear the same shoe everyday.
- Use a strong eau-de-cologne on the toes, as it acts as an antiperspirant and kill odor too.
- Wear cotton or woolen socks, avoid wearing nylon socks altogether.

Enlarged veins usually appear where one has to stand a lot and sometimes wearing high heels. Your feet need a rest. Avoid wearing high heels and ensure that the garters on your nylon stockings are not tight. 'Cracked heels' is very common complaint in women due to lack of moisture and oil. Prevent cracked heel by using glycerin and oil to massage your feet once a week. If the skin is rough, apply a lanolin based cream and a good moisturizer all over to keep skin moist.

When one walks around a lot in the sun, the feet acquire a lot of tan. Bleaching can help you get rid of it. Do not expose your feet too much to the sun. Swollen feet happen if one is not used to standing or sitting for too long. Avoid feet hanging down and wearing tight shoes. Wash your feet with hot soapy water. Keep your legs up in the air along the walls for at least five minutes daily. This cures swelling on the feet. Bunions are changes that take place in the bones because of pressure of the shoes on the toes. It is best to prevent such condition from developing.

Feet are more prone to fungus infection, because the fungus infection thrives in a moist and airless atmosphere where the sun doesn't reach. Switch over to open shoes or sandals without socks. Use an anti-fungus cream, especially between the toes-a breeding place for the infection Here are few of common nail irregularities and blemishes seen among women:

- Bruised nails: darker, purplish spots due to injury and the bleeding in the nail bed.
- Blue nails: Caused by poor blood circulation or heart disorder.
- Corrugation or wavy ridges: An uneven nail growth of nails due to illness or injury.
- Eggshell nails: More flexible than normal nails having thin white plate caused by a chronic illness.
- Furrows: Nails run lengthwise or across as a result of illness or an injury to nail cells near matrix usually caused by pregnancy or stress.
- Hangnail (agnail): When the cuticle splits around the nail caused by dryness of cuticle, cutting off or carelessness in removing the cuticle.
- Leuconychia: White spots on the nails usually caused by injury to nail base.
- Onychauxis (hypertrophy): An overgrowth of nail in thickness rather than length due to a local infection.

- Onycha trophia: loss of nail's luster. It becomes smaller and sometimes shed entirely due to injury or a disease.
- Onychophagy (bitten nails): disorder as a result of nervous habit that prompts the individual to chew the nail or harden the cuticle.
- Onychorrhexis: split or brittle nails caused by injury, vitamin deficiency, illness and exposure to strong soaps.
- Pterygium: The cuticle growth that adheres to the base of the nail caused by circulatory problems.
- Treating cuts: causes accidentally during a manicure. Apply antiseptic immediately. Do not buff or apply nail polish on it.

Dandruff (seborrheic dermatitis)

Scalp irritation?

Thick scale, despite regularly use of dandruff shampoo?

Yellow crusting?

Red patches along the neckline?

Itchiness?

If the reply is yes, you are suffering from hair dandruff. There are many possible causes of dandruff, including a yeast infection of the scalp or hormone imbalances. If all the treatments to cure dandruff fail, consult a dermatologist for proper diagnosis and medical treatment. If you have dandruff, do not use dandruff shampoos. Instead treat your scalp with the essential oils of aromatherapy. Dandruff is not a hair problem, but a skin problem. The flaking and itchiness are the result of an over-production of a substance called sebum from the glands in the scalp. These glands are usually hyperactive because of excessively dry hair. Hair shampoos available in the market for the treatment of dandruff and strong medications to control it, however, may provide a temporary relief but they don't do anything to address the underlying disorder such as dryness and poor health of the scalp. Such dandruff shampoos and strong medicines destroy the scalp's delicate balance of water and oil, which irritate the glands. The following natural ways stop flaking:

- Aromatherapy helps to eliminate dandruff. Collect the following ingredients:

Unscented mild shampoo	2 tablespoons
Tea tree oil	10 drops

Cedar wood oil	8 drops
Pine oil	6 drops
Rosemary oil	6 drops
Clary sage oil	4 drops
Lemon oil	4 drops

Mix above ingredients. These essential oils encourage body's system to heal the problems that cause dandruff. Tea tree oil is an antiseptic helping to normalize the bacteria on the scalp. Rosemary and cedar wood oil increase circulation to the scalp. Pine oil encourages elimination of toxins from the skin of the scalp. Clary sage helps regulate and balance oil production and lemon encourages elimination of toxins and promotes internal cleansing. Use shampoo several times a week.

- Massage: Dandruff is a symptom of a body-wide condition of 'vatta' or dryness. Massaging the scalp twice a week with warm sesame oil combats the excessive dryness. It is also very calming and soothing to the system, which is important, since dandruff is often caused by anxiety. Massage the oil into your scalp before sleep for about ten minutes. Then wrap your head in a hot towel and steam for ten minutes. Wash the hair next morning.
- Vitamin E: helps to balance the oils on the scalp and relieve dryness (recommended dose: a capsule of 400 international units a day).
- Zinc: help your scalp heal from dandruff. This mineral rebuilds skin (recommended dose 15-20 milligrams daily).
- Salenium relieves flaking and itching due to dandruff (recommended dose 200-microgram supplement daily)
- Eucalyptus rinse help fight infection due to dandruff. To make a rinse , put 4 teaspoons of dried leaves in half liter boiling water and stir. Then cover, remove from heat and steep for an hour. Strain the liquid and add to it 1 tablespoon of apple-cider vinegar. After taking a shower, pour the rinse very slowly over the hair, but do not rinse it out, just let it dry.

Depression

Depression is a common disorder among women. Here are few symptoms seen in depressed person:

- Persistent sad, anxious or empty feelings.
- Feeling of hopelessness.
- Feeling of guilt, worthlessness and helplessness.
- Loss of interest or pleasure in activities, including sex.
- Sleep disturbances including insomnia, early morning waking and/or oversleeping.
- Eating disturbances, loss of appetite and weight loss or gain.
- Decreased energy and fatigue.
- Thoughts of death or suicide or suicide attempts.
- Restlessness and/or irritability.
- Difficulty in concentrating and making decisions.

Treating measures:

- Get yourself involved in physical activities and light exercise.
- Try to find out solution and create a safe environment.
- If talking about your problems to someone leads to tears, let them flow.
- Avoid making decisions during the depression period.

Dry skin or dry hair

If your skin feels tight, looks dull and flaky-it is a dry skin. A dry skin is prone to wrinkles and premature ageing. If your skin has become widespread and uncomfortable and there is no improvement after two weeks of self-care, see a dermatologist for diagnosis and treatment. The following steps should be adopted to treat a dry skin:

- Aromatherapy treatment: A warm facial compress, using essential oils greatly benefits a dry skin. Fill a basin with lukewarm water and add to it two to three drops of one of three essential oils: lavender, rose or neroli.
- Do not apply soap to wash the facial skin. Use a washing gel.
- Follow each bath with a moisturizer.
- Drink 7 to 8 glasses of water a day to keep the skin hydrated and prevent dryness.
- Use oatmeal as a soap substitute. Oatmeal is a soothing agent.

- Beta-carotene taken with lunch and dinner is a nutrient diet for soft, smooth, disease-free skin. (Normal dose 15 milligrams a day taken half twice each with lunch and the dinner).
- Mineral Zinc (15 milligrams daily dose) is an important nutrient for the repair of damaged skin tissue. Zinc deficiency can cause dry skin.
- Vitamin B complex (100 milligrams a day) cures a dry skin and other skin diseases.
- Vitamin C (1,000 milligrams a day) helps immune system, which leads to healthier skin.
- Vitamin E capsules (400 international units a day) is a strong nutrient for the skin, which helps replace cells on the skin's outer layer.

Dry Hair: Like skin, dry hair look lifeless, lacking luster and may be brittle with split ends. The hair becomes dry as a result of too much sun exposure, excessive use of hair dryer or chemical treatments such as bleaching, coloring and perms. When hair becomes dry, the outer layer called cuticles peel off from the central shaft. Use hair conditioner to lubricate the hair and prevent static electricity. Beer is a wonderful hair setting lotion to give a crisp, healthy, shiny look to dry hair.

Oily Hair and Skin

Oily hair is caused by overly oily scalp and one common cause of an oily scalp is a high-fat diet. The hair is fed through hair bulbs in the scalp, which are intertwined with sebaceous glands and produce oil, also known as sebum. A diet full of fried foods and saturated fats can trigger over-production of sebum. Those women with fine hair have as many as 1,40,000 oil glands on their scalp. Redheads have an average 80,000 to 100,000 hair on the scalp. To decrease the oil production from the scalp and reduce oiliness the following remedies are suggested:

- Rinse hair with lemon water after shampooing. Squeeze juice of two lemons into two cups of soft water. Apply this liquid evenly to your hair and massage gently. Leave it on for five minutes, then rinse with cool to tepid water. Blot your hair dry with a towel.
- Use of herb horsetail is an effective remedy for oily hair. Boil

one cup of distilled water, adding to it 2 tablespoons of dried powder of horsetail. Use liquid as a last rinse after shampoo.

- Aromatherapy helps to cut the oil in hair. Add 3-4 drops of rosemary, lavender, eucalyptus, cypress or lemon oil in rinsing water. All these oils are astringent and cleanse and tone the sebaceous glands.
- Massage your scalp during the shampoo (never between the shampoo).
- Don't over-brush your hair as brushing from the roots carry oil from the scalp to the ends of hair.
- Learn to relax. When you are under stress, the body produces more androgens, which produce excessive oil.
- Apply astringent to the scalp, which helps slow down oil secretion from the scalp.

An oily skin having medium to large pores on the skin have the following symptoms:

- Have blackheads and acnes.
- Is prone to skin blemishes.

Treatment to get rid of oily skin:

- Aromatherapy treatments can be very beneficial for a oily skin to help balance glandular activity, improve circulation and detoxify.
- Steaming helps to deep-clean oily skin. Steam the face once a week. Start the face with cleaning, followed by steaming, next rinse with warm water and finally splash with cool water and pat dry.

Fatigue

In today's busy, stressed life, fatigue among women is common problem. The following conditions can cause very serious fatigue:

- Low thyroid function.
- Mononucleosis.
- Illness including hepatitis, thyroid diseases and cancer.
- Overwork.

The following measures prove helpful to fight fatigue:

- Eating well. Focus on food and drinks that power you with high-octane energy fuel. Avoid high-fat food in the evening.
- Have sufficient rest. Try to go to bed and get up at the same time every day, since the body craves regularity.
- A good restful sleep in a cool, dark, quiet room. Sleep on your side, you will breathe easier and reduce snoring.
- Warming up. Give yourself an extra 10-15 minutes in the morning for light exercise, before you start the day.
- Eat a three-piece breakfast containing carbohydrates, proteins and fats- that will over-activate your insulin and blood sugar will be controlled.
- Eliminate fatigue factors, which affect energized lifestyle.
- Do not have coffee after a meal, which can disturb sleep.
- A brisk 10 minutes walk can energize you for hours. You can walk anywhere, any time. Add some weight lifting or stretching postures in your daily program to tone up and keep your muscles loose.
- Gentle yoga exercise and Chinese exercises of tai chi help build your energy.
- Avoid watching TV as far as possible, which makes one lethargic. Try reading instead that energizes.
- Think positive, be motivated and be confident. These thoughts affect your energy level.
- Breathe deeply, that makes you relaxed and energized.
- Avoid sleeping pills.
- The color on the walls of your house leaves good effect on your mind. Dark colors make you feel fatigued. Red color is good for short-term energy stimulation. Green color is good at eliminating fatigue.
- Light music helps fighting fatigue.

Hair Loss

Hair loss in women is difficult to diagnose and can be caused by many factors as below:

- Often have recurrent high blood pressure

- Alopecia areata (baldness on the scalp in patches).
- Hormone imbalances.
- Effect of menopause.
- Shortage of dietary protein and amino acid deficiency.
- Intestinal parasites.
- Damage from hair treatments.
- Stress and sudden shock.
- After-effect of a fever.
- Effect of childbirth.

Consult a doctor for suitable treatment, if hair continues falling even after a treatment. The following measures are suggested:

- Aromatherapy: Essential oils such as jojoba oil, rosemary oil, lavender oil, lemon balm and cedar wood oil helps fighting hair loss. Massage the mixture into the scalp with your fingertips. Leave it on for 30 minutes or overnight, then shampoo in the morning. As a final rinse, add one drop of lavender oil and one drop of rosemary oil to ½ liter water and pour it over the head.
- You may consult an experienced beauty therapist for a suitable advise to maintain your hair.

Fissures (ulcers)

Fissures, the painful ulcers or the breaks in the skin, many times develop at the corners of the mouth. The similarities between anal fissures and hemorrhoids are superficial, which usually grip a female. Hemorrhoids generally are the swollen veins, where as fissures are more or less ulcers. Fissures generally occur in the anus due to passing of a large, hard stool. The fissures often burn, sting and bleed. If the fissures don't heal within four to eight weeks, consult a doctor. Sometimes, a sore that doesn't heal is a warning sign of cancer. If you notice a mucous discharge from your anus, consult your doctor immediately. The following precautions should be taken in case of suffering from fissures:

- Try to avoid hard stools. Adapt to a diet high in fiber and fluids. Drink six to eight glasses of water a day. Eat fruit, vegetables and whole grains. Remember, constipated stools worsen anal fissures.
- A petroleum jelly inserted about ½ inch into the rectum may help the stool pass without damage.

- Keep area around the anus dry. Sprinkle talcum powder.
- In case of itching do not scratch fissures.
- Vitamin cream helps in reducing the inflammation due to fissures.

Gingivitis (Gum Disease)

Here are few warning signals if you suffer from gingivitis. You must see a dentist immediately when you find:

- Bleeding gums.
- You have bad breath that doesn't go away within 24 hours.
- Your mouth feels out of alignment when you shut it.
- Pus forms between your teeth and gums.
- Your teeth becomes loose or fall out.

Precautions:

- Brush correctly. Have two tooth brushes-use alternatively.
- Apply a power tool. Electric rotary toothbrush removes 98% of plaque against about 49% removed in case of hand brushing.
- Try gum massage. Grip your gums between your thumb and index finger. And rub, this will increase blood circulation to your gums.
- Vitamin C doesn't cure gingivitis, but it can help check bleeding gums.
- Use a good quality mouthwash.
- Women smokers should avoid excessive smoking and drinking. These drain body of vitamins and minerals.
- Scrape your tongue to remove the bacteria and toxins accumulated there.
- Mix together equal quantity of hydrogen peroxide (3% solution) and water. Apply for 30 seconds (Do not swallow) to finish bacteria.
- Eat raw vegetables, it will keep gingivitis away.

Gout

Gout is a type of arthritis causing throbbing pain that often strikes at night turning the skin red, hot, leaving the affected joint swollen and tender. Gout is caused by uric acid crystals, which settle in joints. Often the big toe is the prime target of its effect. Doctors usually inject very toxic drug to stop pain by dissolving uric acid crystals or prescribe ibuprofen (800-milligram) for relieving pain. The following curative measures are suggested to treat gout:

- If the affected joint is not too tender, try applying a crushed ice pack placing on the painful joint for about ten minutes.
- Avoid taking high-purine foods (include high protein animal products and sweetbread, dry beans, whole-grain cereals and yeast) that contribute to higher levels of uric acid.
- Drink lot of water to flush out excess uric acid from body system.
- Avoid taking alcohol if you have a history of gout. Alcohol increases uric acid production in the body, which get deposited on joints.
- Eating cherries prevents production of uric acid.
- Vitamin B 6 helps distribute water in the body to keep its all tissues hydrated, which helps prevent uric acid from turning into crystals.
- Taking a tablespoon of apple cider vinegar in the morning daily is very effective to prevent gout attacks.
- Mix charcoal into a bath and soak affected foot in it for 30 to 60 minutes. Mix ½ cup of charcoal powder in water.
- Persons with high blood pressure should control the blood pressure when they suffer from gout.

HIV and AIDS

HIV (human immunodeficiency virus) is the virus that causes AIDS-a disease that destroys the immune system and ravages the body. In fact, there is no cure for AIDS, no way to eradicate HIV. An HIV infection is extremely complicated to treat. There are few natural techniques suggested to HIV/AID patients.

- Meditation, prayer and yoga relax the body and decrease stress and uplift emotional and spiritual healing.
- Infection and skin problems are common in people with HIV. However, essential fatty acids abundant in cold-water fish, flaxseed oil and borage oil help keep the skin healthy.
- Protein, feeds the immune system. HIV attacks the immune system severely, thus HIV patients need protein as maximum

as possible. Barley, peanut butter, beans, nut, pasta and eggs are rich sources of protein.

- Garlic contains ample quantity of allicin - a powerful compound to fight and kill HIV bacteria. The garlic can be taken in three doses of 3 gm. each three times a day at morning, noon and evening.

An Anti-HIV multivitamin/mineral supplement nutrient program recommended daily by the experts is as below:

Vitamin A/ beta-carotene:	10,000 to 20,000 international units.
B Vitamins (thiamin, riboflavin, Pantothenic acid and B 6):	50 to 100 milligrams.
Vitamin B 12:	500 to 1000 micrograms.
Vitamin C:	250 to 1000 milligrams.
Vitamin E:	150 to 400 international units.
Iron:	9 to 18 milligrams.
Zinc:	10 to 25 milligrams.
Calcium:	50 to 250 milligrams.
Magnesium:	25 to 125 milligrams.
Selenium:	100 to 200 micrograms.

Hypoglycemia (Low blood sugar)

This disorder causes several symptoms as below:

- Cravings for sweets
- Irritability.
- Fatigue.
- Dizziness.
- Headaches.
- Poor memory.
- Heart palpitations.
- Shakiness.
- Blurry vision.
- Depression.
- Frequent anxiety or nervousness.

The following curative measures are recommended to treat low blood sugar:

- A diet containing maximum protein, lesser carbohydrates should be taken by the patient. This diet includes white sugar and flour that strengthens spleen and pancreas.
- A diet containing too much fatty, fiber free red meat and too many refined carbohydrates can cure hypoglycemia.
- The following vitamins and minerals supplement nutrients help cure hypoglycemia. In addition to your daily vitamin/mineral supplements, the following individual supplements are taken strictly in consultation of your doctor.

Vitamin C:	1,000 milligrams.
Bioflavonoids:	1,000 milligrams.
Magnesium:	200 milligrams.
Vitamin E:	400 international units.
Chromium:	200 to 400 micrograms.
Coenzyme Q 10:	100 to 200 milligrams.
Standardized milk extract:	250 to 500 milligrams.

Hepatitis C

An extremely serious life-threatening liver disorder caused by viral infection is called hepatitis C. It damages the liver with increased risk of liver failure or a cancer. A patient suspected to have hepatitis C should see a doctor immediately at the first sign of symptoms. The patient with hepatitis C, have a risk of hepatitis A and hepatitis C infections. The symptoms of hepatitis C include:

- Jaundice (yellowing of the skin or whites of the eyes).
- Pain in lower right abdomen.
- Loss of appetite.
- Dark colored urine.
- Nausea.
- Chills and fever.

Herbs play an important role to protect liver and cure hepatitis C. The important herbs include turmeric, anti-choke leaf, gentian and ginger. Each of the herb is taken in different ways to cure liver disorder as below:

- Lemon balm: Make tea by adding 1 teaspoon of dried or fresh herb to a cup of boiling water. Steep for 10-15 minutes, strain and drink. Drink two to three cups a day.
- St. John's wort: Take 300-milligram capsule of this herb twice a day.
- Garlic is very effective herb taken in any form-in capsule, fresh cloves or cooked. Take two to three capsules (3,000-4,000 micrograms of allicin each) daily in consultation with a doctor.
- Hepatitis C is a chronic disorder having conditions such as fatigue, nausea and diarrhea. However, hepatitis C can be cured with acupressure treatment pressing pressure points LV on feet and the waist.
- The following anti-hepatitis C diets should be avoided:
    1. Red meats are loaded with antibiotics, growth hormones and steroids, which harms the digestive process, stress the liver and is harmful for gall bladder and pancreas.
    2. Dairy foods, which add strain on the liver.
    3. Alcohol is a liver-harming product.
    4. Caffeine stimulates and stresses the liver. Avoid tea, coffee and colas.
    5. Drink only distilled water. Tap water contains chlorine, fluorides and inorganic chemicals.
    6. Fruit juices are high in concentrated sugar, which is harmful for liver and stresses the digestive process of body and disturbs pancreas.

Headaches

Headaches are of many types and can have symptoms of different health problems. The majority of cases of headache are classified as muscle contraction. These are known as tension headaches. Migraine is most common form of headache that most often strikes women. It causes severe pain in one side of the head. This type of headache is accompanied by nausea and vomiting. It may cause symptoms of dizziness and blurred vision. Tension headache is a throbbing forehead, dull pain on both sides of the head. There are many headaches that trigger from foods, stressful conditions and due to hormones. The headaches are usually accompanied by neurological symptoms such as general weakness, dizziness, numbness, blurred vision and memory loss. Tension is the prominent cause of headache.

Treatment: There are several factors such as proper diet, nutritional supplements, stress management recommended for the treatment of chronic headache as described below:

- Exercise is a useful measure to prevent headache.
- Aspirin is an anti-inflammatory drug to cure headache. But overuse of it may cause more pain. Aspirin should be used in the beginning of the headache.
- Acupressure treatment, when rubbing between thumb and forefinger, can help relieve headache pain. Remember, pregnant women should not practice acupressure treatment because it may cause premature contraction of the uterus.
- In case of severe headache, exercise will prove helpful in curing it.
- Hot shower and putting heat on the neck relieves headache.
- Breathing deeply relieves tension.
- Tying a tight cloth (headband) around the head decreases flow of blood to the scalp, will prove beneficial for relieving headache.
- Skipping or delaying meals can cause severe headache. It causes muscle tension and blood sugar level drops.
- High salt diets can cause severe migraine.
- Excessive noise triggers tension resulting in headache.
- Do not chew gum; it tightens muscles, cause tension resulting in headache.
- Alcoholic drinks are harmful, causing headache.
- Avoid taking chocolate; it contains tyramine, which cause headache.
- Rub peppermint oil on temples. Dilute one part peppermint essential oil in two parts almond oil or any other carrier oil. Other essential oils such as lavender oil or roman chamomile relieve tension, curing headache.
- Vitamin B-6 stabilizes the brain's serotonin, preventing headache.
- Ginger water cures headache. Put I teaspoon ginger in four glasses of water and drink throughout the day.
- Constipation causes headache. Try to relieve constipation and change your eating habits accordingly.

- Low blood sugar triggers headache. To keep blood sugar level balanced, have at least three meals a day.
- Regular practice of meditation helps to relieve migraine.
- Eliminate foods giving you headaches. To check, include one of the following foods at a time to your diet and watch its reaction giving you headache
    1. Packaged meat and fish.
    2. Vinegar.
    3. Pickled and fermented foods.
    4. Cheese.
    5. Products high in yeasts (including coffee, cake and bread).
    6. Citrus fruits.
    7. Chocolate.
    8. Sour cream and yogurt.
    9. Caffeine.
    10. Alcoholic beverages.
- Vitamin E (recommended daily dose 400 international units) helps to stabilize estrogen levels and prevent migraines, generally causing during periods.
- Calcium supplements can help decrease the frequency of menstruation, resulting in frequent migraines.
- Nearly 40% women having migraines as a result of hormonal changes during periods suffer low blood levels of magnesium mineral, which generally causes migraines. Start taking 200 milligrams magnesium supplement a day and gradually increase to 400 milligrams a day. (You may consult a doctor).
- High altitudes trigger headache. Vitamin C maintains the level and relieves headache. Take 3,000 to 5,000 milligrams of vitamin C a day on high altitudes in consultation with a doctor.

Leg Cramps

Leg cramps in the calves or feet commonly occur in women, especially in late pregnancy when she is resting or asleep. Cramps are usually caused by the following factors:

- Fatigue in calf muscles.
- Pressure on the nerves to the legs.

- Impaired circulation.
- Calcium-phosphorus imbalance in the blood.

Relieving Factors: Cramps are relieved by the following measures:

- When the muscle is slowly and gently stretched.
- Gently stretch calf muscles. Keep knees straight, ankles bent and heels resting on the floor. When the leg cramp is severe you may need help.
- A foot cramp, which usually tightens the muscles of the arch and curls the toes can be relieved by stretching out toes. To prevent cramping do not curl your toes.

Reduce your Heart/ Cardiovascular risk

Symptoms if you are likely to have a heart attack?

- Feeling of an uncomfortable pressure, fullness, squeezing or pain in the chest that may last for more than a few minutes.
- When the pain spreads to your shoulders, neck or arms. This may first appear in the arms, shoulders or back.
- Feeling of light-headedness, nausea or sweating.
- When shortness of breadth occurs.
- Feeling of fatigue without pain.
- Difficulty in breathing.
- Abdominal pain or indigestion.

How to reduce risk of heart trouble?

- Aerobics Exercises: A regular exercise program 30 minutes a day strengthens the heart and lungs.
- Improve your cholesterol level.
- Have a regular check over high blood pressure.
- Ensure regular check over your overweight.
- In case of women over 50, vigorous exercises are not advised, but involve in moderate activities such as household work, morning or evening walk and even gardening activities improve fitness of your heart.

- Women physical unfit or after the age 50 should check with the doctor before starting any exercise program.
- Stretch for five minutes before and after exercising.
- When you start to feel pain or pressure in the chest or along the left side of the neck, arm or shoulder, stop exercising. Consult the doctor and have done thorough check-ups and tests.
- The sports such as jogging, cycling, jumping rope, walking, swimming and playing games (tennis and badminton) condition your heart.
- Heart patients should strictly avoid smoking. According to studies conducted by WHO, every cigarette shorten life by six minutes. A non-smoker has healthy lungs. A cigarette smoker have five times greater risk of a stroke as compared to a non-smoker. A smoker is likely to have five to six times more risk for a heart stroke. Avoid smokers and smoking situations (after the meals, drinks, visiting parties and clubs etc.), which make you feel like smoking.
- In case you are a smoker, don't inhale so much.
- Drink lot of water to flush nicotine from your system.
- Practice yoga and meditation for healthy heart.
- Improve your diet. Eat a diet rich in fruits, vegetables, whole grains which include breads, cereals and rice. In case of non-vegetarians, eat skinless chicken and red meat. Avoid fried food and meat (liver and kidney). Do not take egg yolks, butter and saturated fats.
- For cooking use sunflower or olive oil instead of butter and ghee. Use lemon or vinegar over salad for dressing.

How to avoid cardiovascular risks?

- Reduce stress. When in stressful condition, symptoms such as clenched fists, excessive smoking, constant lip biting, sleeping too much or lack of sleep take place.
- Stop worrying. Keep a sense of humor.
- Practice calming techniques including light exercises, meditation, yoga or tai chi.
- Control blood pressure. Get your blood pressure checked once a week or at regular intervals, as high blood pressure usually

has no symptoms. There are few ways as below to lower blood pressure:

1. Keep your weight normal (as required).
2. Have a low-fat, calcium-rich diet.
3. Reduce intake of salt.
4. Avoid alcoholic beverages
5. Do not smoke.

- Switch to a low-fat diet to lower cholesterol build up in the body. Add more calcium to your diet. Avoid foods high in sodium, which include canned soups, canned vegetables, shellfish and pickled meals.
- Check diabetes, which has the following symptoms (consult a doctor):
  1. Excessive thirst.
  2. Excessive urination.
  3. Weight loss.
  4. Dehydration and weakness.
  5. Leg cramps.
  6. Blurred vision.

Health hints for men and women

- Blood Pressure (Hypertension): Detect hypertension- a common risk factor for heart disease after the age 35+. It should be tested once a year or more often if it is 140/90 or higher than this.
- Cholesterol Test: Check if cholesterol content of blood is high, especially after the age 35+. It should be tested after every 3 to 5 years or as and when directed by the doctor.
- Dental Examination: Have a regular check for cavities, gum diseases and other oral problems usually arising after the age 18+. Get tested by a dentist once in a year or two years.
- Eye Examination: Check for the problems including cataracts and glaucoma. Eyes must be tested when an eye problem is suspected or as and when directed by the doctor during the age 18 to 40. Eyes must be tested after every 2-4 years during the age 41-64 and tested after every 1-2 year after age 65+.
- Prostate Cancer: Prostate Specific Antigen (PSA) blood test is taken to detect a prostate cancer in men usually after the

age 55+. As an early detection helps to cure the disease, a doctor should be consulted as and when there is any urinary/ kidney problem takes place.

- Testicular Examination: Self examine painless lumps to detect testicular cancer common in males. Have a complete physical examination on detection of lumps.

Serious sleeping troubles in women (chronic insomnia)

Some of the symptoms include disturbed sleep, psychiatric disturbance, breathing problems or leg movements during night. Usually sleeping pills are recommended as the best treatment for insomnia. Sleeping pills, however, are effective for short term treatment, but these become ineffective with regular use and can cause many side effects. There are several steps to a good night's sleep.

- Avoid stress. Choose a quiet place not to be disturbed by noise during sleep.
- Sleeping pills are a nightmare. These medications can interfere with normal brain functioning, causing poor sleep. Moreover, the brain become accustomed to the drugs and in the long run such drugs become un-effective.
- For relaxation focus your mind on various organs of your body such as your hands, feet, thighs, stomach, chest, shoulder, neck, face and forehead. You will find a good result.
- Monitor your breathing. Place one hand on your stomach and the other on your chest. Deep abdominal breathing is more relaxing than shallow chest breathing. Deep breathing relaxes muscles.
- High carbohydrate diet eaten before bedtime can increase serotonin (a brain chemical) that promotes sleep.
- Do not sleep more than required. Newborn babies sleep up to 18 hours a day. A 10 years old child needs 9-10 hours sleep. An adult requires sleep between 7-8 hours. Sleep depends on individual's requirement. A few need 5-6 hours sleep, whereas others of the same age group need up to 9-10 hours sleep. If you are not getting sleep, read a magazine or a book.
- Avoid stimulants such as coffee, colas and chocolates that contain caffeine.
- Take a warm bath before retiring to bed, which will make it easier to fall asleep.

- Try sex before sleep. Sexual activity help enhance sleep. Remember, if sex causes anxiety and problems, you will not enjoy good sleep.
- Acupressure treatment helps for a good sleep. Consult an acupressure expert to suggest a suitable treatment.

Menopausal Problems

Menopause-usually around the age of 50 is called 'The Change' when functioning of ovaries to produce eggs, the swelling and bursting of the egg sac, release of the hormones (estrogen secretion), monthly menstrual shedding of uterine cells and blood becomes irregular and slowly comes to a halt. Following are the symptoms of menopause:

- Hot flashes and sudden chills.
- Lowered sexual desire.
- Vaginal dryness and loss of sex drive.
- Emotionally upset.
- Insomnia (sleeping problems).
- Depression.
- Memory loss and sudden change in the mood.
- Night sweating. Sometimes, the sweating is so high you may have to change the bed sheet.
- Vaginal bleeding. In this condition see doctor immediately.

The following measures make better outlook of life during menopause:

- Make life an adventure. Find a new hobby and change in the career.
- Daily exercise should be a part of your daily life. Walking, jogging, bicycling, jumping rope, dancing, swimming or any other daily exercise can relieve menopausal disorders. Yoga aids relaxation and reduces stress.
- Hot flashes are body's response to lower estrogen levels and more than 75% women usually have hot flashes lasting between two to three minutes. During excretion of hot flashes, heat is produced in the body, the face reddens and there is excessive sweating.
- Nutrients can help control or completely eliminate hot flashes. Vitamin A is as effective as estrogen (recommended daily

dose 400 to 1200 international units as advised by your doctor). In case of night sweats, have two doses during the night as per suggestions of your doctor.

- Vitamin E helps in case of vaginal dryness.
- Learn meditation or yoga or sit quietly, eyes closed to relax your mind.
- Alcohol triggers hot flashes. Similarly cut down caffeine containing beverages that stimulate production of the stress hormones and trigger hot flashes.
- Wear fiber clothes. Synthetic fiber trap heat and produce perspiration during a hot flash.
- Drink lot of water or juice, especially after exercising to check body temperature.
- Eat small meals-minimum three meals a day. Even five to six small meals a day will help your body regulate temperature more easily.
- Vitamin B complex helps to reduce stress in menopausal women.
- The herb sage works very well if menopausal woman have hot flashes throughout the day and sweat during night. Drink a sage tea.
- Hydrotherapy treatment is very helpful for menopausal women. The body expels toxins during menstruation. When menstrual cycle decreases or stops the body requires another outlet for the toxins, so it starts sweating or has hot flashes. It is advised to have sauna (steam) bath to release toxins from the body. In case a sauna or steam room is not possible, take a hot bath for 10-20 minutes a day.
- Valerian and lavender herbs help better sleep. Take 300 to 500 milligrams valerian extract one hour before retiring to bed at night. Dabbing a few drops of lavender essential oil on your pillow before sleep can help you a sound sleep.
- Acupressure therapy relieves insomnia and anxiety in menopausal women. Stimulate two pressure points on the feet for 1 to 3 minutes each with your middle and index fingers.
- Women passing through their menopausal period if stay sexy and have regular intercourse once a week or once a fortnight, have few or no hot flashes or night sweating as compared to

those women who doesn't indulge in sexual intercourse at all. Having frequent sex helps moderate drop in estrogen levels, which reduce hot flashes. A study reveals that regular sexual activity stimulates the functioning of ovaries.

- Vaginal dryness from a lack of estrogen decreases interest in sexual intercourse among menopausal women. Lubricants suitable for vaginal dryness include vaginal jelly, vegetable oil and unscented cream or oil.
- Vitamin E can be used to massage as a lubricant. Break open vitamin E capsules and mix to the lubricant.

Anemia

Anemia-an iron deficiency, is a problem that affects every one out of five women not only in India but all over World. Anemia is a condition in which the blood has too few red cells, which results in a lessened ability of the blood to supply oxygen to the tissues resulting in weakness, lassitude and pallor. Iron-deficiency anemia may cause the following symptoms:

- Dizziness.
- Loss of appetite.
- Diarrhea.
- Abdominal pain.
- Pale complexion.
- Palpitation of the heart.
- Shortness of breath.
- Feeling of weakness.
- Frequent headache.

The blood needs iron to produce red blood cells. Women who don't get enough iron in their diets or who have heavy menstrual periods may have insufficient levels of either red blood cells or hemoglobin-the oxygen carrying protein in red blood cells. Women whose hemoglobin level decline feel tired and weak. If you have excessively heavy or lengthy menstrual flow or your menstrual period lasts for more than seven days, you should consult a doctor. If you are having rectal bleeding, you need to see a doctor. Improve your diet and lifestyle.

How to find that you are anemic?

Press your unpolished fingernail against the nail bed for few seconds. The area will turn white. Then stop pressing, if the nail area turns pink very slowly and takes time, you have anemia. By having a complete blood count performed by a competent laboratory, it can be observed that a man or a woman is anemic. Skin color cannot confirm that he or she is anemic. Many people who seem, to be pale have normal red blood cells and are not anemic at all. However, it is common for females in the age group that menstruate. The loss of blood during periods must be replaced by new blood produced in the bone marrow. This required that the woman have enough iron in her diet. In case of un-sufficient iron contents in diet she may become anemic.

What is blood?

Blood is the fluid circulating through blood vessels. It contains red blood cells, platelets and a pale yellowish liquid known as plasma. Plasma acts as a fluid medium for the suspension of blood cells, transports dissolved nutrients to the tissues, carries waste products from tissues to the organs. The red blood cells contain hemoglobin and red pigment of the blood. The oxygen is thus carried to all the tissues of the body. The white blood cells known as leukocytes, which act as body's defense again infection and combat fighting against bacteria and viruses. They also produce proteins called antibodies, which fights infection. Platelets are circulating cells that prevent and stop bleeding.

Few home remedies for anemic women

- Have iron-rich food. Good sources of iron include whole grains such as barley and oats, beans and peas, seeds and nuts, fruits and vegetables.
- Calcium rich foods put more iron in your body. Dairy products decrease iron absorption in women with anemia, whereas increase your intake of beans, peas, soybeans, sesame seeds, soups and leafy green vegetables. Inadequate diet is one of the most common cause of anemia.
- Vitamin C is acidic and helps the body to absorb iron contents. Squeeze the juice of a lemon into a glass of water and drink before meals. Alternatively, take vitamin C (1,000 to 2,000 milligrams a day with each meal).

- Remember, alcoholic beverages (wine and beer) deplete the body of vitamin B complex and minerals, which can worsen anemia. Reduce your sugar intake, which also depletes the body of vitamin B complex.
- Delete caffeine (products such as coffee, black tea, soda, chocolate etc.) from your daily diet, which depletes the body of vitamin B complex.
- If the anemia results from iron deficiency, iron pills are suggested. But if the anemia is associated with vitamin B-12 deficiency, the vitamin must be administered by injection.

Types of anemia

- Sickle-cell anemia: Usually characterized by a chemical abnormality of the hemoglobin, which results in the sickle-cell shape of the cells. The cells do not survive and circulate and the patient becomes anemic. In this case a severe anemia is present and children (including older children) with this condition are usually jaundiced, may have long, thin arms and legs and a protruding abdomens as a result of blood not circulating thoroughly in the body. To treat sickle-cell anemia, blood transfusions are given to restore red cells. Doctors recommend antibiotics to protect against infection. Good nutrition, plenty of fluids and vitamins help to improve condition. A female or a male suffering from sickle-cell anemia may get marry but they need genetic counseling before having a child.
- Deficiency anemia: Usually caused by lack of a substance necessary for the formation of blood.
- Pernicious anemia: It results from vitamin B-12 deficiency. Such women should take vitamin B-12 throughout the life.
- Iron-deficiency anemia: It is caused by acute or chronic loss of blood. Such anemia can be treated by blood replacement by giving iron pills, which produce red blood cells.
- Congenital anemia: This type of anemia occurs in women born with defective blood in the body. Blood cells usually are destroyed in the body.
- Hemolytic anemia: This diseased type of anemia has cells destroyed rapidly and run in families due to inherited defects in the blood.

Anger

Most of the women involved in day-to-day family problems suffer from anger, which must be released. In fact anger is a feeling in the body that needs to be released. There are few signs such as weeping, screaming and yelling, which help you release anger. The physical signs that your anger is based on include emotional experiences such as a dry mouth, a knotted stomach, sweating, cold hands and a lump in your throat. The following precautions help to release anger:

- Feel relaxed at a where you can be alone and undisturbed.
- Sit in a car, close the windows and scream as loudly as you can to release anger.
- Any form of exercise releases anger. Ride a stationary bicycle as hard as you can.
- Breathing release anger. Breathe slowly and deeply through your nose.

Constipation

Constipation is not serious. However, you must consult a doctor in case the symptoms are severe giving signals for a serious underlying disorder, last longer than three weeks or so, there are signals of an intestinal obstruction and if you find blood in your stool.

Solutions to relieve constipation:

- Fiber in your diet: A daily consumption of 20 to 35 gm. of dietary fiber for adults and minimum 30 gm. for those suffering from constipation is required. Foods such as green peas, apple, bran cereal, oatmeal, dried beans and nuts are rich source of fiber.
- Go to the gym. Exercise is good for your bowels and combat constipation.
- Six to eight glasses of liquid, preferably water should be a part of daily diet in adults.
- Improve your bowel habits. The most natural time to go to the toilet is after a meal. Sit on the toilet for ten minutes.
- Beware of certain foods. Milk can be extremely constipating to some, while it gives others diarrhea. People who suffer from frequent constipation must avoid foods such as beans, cauliflower and cabbage, which tend to produce gas.

- Avoid large meals that distend the digestive tract and worsen constipation.
- Herbs such as aloe juice, dandelion root and plantain seeds are very useful to treat constipation.
- First thing in the morning should be juice of a lemon mixed to half glass of warm water.
- Healthy oils such as olive, canola and other monounsaturated and polyunsaturated oils act as digestive lubricants helping out in clearing out constipation.
- Massage your colon- the final section of the digestive tract, where constipation takes place. It is highly effective method of helping your elimination. Use the fingertips of both hands to massage abdominal area on right side, and moving in a circular massaging motion pressing till the hands reach just above your belly button. Continue to massage down to your hips in the same way.
- 'Triphala' is a laxative herb to rejuvenate your digestive tract. Take one tablespoon three times a day.
- Magnesium deficiency contributes to constipation. This mineral relaxes the intestinal muscles.
- Make a regular routine of waking up five to ten minutes earlier in the morning and spending five minutes on the toilet, even if you feel that you need not to go to the toilet.

Polycythemia vera

A condition in which the body produces excess red blood cells, which thickens and tends to clot within the blood vessels. The cause of this disorder is unknown. The signs and symptoms of this disorder are as following:

- Complain of weakness.
- Headache.
- Hemorrhages in the skin and mucous membranes.
- Blue-red flush to the skin.
- Enlarged spleen.
- Blood count showing excess of red blood cells.

It is treated by frequent bleedings by the patient or administering drugs to reduce red blood cells as prescribed by the doctor.

Blood Poisoning

A condition in which the bacteria are present in the blood. If the bacteria are present for a short duration, the condition is called bacteremia. Sometimes, neglected or badly treated abscess or other infection causes blood poisoning. If untreated, the blood poisoning may spread to the tissues under the skin, the lungs, the liver and the brain.

Leukemia

Leukemia is a malignant disease of the blood forming tissues, wherein abnormal white blood cells are found in the blood stream. Leukemia is of various kinds according to the type of cell. Leukemia is a form of cancer (known as blood cancer). The cause of leukemia is unknown, but it occurs frequently in people exposed to radiation and certain chemicals. The leukemia is of two types:

- Acute type.
- Rapidly progressing.

Leukemia having white cell, begin in the bone marrow. Following are the symptoms of the leukemia:

- Loss of weight.
- Loss of appetite.
- Excessive weakness.
- Fatigue.
- Slight fever.
- Excessive bleeding after a minor injury.

Drugless Healing Therapies

Acupressure	It is a branch of traditional Chinese medicine that flow throughout the body to give life-energy. Acupressure is particulariy effective for treating problems with the soft tissues such as muscles, tendons and ligaments to leave a curative effect for back pain, joint problems such as arthritis, gynecological and all body disorders. There are various pressure points on

the body, which provide relief. Press each point for 20 to 40 seconds Given here are various pressure points on the body as shown in the sketches. Each pressure point has specific relation to treat a body organ listed below:

BL: Bladder
CV: Conception vessel
GB: Gallbladder
GV: Governing vessel
HE: Heart
KI: Kidney
LI: Large intestine
LU: Lung
LV: Liver
PE: Pericardium
SI: Small intestine
SP: Spleen
ST: Stomach
TB: Triple burner
TW: Triple warmer

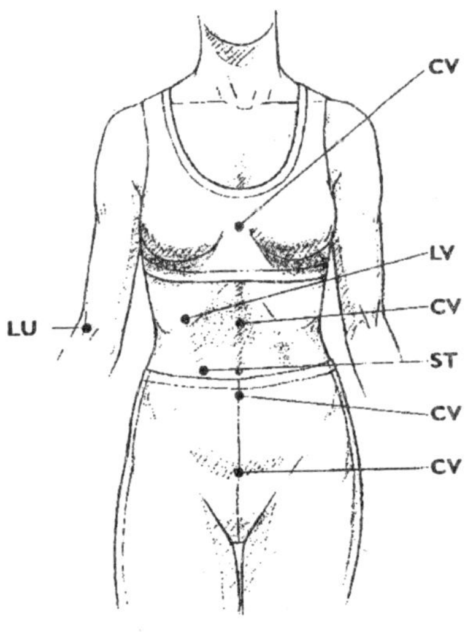

Illustration 1: Pressure points on the front of body.

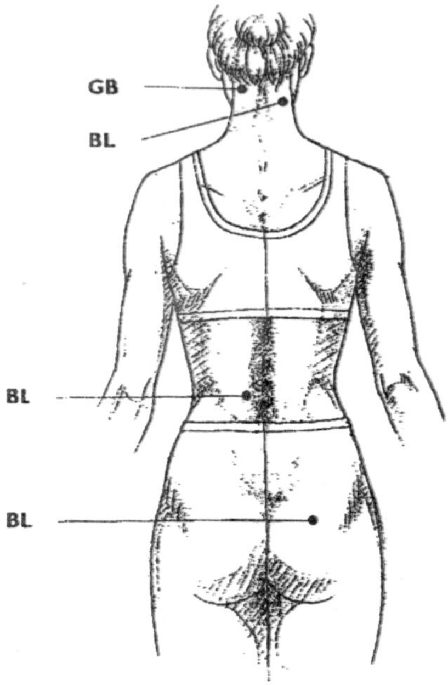

Illustration 2: Pressure points on the back of body.

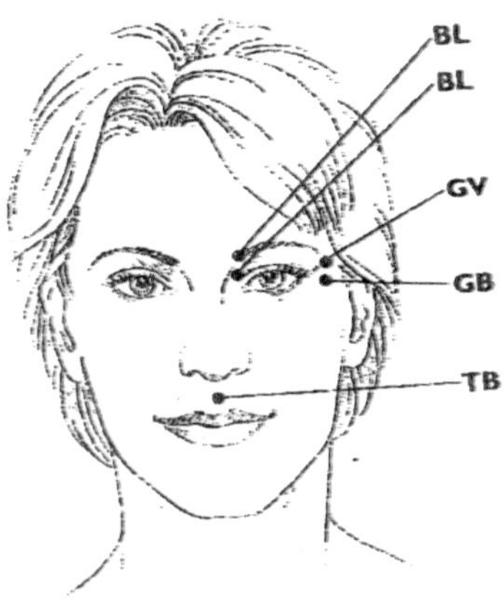

Illustration 3: Pressure points on the face.

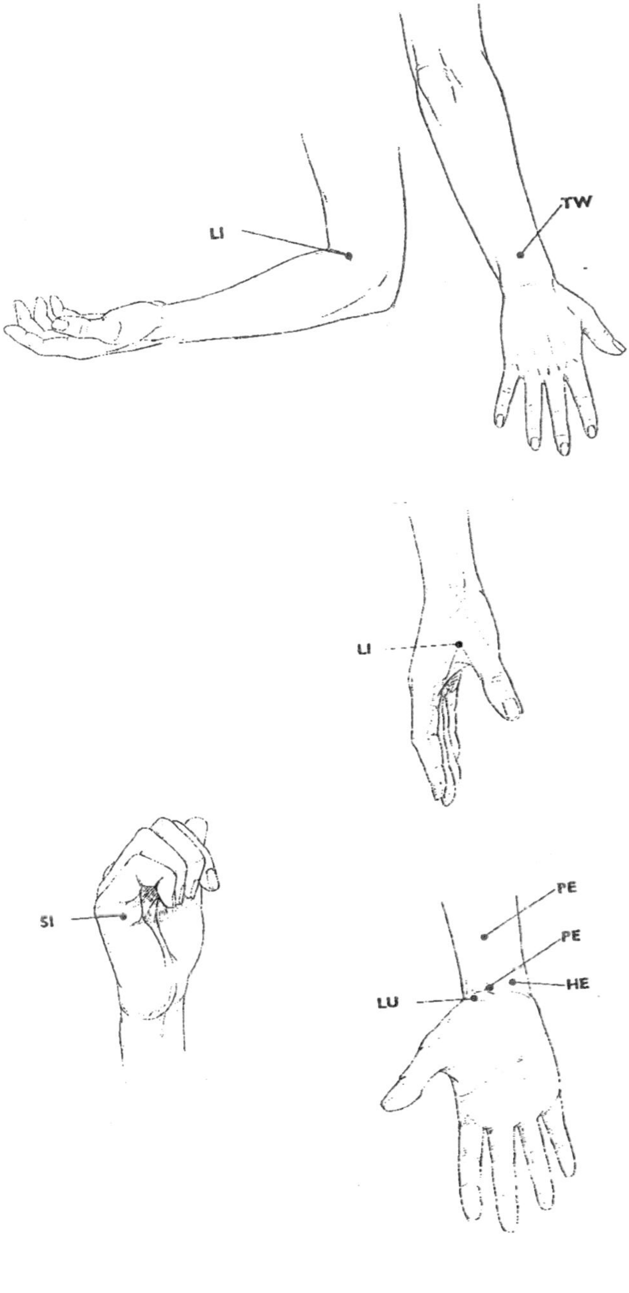

Illustration 4: Pressure points on hand and arms.

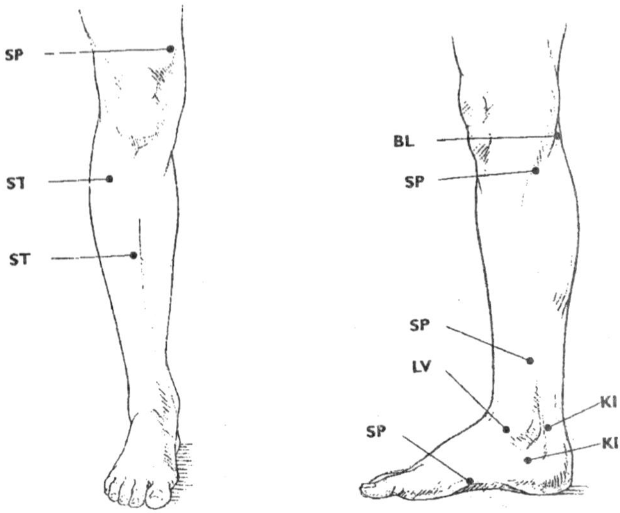

Illustration 5: Pressure points on leg.

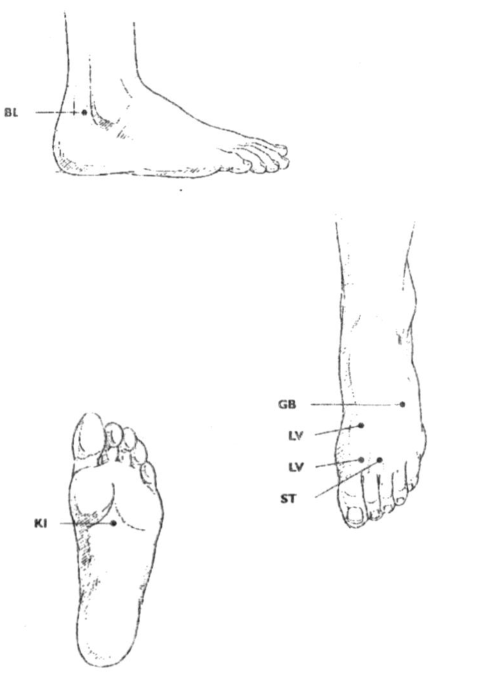

Illustration 6: Pressure points on feet.

Aromatherapy

It is a therapy in use of aroma oils for physical, mental and emotional healing. Aroma oils are distilled from herbs and flowers. Essential oils are volatile, which evaporate quickly in to the environment. Aroma oils enter the body by inhalation or massage on the skin, which are absorbed in to blood stream. Aromatherapy is very useful for:

1. Digestive complaints.
2. Skin problems.
3. Burns.
4. Infections.
5. Stress and emotional upset.
6. Hormone imbalances.
7. Respiratory complaints.
8. Relieves menopausal women.

Women undergoing pregnancy should avoid use of essential oils during the first trimester of pregnancy.

Ayurvedic Treatment

It is an ancient system of natural healing, also known as 'Science of Life', which includes wide range of treatments such as use of diets, herbs, massage, exercise, meditation, yoga, music therapy, juice therapy, aromatherapy etc. There are three categories or 'doshas': vatta (space and air), pitta (fire and water) and kapha (earth and water). Ayurveda treatments are aimed at restoring balance in the body emphasizing the psychological, social and spiritual causes of disease. This therapy is very useful in healing diabetes, arthritis, anemia, allergies and other problems involving immune system.

Flower Essences	These are liquid extracts prepared from wildflowers or garden blossoms. They heal several body disorders and are used to calm, stabilize and energize when a person is undergoing stress.
Herbal Therapy	A technique for use of medicinal plants for health and healing. Plants contain a variety of properties, which heal a disease. Herbal therapy is recommended for treating chronic conditions such as skin diseases, cardiovascular disease, diabetes, memory problems, arthritis and acute illness.
Hydrotherapy	Hydro means 'water'. Hydrotherapy is a technique in which water is applied to the body in order to stimulate and control the flow of blood and lymph. Hydrotherapy helps nourish the cells and promote the regeneration of tissues, which allow the body to heal from illness. Hot water causes arteries and veins to expand and bring additional blood and lymph to the area. Cold water makes the arteries and veins to constrict pushing away blood and lymph. This process brings fresh oxygen and expels toxins and waste products. Hot and cold water bath helps stimulate the nervous system of abdomen, lungs and heart. It relieves infection and inflammation.
Magnet Therapy	The therapy achieves a healing effect by putting permanent magnet on the skin or treatment with a medical device, which emits an electromagnetic field. Magnetic therapy includes the following health remedies: 1. Relieve pain. 2. Reduce inflammation.

3. Help healing bones and injured soft tissues (muscle, ligaments and tendons).
4. Back, neck and shoulder pain.
5. Arthritis.
6. Headaches and post-surgical pain.
7. Fibromyalgia.
8. Sprains, fractures and other muscle or bone injuries.
9. Diabetic neuropathy.
10. Insomnia.
11. Drug addiction.
12. Depression, anxiety and high blood pressure.
13. Osteoporosia, glaucoma and neurological disorders such as Parkinson's disease, Alzheimer's disease and epilepsy.

Pregnant women or someone who has a pacemaker or other implanted electrical device should avoid magnetic treatment without consulting a doctor.

Massage Therapy

A technique in which muscles and other soft tissues are pressed, rubbed and manipulated. Massage is helpful in the following ways:

1. It is effective for any type of pain in the body including back, neck, shoulder and headache.
2. Relieves tense muscles of head, face and neck.
3. Cures bursitis, tendonitis, strain injuries and sports injuries.

Music Therapy

Helps to promote healing of body, mind and spirit. It provides the following curative measures:

1. Music stimulates relaxation, known as rhythm entertainment.
2. Calms stress-related conditions, including muscle pain, tension headaches, high blood pressure (hypertension).
3. Insomnia, depression anxiety and fatigue.

Reflexology

Reflexology therapy includes specific touch techniques on various points on the body usually on feet, hands, ears, abdomen and back. Each of these points corresponds to a specific part of the body. By using touch techniques on these areas you can help maintain or improve the health of corresponding areas in the body. Using reflexology by pressing various points, stimulate specific sensory nerves, which send message to the brain, which further send relief message to the corresponding area of the body to produce relaxation. Reflexology improves blood flow and increases supply of oxygen and nutrients to the areas of the body for reducing the accumulation of stress. Reflexology reduces stress in areas such as neck, shoulders, lower back and inside the body such as in the lungs, heart, kidneys and intestinal tract.

You should not have reflexology treatment in case:

1. of the area in which the skin is broken.
2. on the area , which has infection.
3. on the area where a fracture is healing.

4. you have had reconstructive surgery.
5. in case of women who are in the first trimester of pregnancy, as reflexology stimulates the uterine points.

Relaxation Therapy

This therapy aims a calm, rested state of mind that relieves tension and stress. Deep breathing calms and balances the nervous system. It is best used for common stress-related complaints such as

1. High blood pressure.
2. Insomnia.
3. Headaches.
4. Fatigue.
5. Irregular heartbeat (arrhythmia).
6. Digestive problems.
7. Allergies.
8. Skin disorders.
9. Anxiety.
10. Depression.
11. Chronic anger or hostility.

Vitamin & Mineral therapy

By supplementing your diet with vitamins and minerals help prevent disease, relieve symptoms and speed healing. Vitamins and minerals act as natural medications. Vitamin A and B provide nutrients. Vitamin C helps relieve symptoms of angina, diabetes, menopausal discomfort, premenstrual syndrome, prostate problems, shingles, varicose veins and many other health and skin problems.

Yoga

A ancient form of physical and mental technique to purify and vitalize the body and mind. Yoga therapy can be very effective in treating all types of muscle and skeletal problems such as neck and shoulder pain, lower-back disorders, to treat fibromyalgia, arthritis, high blood pressure, insomnia, diabetes, asthma, digestive problems, overweight and common complaints of aging. Consult your doctor while practicing yoga during pregnancy.

Acupuncture Therapy

Acupuncture-a basic Chinese concept to treat diseases entails a flow in the body to imbalance the system with the help of needles. There are five fundamental substances in Chinese philosophy such

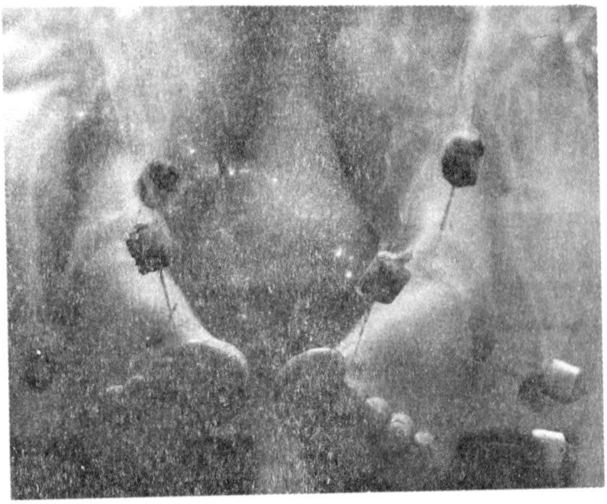

as Chi, blood, jing, shen and other fluids, which include sweat, saliva, gastric juices, urine etc. The most important substances are Chi and blood, which circulate in the channels called meridians. The diseases of internal organs in human body are associated with "tender points' or also known as 'trigger points' at the surface of the body. The tender points are either pressed by massage, freezed or a needle is injected into a trigger point, which spreads sensation in the tissues, stimulates the nerves and cure particular limb or organ associated with tender points. There are nearly 300 tender parts on the body. For example, some of the common tender points are described below:

- Heart disease (angina) is associated with the muscles on the front and back of the chest and arms.

- Backache is associated with back and buttock muscles.
- Painful neck is connected with the muscles on the top of shoulders.
- Menstrual disorders in females are associated with the tender areas on the inside of the shins.

The traditional acupuncturists study the pulse and identify the acupuncture points to select the treatment, its duration and frequency according to the anatomy of the body. The duration of treatment varies from patient to patient. The frequency of treatment needed vary from case to case. Usually, within a few seconds of needle is inserted the patient feel deeply relaxed even drowsy causing sensation in the related limb being treated. Avoid acupuncture treatment during pregnancy. The commonest type of disorders treated by the acupuncture are following:

- Painful conditions of the muscles and joints in the body.
- Spondylosis (wear and tear in the spine).
- Backache.
- Gynecological disorders, especially menstrual problems.
- Menopausal symptoms.
- Allergic disorders, including hay fever and nettle rash.
- Headaches and migraines.
- Pain from cancer.
- Psychological tension.
- Stress and emotional release.
- Asthma.
- Skin diseases, such as eczema and psoriasis.
- Nausea, fatigue and lack of energy.
- Viral infections.

Pressing on appropriate areas of the body, too, helps to some extent, but it is less effective as compared to needling. The main risks when needling include infection and damage to the internal organs. The most serious type of infection that may occur is hepatitis, which can be transmitted from one person to another through blood. Even boiling needle doesn't eliminate the risk of transmitting hepatitis infection. Autoclaving is more effective means of sterilization.

Index